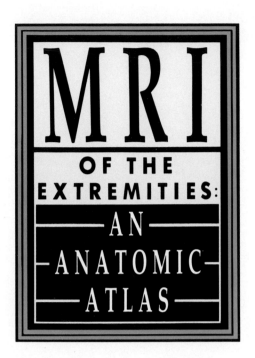

MRI
OF THE
EXTREMITIES:
AN ANATOMIC ATLAS

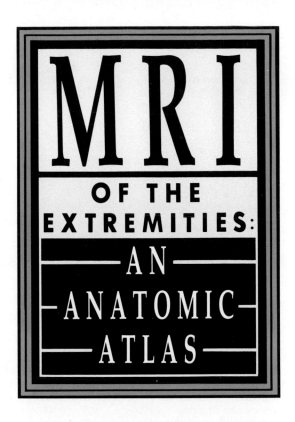

MRI
OF THE
EXTREMITIES:
AN
ANATOMIC
ATLAS

HEUNG SIK KANG, M.D.

Assistant Professor
Department of Radiology
College of Medicine
Seoul National University
Seoul, Korea

DONALD RESNICK, M.D.

Professor of Radiology
University of California, San Diego
and
Veterans Administration Medical Center
San Diego, California

With the technical assistance
of
DEBRA TRUDELL

1991
W.B. SAUNDERS COMPANY
Harcourt Brace Jovanovich, Inc.
Philadelphia   London   Toronto   Montreal   Sydney   Tokyo

W. B. Saunders Company
Harcourt Brace Jovanovich, Inc
The Curtis Center

Independence Square West
Philadelphia, PA 19106

Library of Congress Cataloging-in-Publication Data

Kang, Heung Sik.
 Magnetic resonance imaging atlas of the extremities / Heung Sik Kang, Donald Resnick.
 p. cm.
 ISBN 0-7216-3071-5
 1. Extremities—Magnetic resonance imaging—Atlases.   I. Resnick, Donald.
II. Title.
 [DNLM: 1. Extremities—anatomy & histology—atlases.   2. Magnetic Resonance Imaging—atlases.   WE 17 K16m]
 QM548.K36   1990
 617.5'807548—dc20
 DNLM/DLC   90-8571
 for Library of Congress   CIP

Editor: Lisette Bralow
Designer: Paul Fry
Production Manager: Carolyn Naylor
Manuscript Editor: Wendy Andresen
Illustration Coordinator: Brett MacNaughton
Indexer: Victoria Boyle
Magnetic Resonance Imaging Atlas of the Extremities   ISBN 0-7216-3071-5

Printed in the United States of America.

Last digit is the print number:

To my wife Yeong-Sun
H.S.K.

To Heung Sik Kang,
whose energy, enthusiasm,
and pursuit of excellence
were the major factors in the
production of this atlas
D.R.

PREFACE

Magnetic resonance imaging has been applied with great success to the assessment of a variety of musculoskeletal disorders. The advantages of this technique include an ability to provide sectional images in any plane with excellent spatial and contrast resolution and the capability of revealing considerable physiologic and histologic data. Unlike routine radiography, computed tomography, and scintigraphy, magnetic resonance imaging can accomplish these things without the use of ionizing radiation or radiation-emitting pharmaceutical agents. The accurate interpretation of the images provided by magnetic resonance, however, is not accomplished without difficulty, requiring foremost that the examiner have considerable knowledge of pertinent osseous and soft tissue anatomy. Unless one knows where to look for abnormalities of signal and morphology, missed diagnosis or misdiagnosis will result.

With this atlas, the authors have attempted to demonstrate the anatomic information that is necessary for correct interpretation of magnetic resonance images of the extremities. Although other atlases exist, it was our belief that there was a need for a publication based not on *in vivo* imaging of normal volunteers but rather on cadaveric imaging alone and precise correlation of the anatomic features depicted with magnetic resonance and with specimen photography. An atlas of this type required meticulous preparation and imaging of the cadaveric parts (see Introduction), which proved to be the most challenging aspect of the endeavor.

This atlas is divided into seven chapters: shoulder; elbow; wrist and hand; finger; hip; knee; and ankle and foot. For each region of the body, transverse, coronal, and sagittal planes are illustrated. With regard to the shoulder, coronal oblique and sagittal oblique data, rather than strict coronal and sagittal data, are illustrated because these are the planes most often used in clinical imaging. At each level, two illustrations are provided, with the magnetic resonance image presented before the corresponding sectional photograph, and a line drawing is used to indicate the orientation and location of the section. With the exception of the wrist and hand, the images in the transverse plane are presented as if viewed from the caudal aspect; medial structures are to the reader's right and lateral structures are to the reader's left. The reverse is true for the wrist and hand, and in the elbow, medial and lateral orientations are reversed. In the coronal plane, the images are presented as if viewed from the anterior aspect with medial structures located to the reader's right and lateral structures to the reader's left; the orientation of the coronal images of the wrist and hand is reversed. The images in the sagittal plane are presented as if viewed from the midline; posterior structures are to the reader's right and anterior structures to the reader's left.

In selected instances, we employed a specifically prepared solution that was injected into the articulation prior to magnetic resonance imaging. As described in the Introduction, the solution was composed of ingredients that ensured accurate monitoring with fluoroscopy during the injection procedure, a bright signal with T_1-weighted sequences, and rapid solidification before sectioning of the specimen was accomplished.

With regard to labeling of the illustrations, we have defined as many structures as possible at each level, been consistent in labeling from one level to another, and used the specific terminology that currently is generally accepted. Where controversy or inconsistency exists in the literature, we have employed the designations that most often are used.

The following abbreviations are utilized throughout this atlas:

anterior = ant	posterior = post
medial = med	lateral = lat
superior = sup	inferior = inf
internal = int	external = ext
muscle = m	muscles = mm
nerve = n	nerves = nn
tendon = t	tendons = tt
ligament = lig	ligaments = ligs
artery = a	arteries = aa
vein = v	veins = vv
aponeurosis = apon	joint = j

In the transverse sections of the finger, the following abbreviations also are used:

MC = metacarpal
MP = middle phalanx
PP = proximal phalanx

In the transverse sections of the wrist and hand, the following abbreviations also are used:

P = palmar interosseous muscle
D = dorsal interosseous muscle
1, 2, 3, 4, 5 = metacarpals

In coronal sections of the foot and ankle, one additional abbreviation was used:

I = interosseous muscle

This atlas represents the final product of 12 months of cadaveric preparation, image acquisition, specimen processing, photography, and labeling of illustrations. Although there were moments of considerable fatigue and frustration, we maintained our energy and enthusiasm throughout because of our strong belief that knowledge of anatomy, above all else, is essential to correct analysis of magnetic resonance images. Indeed, we ourselves profited im-

mensely from the information gained during hours of investigation and prob-
ing of the specimens as we traced structures from one level to another, at-
tempting to differentiate among the many muscles (mm) and tendons (tt) we
encountered, to distinguish arteries (aa) from veins (vv), and to identify im-
portant nerves (nn), ligaments (ligs), and other structures. We gained new
respect for the intricacy of human anatomy and derived considerable satisfac-
tion in our increasing ability to identify this anatomy as depicted in the magnetic resonance images. It is our hope that the reader who studies these illustrations also will profit from the experience and that he or she will
understand, more than before, the considerable challenge and splendid op-
portunity provided by the remarkable technique utilizing magnetic resonance.

HEUNG SIK KANG, M.D.
DONALD RESNICK, M.D.

ACKNOWLEDGMENTS

An atlas such as this one requires the assistance of a number of persons to whom the authors are deeply indebted. We would like to acknowledge the cooperation of the Anatomy Department of the University of California, San Diego, in supplying the cadaveric specimens. The extraordinary efforts of Debra Trudell, who assisted in specimen preparation and photography, are indicated by her inclusion on the title page of this atlas. We also would like to thank Cecelia Kemper, Research Assistant at the Magnetic Resonance Institute of the University of California, San Diego; David J. Phillips in the Department of Medical Media at the Veterans Administration Medical Center in San Diego; and Cynde Williams, Sook Hee Yu, and Seung Yeon Kong for secretarial assistance.

H.S.K.

D.R.

CONTENTS

INTRODUCTION

It is the authors' belief that the value of an atlas such as this one lies in the precise correlation of the information revealed by the magnetic resonance images and that provided in the corresponding specimen photographs. To accomplish such correlation, meticulous preparation of cadaveric parts and careful imaging technique were required. In the following paragraphs we summarize our methodology.

SPECIMEN SELECTION

Fresh cadaveric specimens were obtained from the Department of Anatomy, University of California, San Diego. With the exception of the elbow specimen used for the transverse plane, extremities from the right side of the body were employed. After careful inspection and routine radiography, we rejected those cadaveric parts that demonstrated significant abnormalities.

SPECIMEN PREPARATION

The specimens were frozen in anatomic position at $-60°C$ for at least three days. While frozen, they were trimmed with a bandsaw into a size suitable for imaging. A rectangular cardboard box of appropriate size was prepared, the inside of which was covered with a plastic bag to prevent leakage of melted paraffin. The specimen was placed in proper position in the cardboard box. Melted paraffin (Paraplast Tissue Embedding Medium, Mono Jec Scientific, St. Louis, MO) was poured around the specimen. The amount of paraffin that was used was the minimum needed to fix the specimen within the box, as excessive paraffin interfered with proper sectioning of the specimen. Owing to the frozen state of the specimen, solidification of the paraffin occurred quickly. Prior to magnetic resonance imaging, the specimen was thawed at room temperature.

SPECIMEN INJECTION

To better delineate joint anatomy, intra-articular injection of a specifically prepared material was used in selected cases. This material consisted of a solution composed of a 2 mMol concentration of copper sulfate ($CuSO_4$), 15% concentration of iothalamate meglumine (Conray 60), and 15% concentration of gelatin. $CuSO_4$ was chosen owing to its short T_1 relaxation time, providing high signal intensity on T_1-weighted images. Conray 60 was used to facilitate accurate intra-articular placement of the solution during fluoroscopic monitoring. Gelatin was chosen to ensure solidification of the material at room temperature for dissection and photographic purposes. The various ingredients of this arthrographic solution were mixed and heated with a magnetic stir. The solution was injected into two shoulders (for transverse and coronal oblique images), two wrists (for coronal and sagittal images), and one knee (for sagittal images) using a small needle and fluoroscopic control. After injection, the specimens were frozen in anatomic position.

MAGNETIC RESONANCE IMAGING

A 1.5 Tesla GE Signa magnet was used for all images. An extremity coil was employed for the elbow, wrist and hand, finger, knee, and ankle and foot. A head coil was used for the shoulder and hip. Transverse, coronal, and sagittal images were obtained (at 3- to 5-mm intervals) for each joint, with the exception of the shoulder, in which coronal oblique (perpendicular to the glenohumeral joint) and sagittal oblique (parallel to the glenohumeral joint) images were obtained. T_1-weighted sequences (TR = 600 ms, TE = 20 ms) were utilized. The imaging planes were indicated by carefully marking the cardboard box.

SPECIMEN SECTIONING

After obtaining magnetic resonance images, the specimens again were frozen and, subsequently, sectioned with a bandsaw into slices 3 to 5 mm thick. The plane of the sections was parallel to the edge of the cardboard box and to the imaging plane shown by the marks on the box. After each slice, comparison of the section with the magnetic resonance image was employed to ensure that the plane was accurately determined and, if not, minor modifications in the sectioning plane were made. The paraffin was then removed, and sliced specimens were frozen.

SPECIMEN PHOTOGRAPHY

A Nikon FM2 camera with a 55-mm f2.8 lens was employed. Two electronic flash units were used. Before photography, each frozen specimen was cleaned with running water, and the excess water was removed with a cotton towel. Specimens were photographed on a black glass plate using Kodak Ektachrome Daylight 35-mm film.

1 SHOULDER

SHOULDER, CORONAL

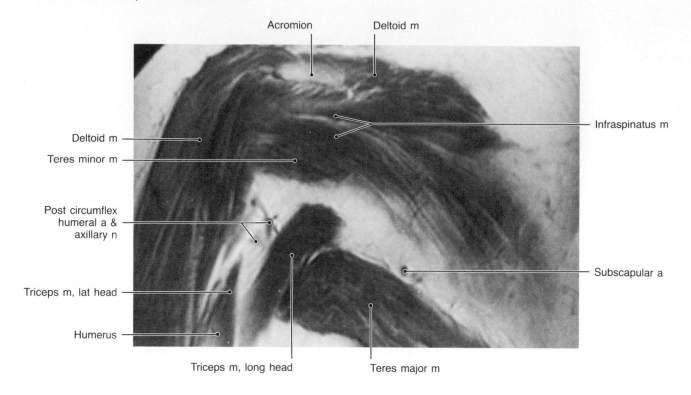

Acromion

Deltoid m

Deltoid m

Teres minor m

Post circumflex
humeral a &
axillary n

Triceps m, lat head

Humerus

Triceps m, long head

Teres major m

Infraspinatus m

Subscapular a

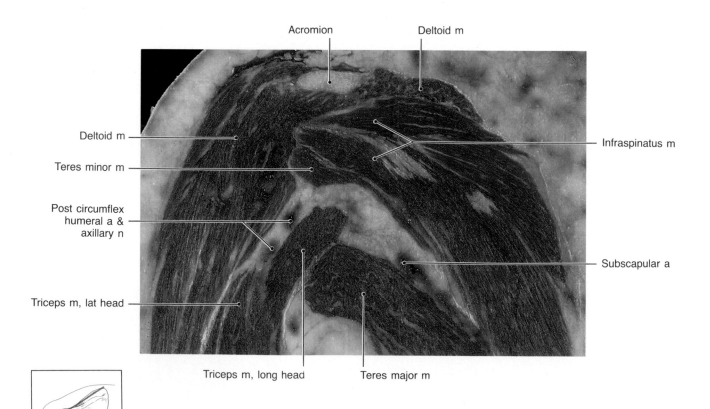

Acromion

Deltoid m

Deltoid m

Teres minor m

Post circumflex
humeral a &
axillary n

Triceps m, lat head

Triceps m, long head

Teres major m

Infraspinatus m

Subscapular a

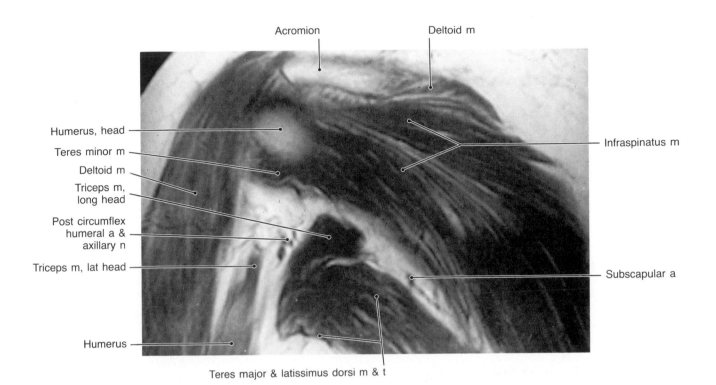

Acromion

Deltoid m

Humerus, head

Teres minor m

Deltoid m

Triceps m, long head

Post circumflex humeral a & axillary n

Triceps m, lat head

Infraspinatus m

Subscapular a

Humerus

Teres major & latissimus dorsi m & t

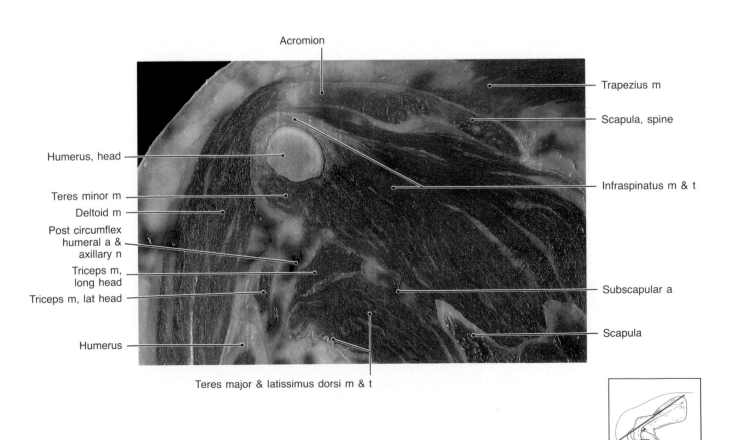

Acromion

Trapezius m

Scapula, spine

Humerus, head

Teres minor m

Deltoid m

Post circumflex humeral a & axillary n

Triceps m, long head

Triceps m, lat head

Infraspinatus m & t

Subscapular a

Scapula

Humerus

Teres major & latissimus dorsi m & t

SHOULDER, CORONAL

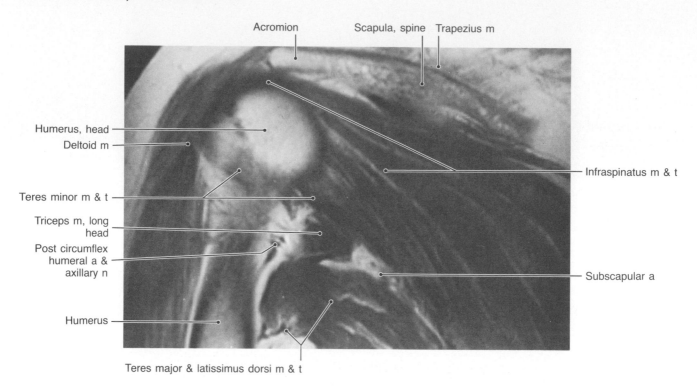

Acromion   Scapula, spine   Trapezius m

Humerus, head

Deltoid m

Teres minor m & t

Triceps m, long head

Post circumflex humeral a & axillary n

Humerus

Infraspinatus m & t

Subscapular a

Teres major & latissimus dorsi m & t

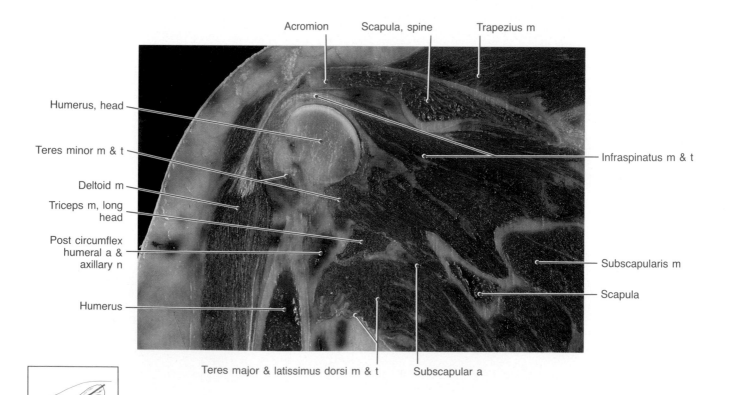

Acromion   Scapula, spine   Trapezius m

Humerus, head

Teres minor m & t

Deltoid m

Triceps m, long head

Post circumflex humeral a & axillary n

Humerus

Infraspinatus m & t

Subscapularis m

Scapula

Teres major & latissimus dorsi m & t   Subscapular a

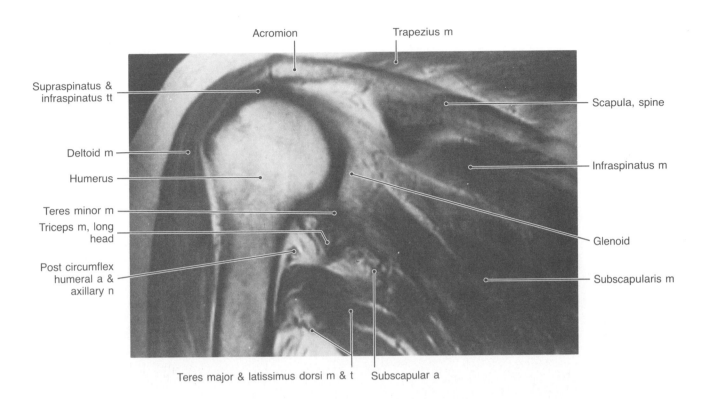

Acromion

Trapezius m

Supraspinatus & infraspinatus tt

Scapula, spine

Deltoid m

Infraspinatus m

Humerus

Teres minor m

Triceps m, long head

Glenoid

Post circumflex humeral a & axillary n

Subscapularis m

Teres major & latissimus dorsi m & t   Subscapular a

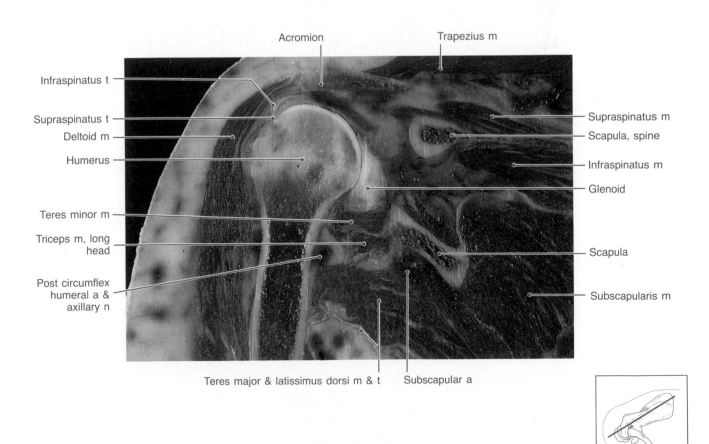

Acromion

Trapezius m

Infraspinatus t

Supraspinatus m

Supraspinatus t

Scapula, spine

Deltoid m

Humerus

Infraspinatus m

Glenoid

Teres minor m

Triceps m, long head

Scapula

Post circumflex humeral a & axillary n

Subscapularis m

Teres major & latissimus dorsi m & t   Subscapular a

SHOULDER, CORONAL

Acromion

Trapezius m

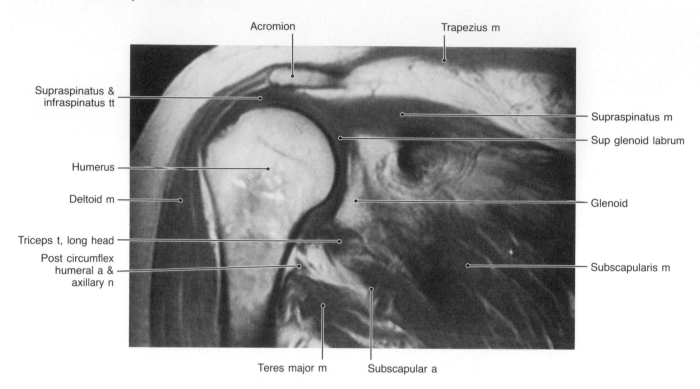

Supraspinatus & infraspinatus tt

Humerus

Deltoid m

Triceps t, long head

Post circumflex humeral a & axillary n

Supraspinatus m

Sup glenoid labrum

Glenoid

Subscapularis m

Teres major m

Subscapular a

Acromion

Trapezius m

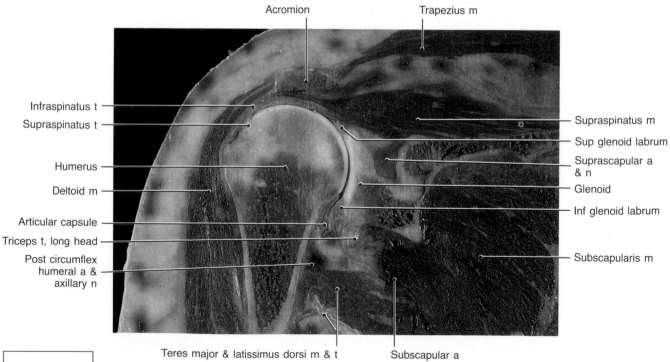

Infraspinatus t

Supraspinatus t

Humerus

Deltoid m

Articular capsule

Triceps t, long head

Post circumflex humeral a & axillary n

Supraspinatus m

Sup glenoid labrum

Suprascapular a & n

Glenoid

Inf glenoid labrum

Subscapularis m

Teres major & latissimus dorsi m & t

Subscapular a

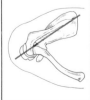

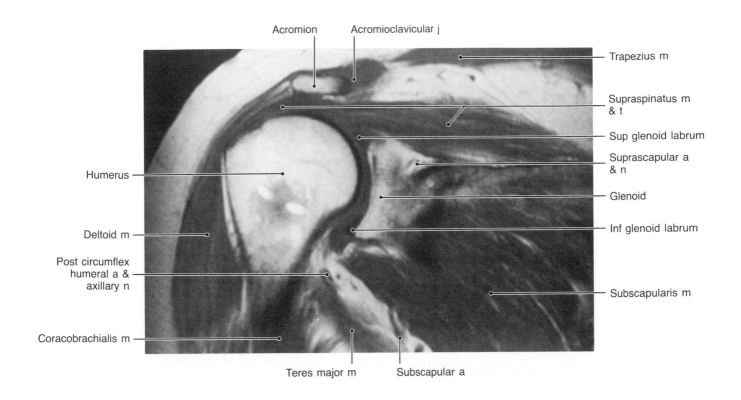

Acromion — Acromioclavicular j

Trapezius m

Supraspinatus m & t

Sup glenoid labrum

Suprascapular a & n

Glenoid

Inf glenoid labrum

Humerus

Deltoid m

Post circumflex humeral a & axillary n

Coracobrachialis m

Subscapularis m

Teres major m — Subscapular a

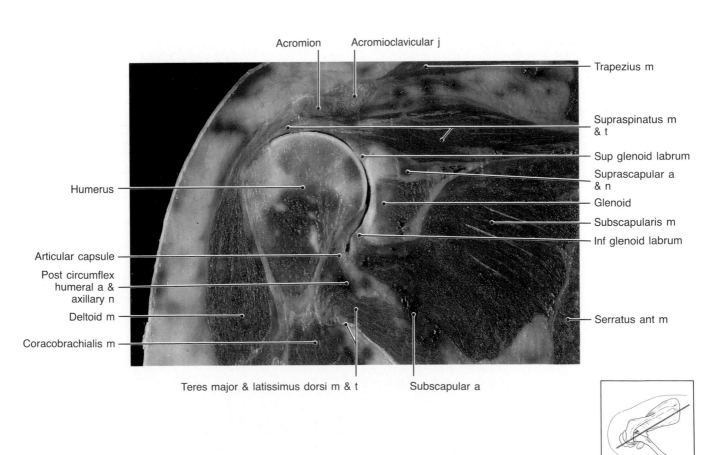

Acromion — Acromioclavicular j

Trapezius m

Supraspinatus m & t

Sup glenoid labrum

Suprascapular a & n

Glenoid

Subscapularis m

Inf glenoid labrum

Humerus

Articular capsule

Post circumflex humeral a & axillary n

Deltoid m

Coracobrachialis m

Serratus ant m

Teres major & latissimus dorsi m & t — Subscapular a

SHOULDER, CORONAL

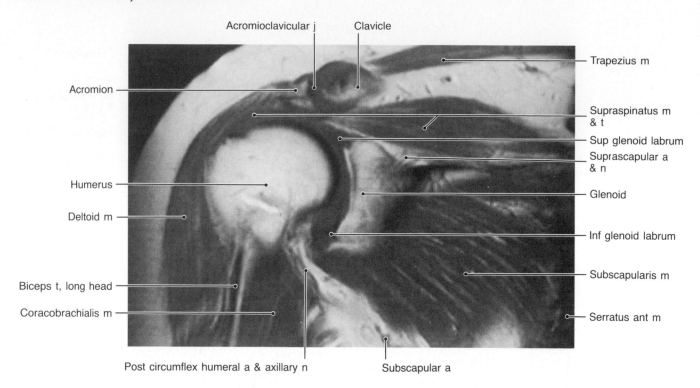

Acromioclavicular j — Clavicle

Acromion

Trapezius m

Supraspinatus m & t

Sup glenoid labrum

Suprascapular a & n

Humerus

Glenoid

Deltoid m

Inf glenoid labrum

Subscapularis m

Biceps t, long head

Serratus ant m

Coracobrachialis m

Post circumflex humeral a & axillary n

Subscapular a

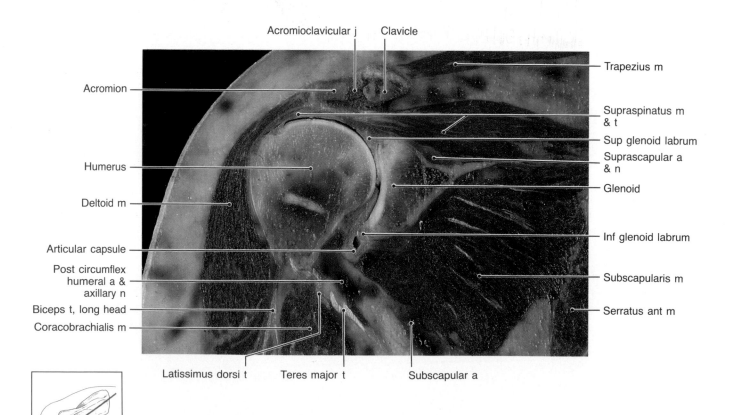

Acromioclavicular j — Clavicle

Acromion

Trapezius m

Supraspinatus m & t

Sup glenoid labrum

Suprascapular a & n

Humerus

Glenoid

Deltoid m

Inf glenoid labrum

Articular capsule

Post circumflex humeral a & axillary n

Subscapularis m

Biceps t, long head

Serratus ant m

Coracobrachialis m

Latissimus dorsi t — Teres major t — Subscapular a

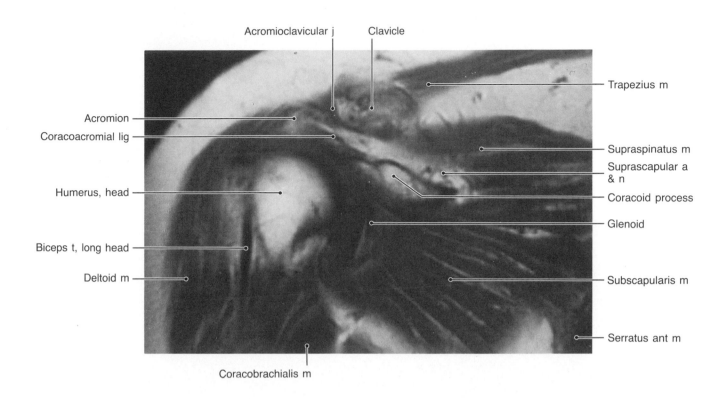

Acromioclavicular j

Clavicle

Trapezius m

Acromion

Coracoacromial lig

Supraspinatus m

Suprascapular a & n

Coracoid process

Humerus, head

Glenoid

Biceps t, long head

Deltoid m

Subscapularis m

Serratus ant m

Coracobrachialis m

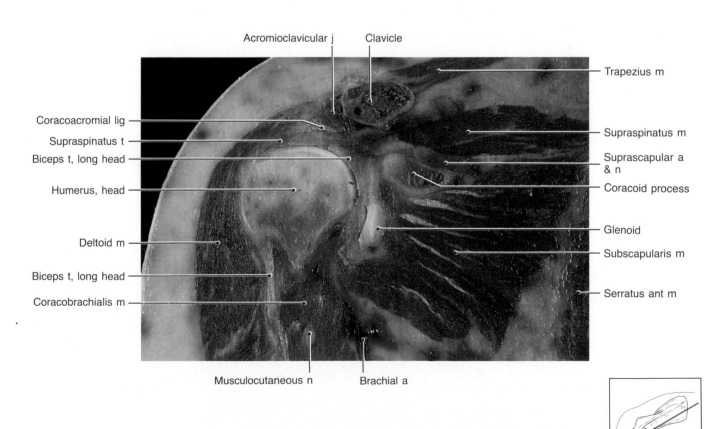

Acromioclavicular j

Clavicle

Trapezius m

Coracoacromial lig

Supraspinatus t

Biceps t, long head

Humerus, head

Supraspinatus m

Suprascapular a & n

Coracoid process

Deltoid m

Glenoid

Biceps t, long head

Subscapularis m

Coracobrachialis m

Serratus ant m

Musculocutaneous n

Brachial a

SHOULDER, CORONAL

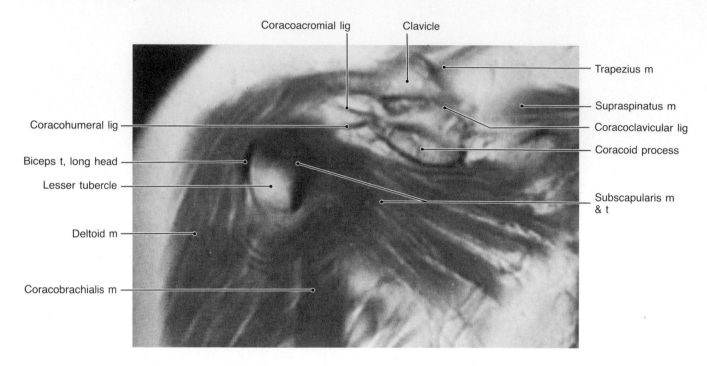

Coracoacromial lig

Clavicle

Trapezius m

Supraspinatus m

Coracohumeral lig

Coracoclavicular lig

Coracoid process

Biceps t, long head

Lesser tubercle

Subscapularis m & t

Deltoid m

Coracobrachialis m

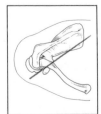

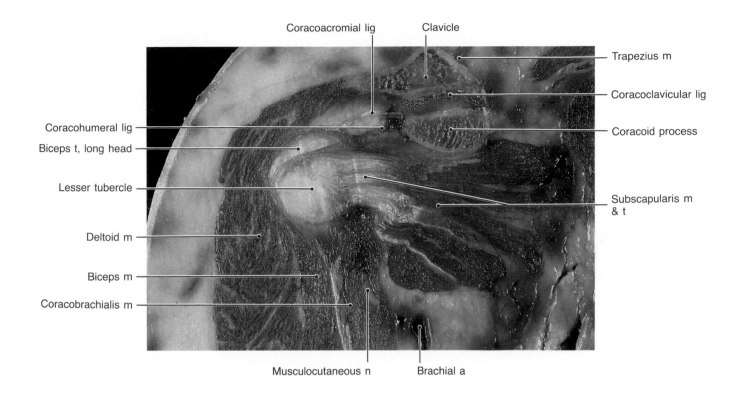

Coracoacromial lig

Clavicle

Trapezius m

Coracoclavicular lig

Coracohumeral lig

Coracoid process

Biceps t, long head

Lesser tubercle

Subscapularis m & t

Deltoid m

Biceps m

Coracobrachialis m

Musculocutaneous n

Brachial a

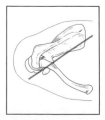

SHOULDER, TRANSVERSE

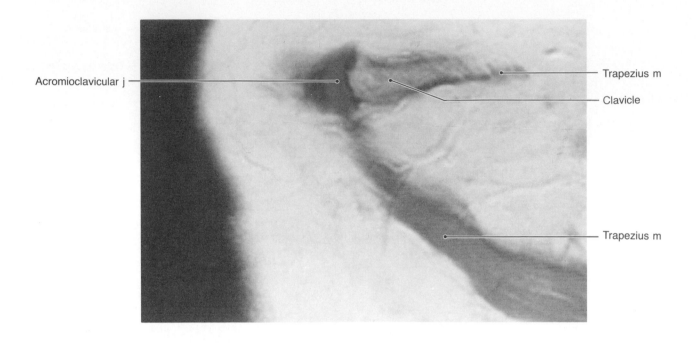

Acromioclavicular j

Trapezius m

Clavicle

Trapezius m

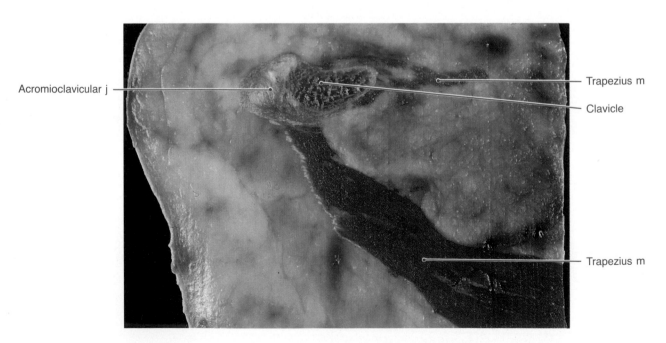

Acromioclavicular j

Trapezius m

Clavicle

Trapezius m

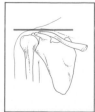

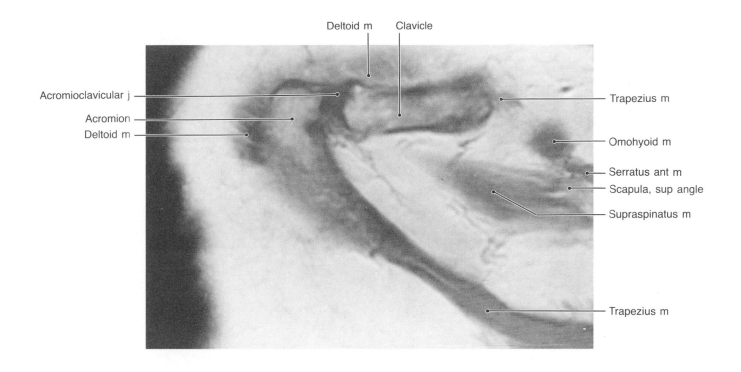

Deltoid m   Clavicle

Acromioclavicular j

Acromion

Deltoid m

Trapezius m

Omohyoid m

Serratus ant m

Scapula, sup angle

Supraspinatus m

Trapezius m

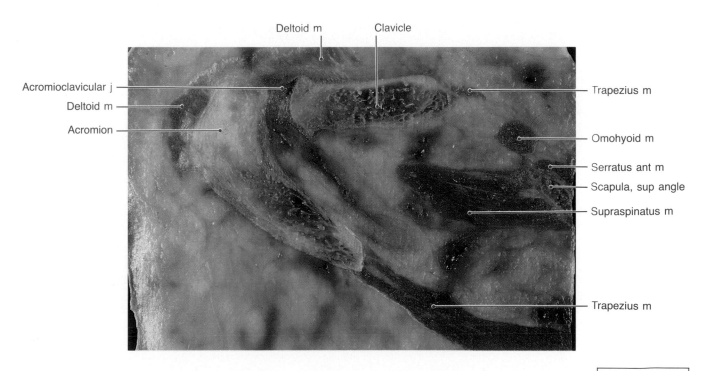

Deltoid m   Clavicle

Acromioclavicular j

Deltoid m

Acromion

Trapezius m

Omohyoid m

Serratus ant m

Scapula, sup angle

Supraspinatus m

Trapezius m

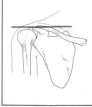

SHOULDER, TRANSVERSE

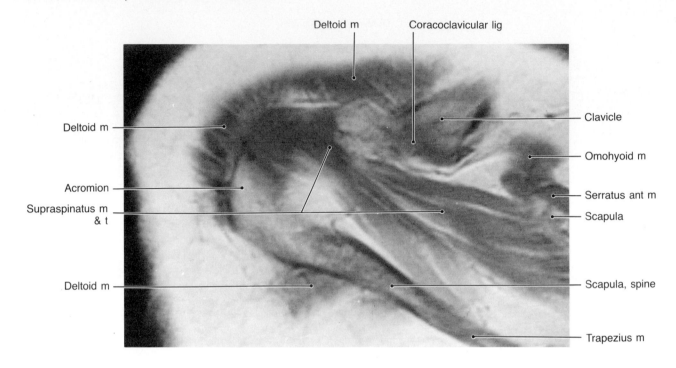

Deltoid m

Coracoclavicular lig

Deltoid m

Acromion

Supraspinatus m & t

Deltoid m

Clavicle

Omohyoid m

Serratus ant m

Scapula

Scapula, spine

Trapezius m

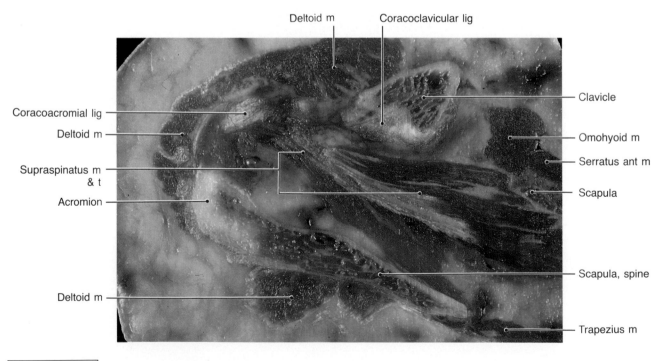

Deltoid m

Coracoclavicular lig

Coracoacromial lig

Deltoid m

Supraspinatus m & t

Acromion

Deltoid m

Clavicle

Omohyoid m

Serratus ant m

Scapula

Scapula, spine

Trapezius m

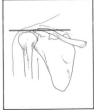

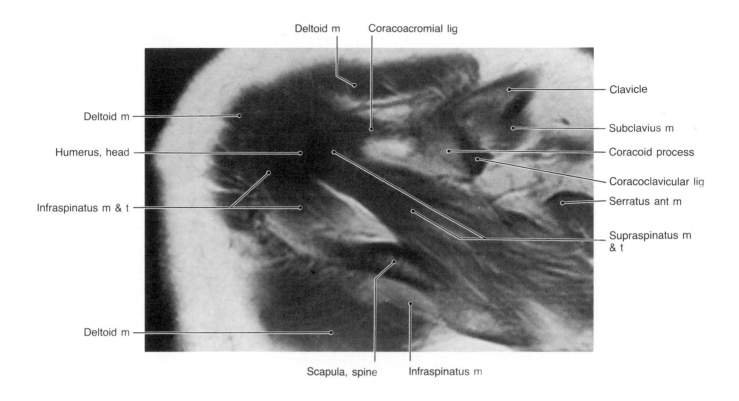

Deltoid m   Coracoacromial lig

Deltoid m

Humerus, head

Infraspinatus m & t

Deltoid m

Clavicle

Subclavius m

Coracoid process

Coracoclavicular lig

Serratus ant m

Supraspinatus m & t

Scapula, spine   Infraspinatus m

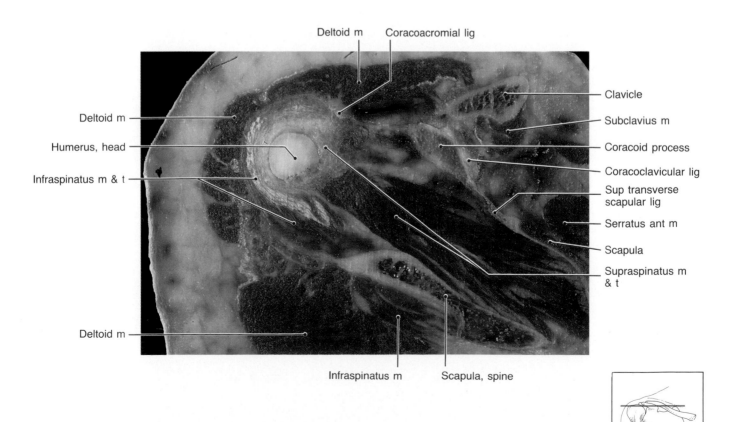

Deltoid m   Coracoacromial lig

Deltoid m

Humerus, head

Infraspinatus m & t

Deltoid m

Clavicle

Subclavius m

Coracoid process

Coracoclavicular lig

Sup transverse scapular lig

Serratus ant m

Scapula

Supraspinatus m & t

Infraspinatus m   Scapula, spine

SHOULDER, TRANSVERSE

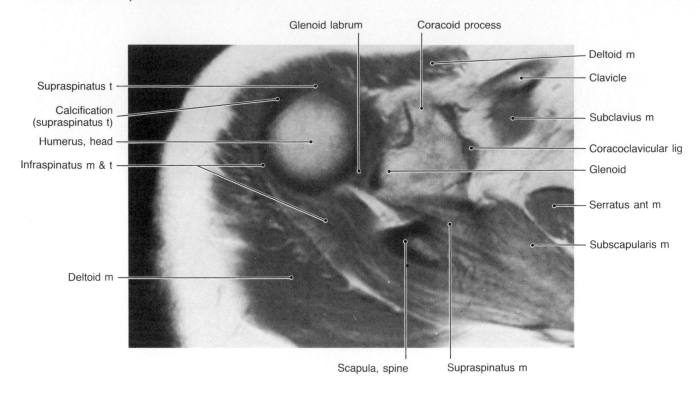

Glenoid labrum   Coracoid process

Supraspinatus t

Calcification
(supraspinatus t)

Humerus, head

Infraspinatus m & t

Deltoid m

Deltoid m

Clavicle

Subclavius m

Coracoclavicular lig

Glenoid

Serratus ant m

Subscapularis m

Scapula, spine   Supraspinatus m

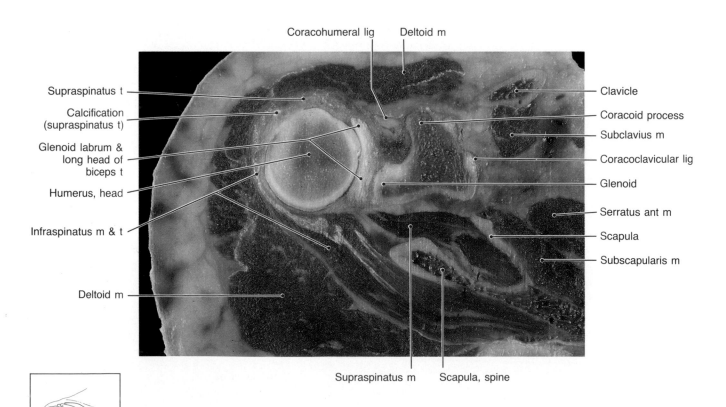

Coracohumeral lig   Deltoid m

Supraspinatus t

Calcification
(supraspinatus t)

Glenoid labrum &
long head of
biceps t

Humerus, head

Infraspinatus m & t

Deltoid m

Clavicle

Coracoid process

Subclavius m

Coracoclavicular lig

Glenoid

Serratus ant m

Scapula

Subscapularis m

Supraspinatus m   Scapula, spine

Coracohumeral lig   Coracoid process

Deltoid m   Clavicle

Biceps t, long head   Pectoralis minor t

Calcification   Subclavius m
(infraspinatus t)

Humerus, head   Ant glenoid labrum

Infraspinatus m & t   Subscapularis m

Serratus ant m

Scapula, spine

Deltoid m

Glenoid   Suprascapular a & n

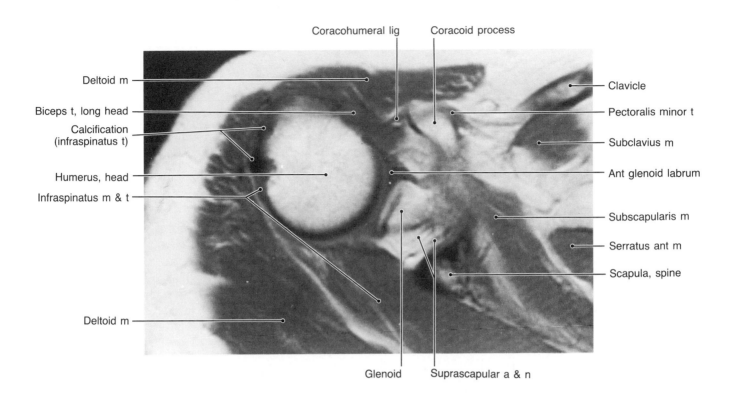

Coracohumeral lig   Coracoid process

Deltoid m   Clavicle

Biceps t, long head   Pectoralis minor t

Calcification   Subclavius m
(infraspinatus t)

Humerus, head   Ant glenoid labrum

Infraspinatus m & t   Serratus ant m

Subscapularis m

Deltoid m

Glenoid   Scapula, spine

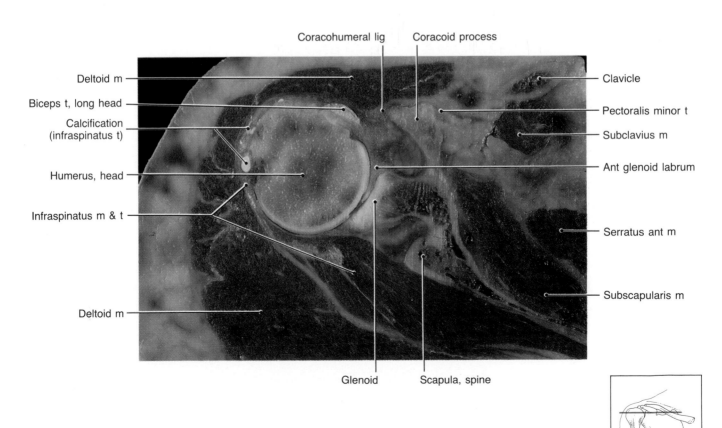

SHOULDER, TRANSVERSE

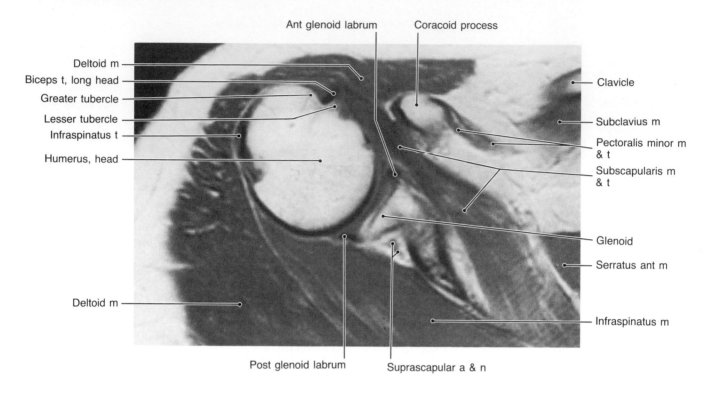

Ant glenoid labrum — Coracoid process

Deltoid m

Biceps t, long head

Greater tubercle

Lesser tubercle

Infraspinatus t

Humerus, head

Clavicle

Subclavius m

Pectoralis minor m & t

Subscapularis m & t

Glenoid

Serratus ant m

Deltoid m

Infraspinatus m

Post glenoid labrum   Suprascapular a & n

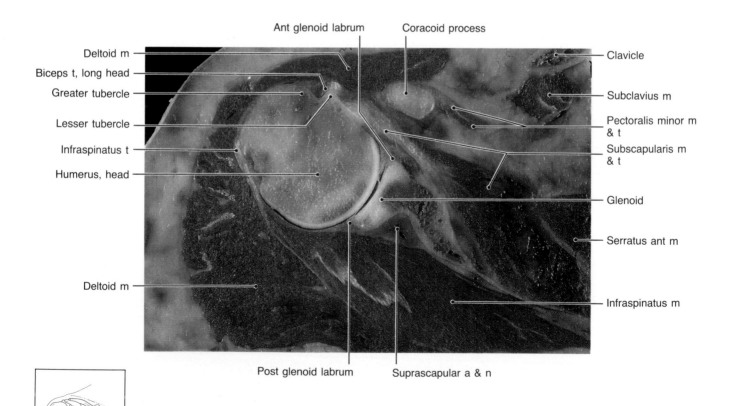

Ant glenoid labrum — Coracoid process

Deltoid m

Biceps t, long head

Greater tubercle

Lesser tubercle

Infraspinatus t

Humerus, head

Clavicle

Subclavius m

Pectoralis minor m & t

Subscapularis m & t

Glenoid

Serratus ant m

Deltoid m

Infraspinatus m

Post glenoid labrum   Suprascapular a & n

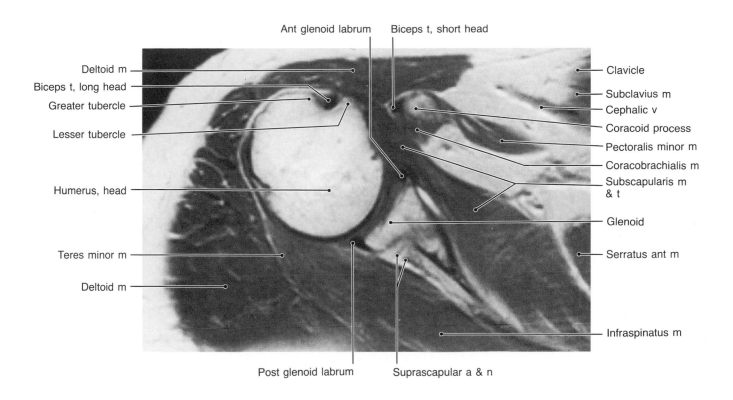

Ant glenoid labrum Biceps t, short head

Deltoid m

Biceps t, long head

Greater tubercle

Lesser tubercle

Humerus, head

Teres minor m

Deltoid m

Clavicle

Subclavius m

Cephalic v

Coracoid process

Pectoralis minor m

Coracobrachialis m

Subscapularis m & t

Glenoid

Serratus ant m

Infraspinatus m

Post glenoid labrum Suprascapular a & n

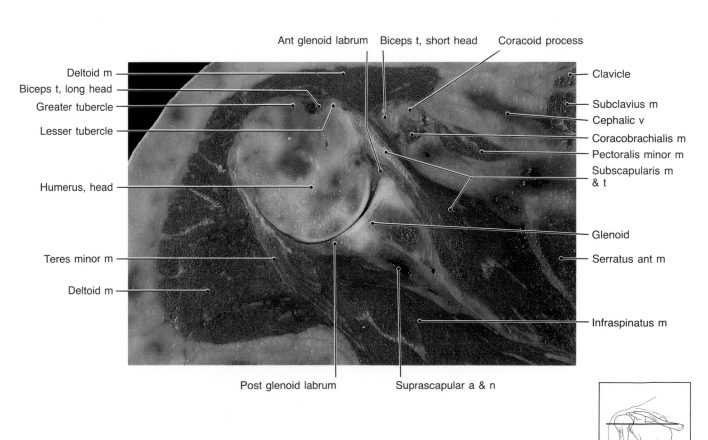

Ant glenoid labrum Biceps t, short head Coracoid process

Deltoid m

Biceps t, long head

Greater tubercle

Lesser tubercle

Humerus, head

Teres minor m

Deltoid m

Clavicle

Subclavius m

Cephalic v

Coracobrachialis m

Pectoralis minor m

Subscapularis m & t

Glenoid

Serratus ant m

Infraspinatus m

Post glenoid labrum Suprascapular a & n

SHOULDER, TRANSVERSE

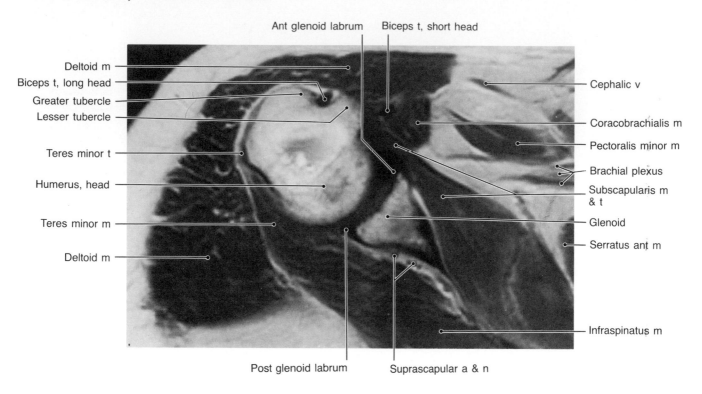

Ant glenoid labrum   Biceps t, short head

Deltoid m

Biceps t, long head

Greater tubercle

Lesser tubercle

Teres minor t

Humerus, head

Teres minor m

Deltoid m

Cephalic v

Coracobrachialis m

Pectoralis minor m

Brachial plexus

Subscapularis m & t

Glenoid

Serratus ant m

Infraspinatus m

Post glenoid labrum   Suprascapular a & n

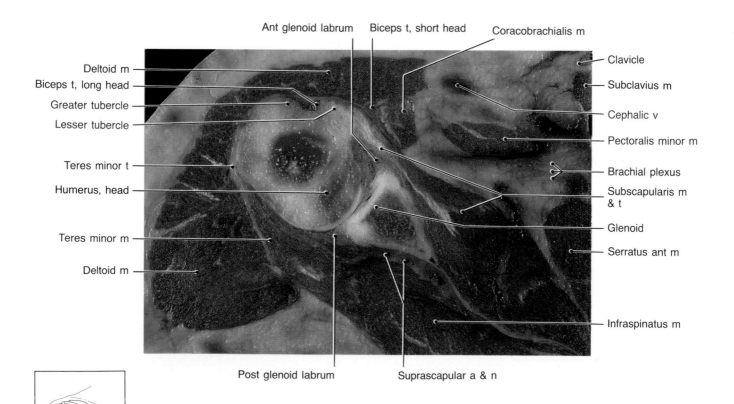

Ant glenoid labrum   Biceps t, short head   Coracobrachialis m

Deltoid m

Biceps t, long head

Greater tubercle

Lesser tubercle

Teres minor t

Humerus, head

Teres minor m

Deltoid m

Clavicle

Subclavius m

Cephalic v

Pectoralis minor m

Brachial plexus

Subscapularis m & t

Glenoid

Serratus ant m

Infraspinatus m

Post glenoid labrum   Suprascapular a & n

Biceps m & t, short head   Coracobrachialis m

Deltoid m

Biceps t, long head

Greater tubercle

Lesser tubercle

Humerus

Teres minor m

Deltoid m

Triceps m, long head

Cephalic v

Pectoralis major m

Thoracoacromial a, deltoid branch

Pectoralis minor m

Brachial plexus

Subscapularis m

Serratus ant m

Infraspinatus m

Glenoid labrum   Glenoid

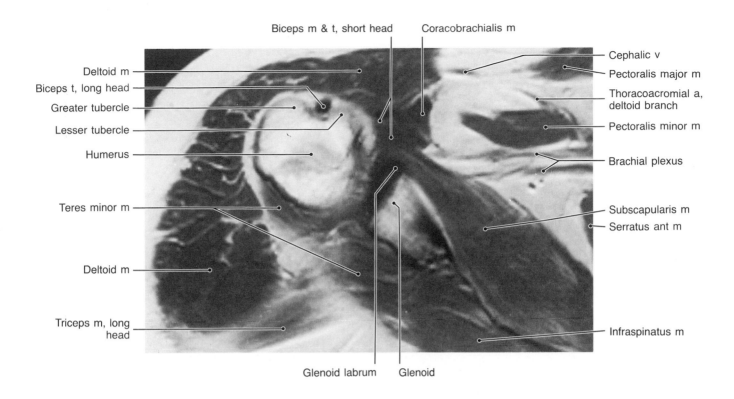

Biceps m & t, short head   Coracobrachialis m

Deltoid m

Biceps t, long head

Greater tubercle

Lesser tubercle

Humerus

Teres minor m

Deltoid m

Triceps m, long head

Cephalic v

Pectoralis major m

Thoracoacromial a, deltoid branch

Pectoralis minor m

Brachial plexus

Ant glenoid labrum

Subscapularis m

Serratus ant m

Infraspinatus m

Post glenoid labrum   Glenoid

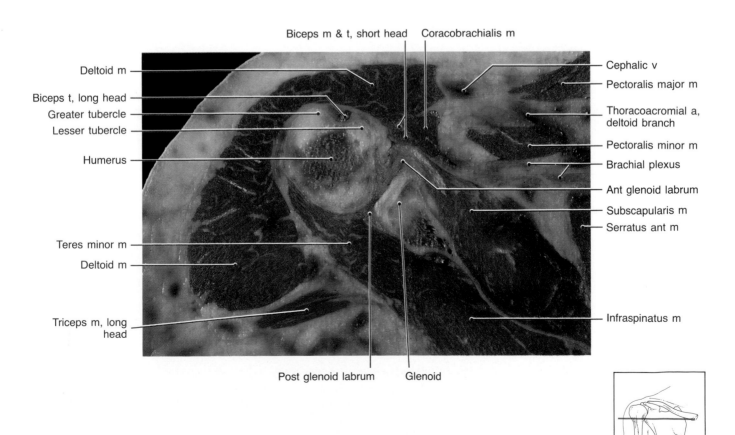

SHOULDER, TRANSVERSE

Biceps m, short head   Coracobrachialis m

Deltoid m

Biceps t, long head

Humerus

Deltoid m

Triceps m, long head

Cephalic v
Pectoralis major m
Thoracoacromial a, deltoid branch
Pectoralis minor m
Axillary a
Brachial plexus
Subscapularis m
Infraspinatus m

Teres minor m   Glenoid

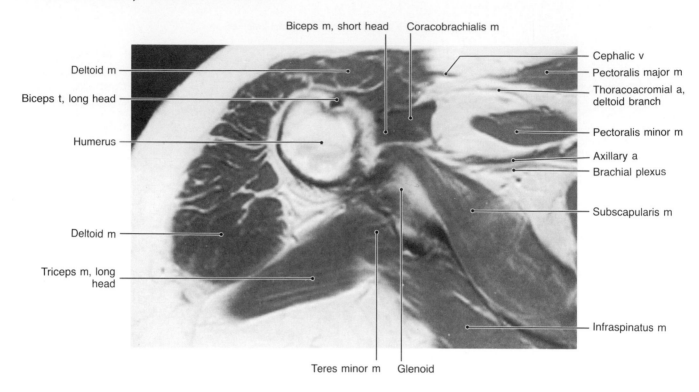

Biceps m, short head   Coracobrachialis m

Deltoid m

Biceps t, long head

Humerus

Deltoid m

Triceps m, long head

Cephalic v
Pectoralis major m
Thoracoacromial a, deltoid branch
Pectoralis minor m
Axillary a
Brachial plexus
Subscapularis m
Infraspinatus m

Teres minor m   Glenoid

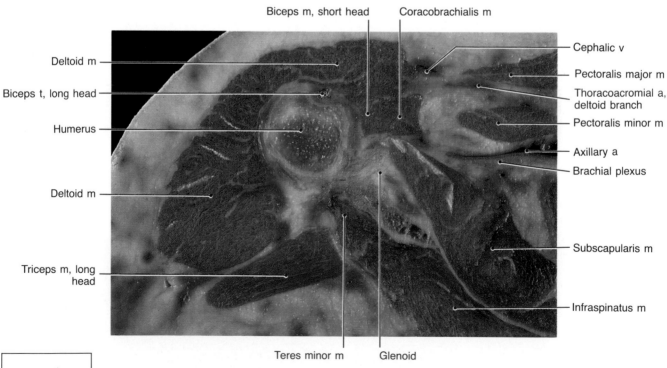

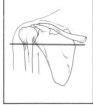

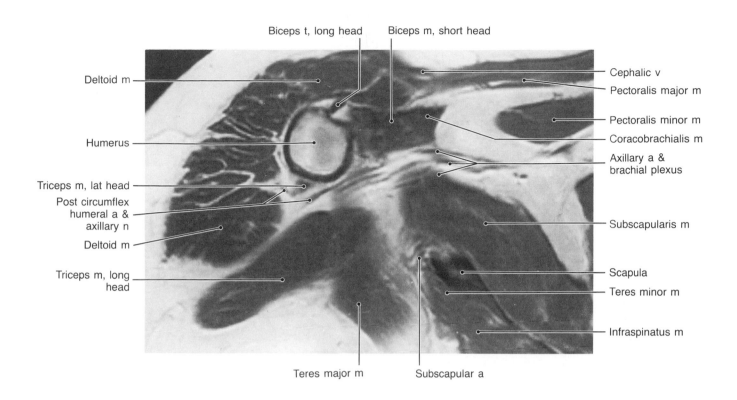

Biceps t, long head
Biceps m, short head
Deltoid m
Cephalic v
Pectoralis major m
Humerus
Pectoralis minor m
Coracobrachialis m
Triceps m, lat head
Axillary a &
brachial plexus
Post circumflex
humeral a &
axillary n
Deltoid m
Subscapularis m
Triceps m, long
head
Scapula
Teres minor m
Infraspinatus m
Teres major m
Subscapular a

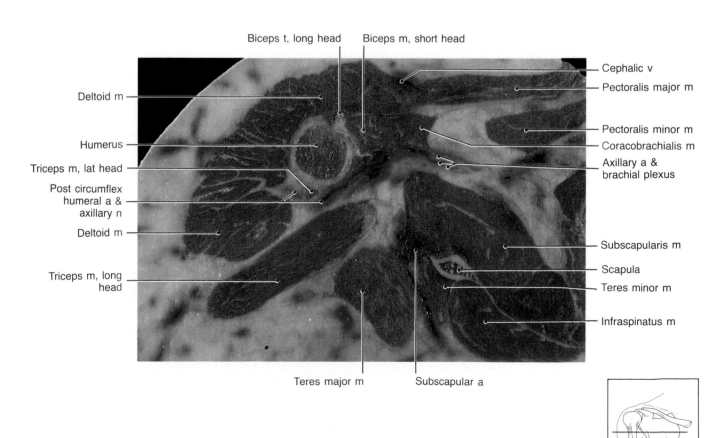

Biceps t, long head
Biceps m, short head
Deltoid m
Cephalic v
Pectoralis major m
Humerus
Pectoralis minor m
Coracobrachialis m
Triceps m, lat head
Axillary a &
brachial plexus
Post circumflex
humeral a &
axillary n
Deltoid m
Subscapularis m
Triceps m, long
head
Scapula
Teres minor m
Infraspinatus m
Teres major m
Subscapular a

SHOULDER, TRANSVERSE

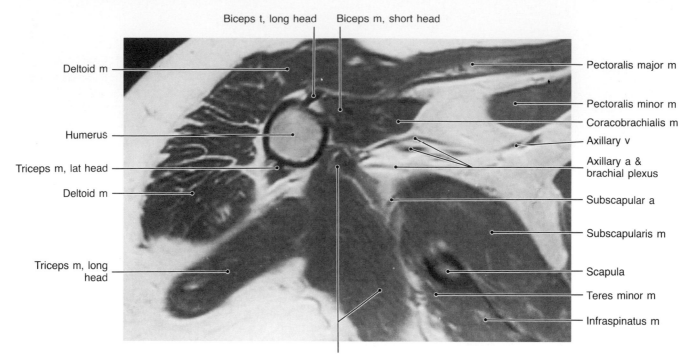

Biceps t, long head

Biceps m, short head

Deltoid m

Humerus

Triceps m, lat head

Deltoid m

Triceps m, long head

Pectoralis major m

Pectoralis minor m

Coracobrachialis m

Axillary v

Axillary a & brachial plexus

Subscapular a

Subscapularis m

Scapula

Teres minor m

Infraspinatus m

Teres major & latissimus dorsi mm

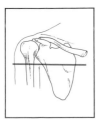

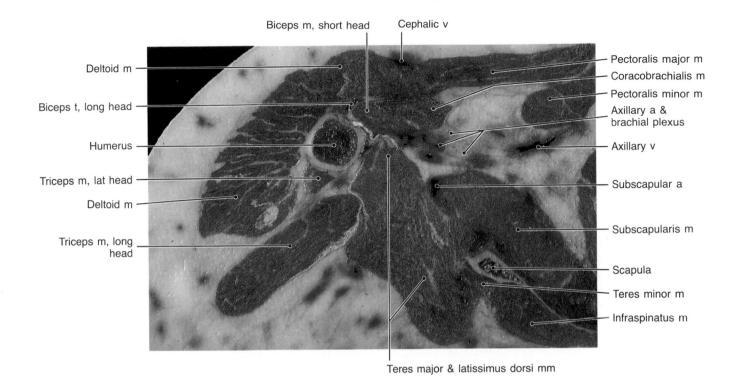

Biceps m, short head

Cephalic v

Deltoid m

Pectoralis major m

Biceps t, long head

Coracobrachialis m

Pectoralis minor m

Humerus

Axillary a & brachial plexus

Triceps m, lat head

Axillary v

Deltoid m

Subscapular a

Triceps m, long head

Subscapularis m

Scapula

Teres minor m

Infraspinatus m

Teres major & latissimus dorsi mm

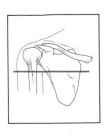

SHOULDER, SAGITTAL

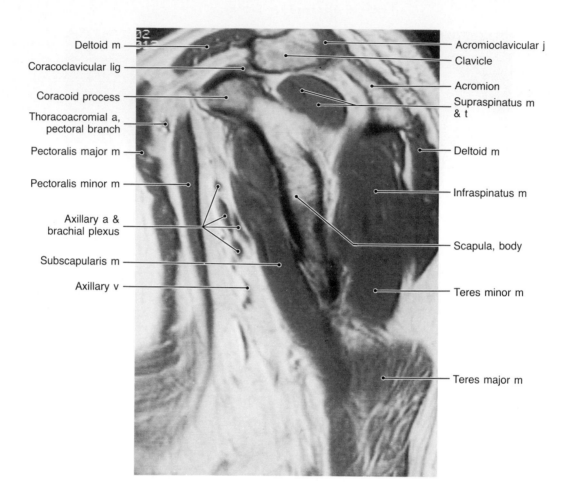

Deltoid m — Acromioclavicular j

Coracoclavicular lig — Clavicle

Coracoid process — Acromion

Thoracoacromial a, pectoral branch — Supraspinatus m & t

Pectoralis major m — Deltoid m

Pectoralis minor m — Infraspinatus m

Axillary a & brachial plexus — Scapula, body

Subscapularis m — Teres minor m

Axillary v —

— Teres major m

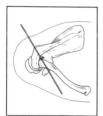

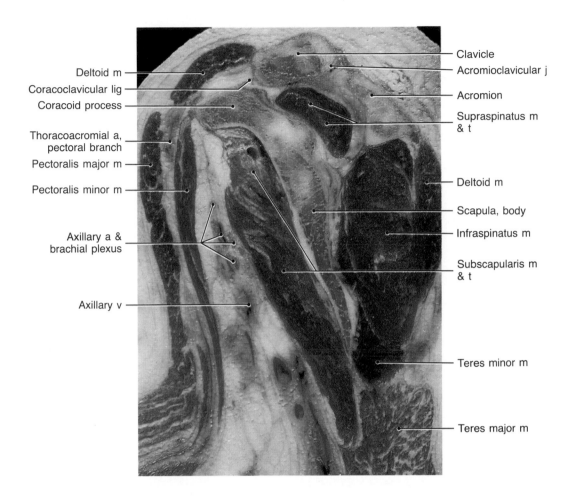

Deltoid m

Coracoclavicular lig

Coracoid process

Thoracoacromial a, pectoral branch

Pectoralis major m

Pectoralis minor m

Axillary a & brachial plexus

Axillary v

Clavicle

Acromioclavicular j

Acromion

Supraspinatus m & t

Deltoid m

Scapula, body

Infraspinatus m

Subscapularis m & t

Teres minor m

Teres major m

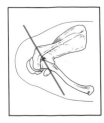

SHOULDER, SAGITTAL

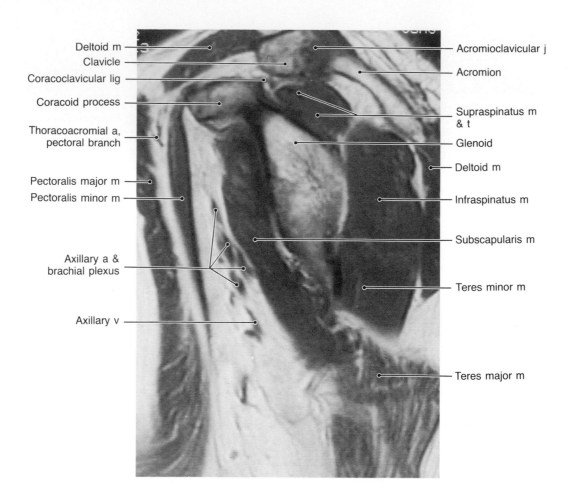

Deltoid m

Clavicle

Coracoclavicular lig

Coracoid process

Thoracoacromial a, pectoral branch

Pectoralis major m

Pectoralis minor m

Axillary a & brachial plexus

Axillary v

Acromioclavicular j

Acromion

Supraspinatus m & t

Glenoid

Deltoid m

Infraspinatus m

Subscapularis m

Teres minor m

Teres major m

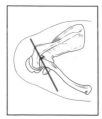

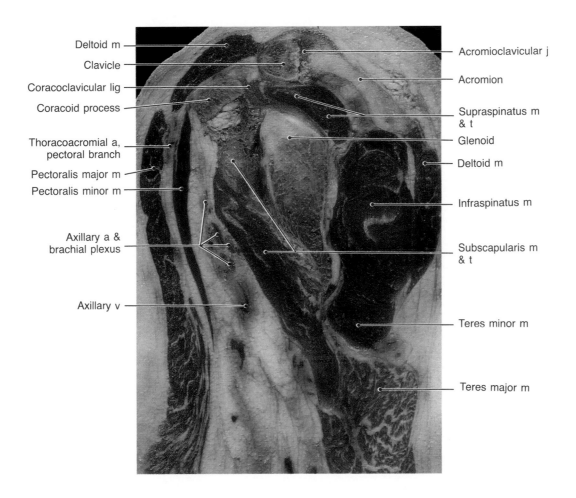

Deltoid m

Clavicle

Coracoclavicular lig

Coracoid process

Thoracoacromial a,
pectoral branch

Pectoralis major m

Pectoralis minor m

Axillary a &
brachial plexus

Axillary v

Acromioclavicular j

Acromion

Supraspinatus m
& t

Glenoid

Deltoid m

Infraspinatus m

Subscapularis m
& t

Teres minor m

Teres major m

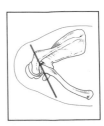

SHOULDER, SAGITTAL

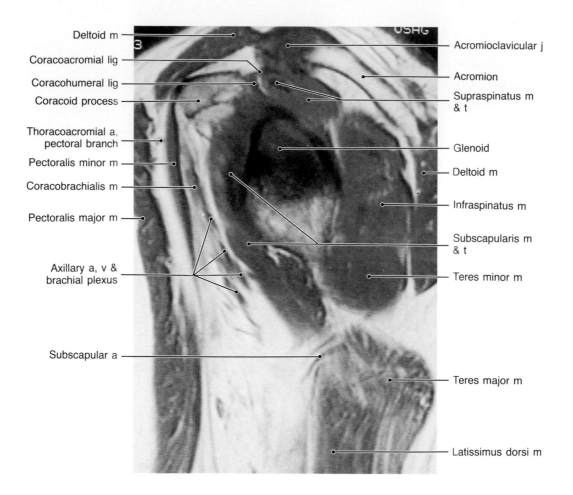

Deltoid m

Coracoacromial lig

Coracohumeral lig

Coracoid process

Thoracoacromial a,
pectoral branch

Pectoralis minor m

Coracobrachialis m

Pectoralis major m

Axillary a, v &
brachial plexus

Subscapular a

Acromioclavicular j

Acromion

Supraspinatus m
& t

Glenoid

Deltoid m

Infraspinatus m

Subscapularis m
& t

Teres minor m

Teres major m

Latissimus dorsi m

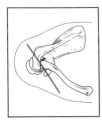

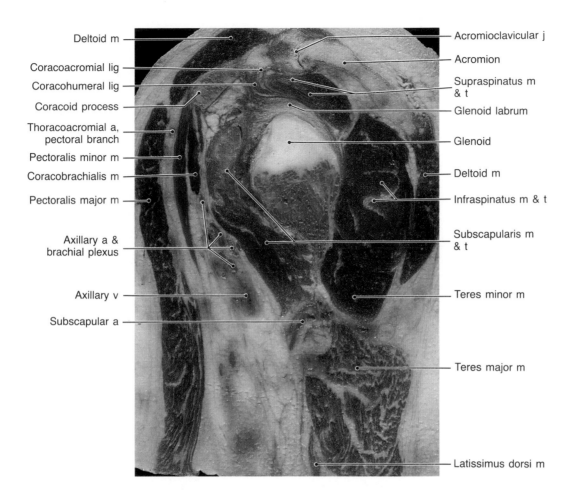

Deltoid m

Coracoacromial lig

Coracohumeral lig

Coracoid process

Thoracoacromial a,
pectoral branch

Pectoralis minor m

Coracobrachialis m

Pectoralis major m

Axillary a &
brachial plexus

Axillary v

Subscapular a

Acromioclavicular j

Acromion

Supraspinatus m
& t

Glenoid labrum

Glenoid

Deltoid m

Infraspinatus m & t

Subscapularis m
& t

Teres minor m

Teres major m

Latissimus dorsi m

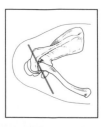

SHOULDER, SAGITTAL

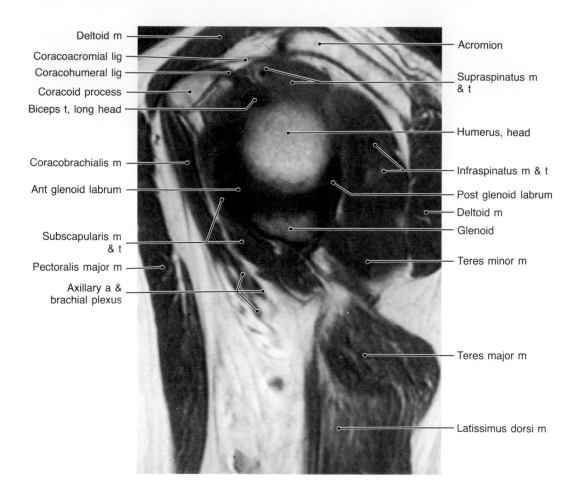

Deltoid m
Coracoacromial lig
Coracohumeral lig
Coracoid process
Biceps t, long head
Coracobrachialis m
Ant glenoid labrum
Subscapularis m & t
Pectoralis major m
Axillary a & brachial plexus

Acromion
Supraspinatus m & t
Humerus, head
Infraspinatus m & t
Post glenoid labrum
Deltoid m
Glenoid
Teres minor m
Teres major m
Latissimus dorsi m

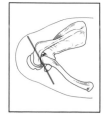

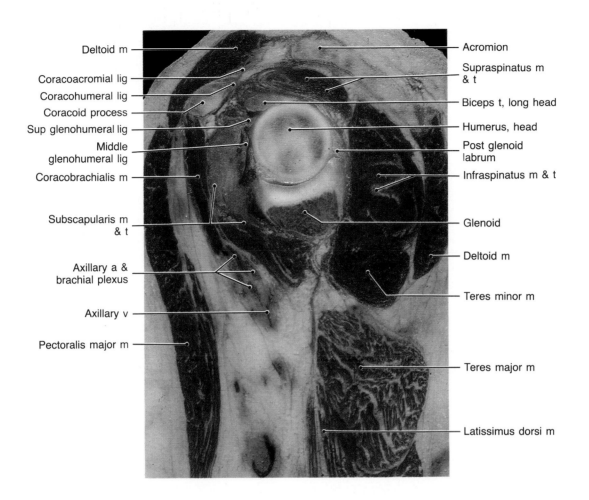

Deltoid m

Coracoacromial lig

Coracohumeral lig

Coracoid process

Sup glenohumeral lig

Middle
glenohumeral lig

Coracobrachialis m

Subscapularis m
& t

Axillary a &
brachial plexus

Axillary v

Pectoralis major m

Acromion

Supraspinatus m
& t

Biceps t, long head

Humerus, head

Post glenoid
labrum

Infraspinatus m & t

Glenoid

Deltoid m

Teres minor m

Teres major m

Latissimus dorsi m

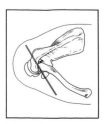

SHOULDER, SAGITTAL

Deltoid m

Coracoacromial lig

Biceps t, long head

Coracoid process

Coracobrachialis m

Subscapularis m & t

Pectoralis major m

Axillary a, v & brachial plexus

Acromion

Supraspinatus m & t

Humerus, head

Infraspinatus m & t

Deltoid m

Inf glenoid labrum

Teres minor m

Triceps m & t, long head

Teres major m

Latissimus dorsi m

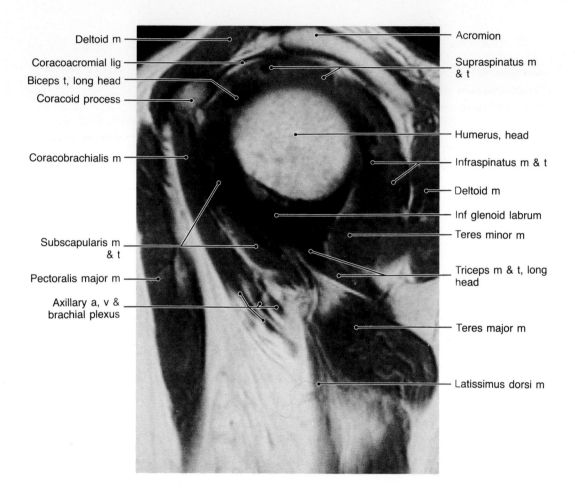

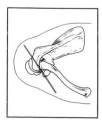

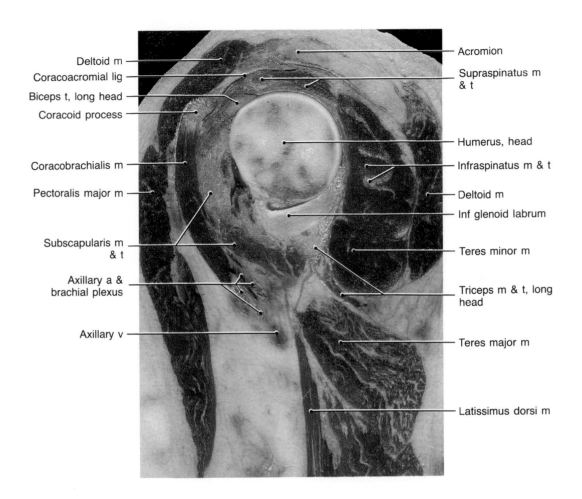

Deltoid m

Coracoacromial lig

Biceps t, long head

Coracoid process

Coracobrachialis m

Pectoralis major m

Subscapularis m & t

Axillary a & brachial plexus

Axillary v

Acromion

Supraspinatus m & t

Humerus, head

Infraspinatus m & t

Deltoid m

Inf glenoid labrum

Teres minor m

Triceps m & t, long head

Teres major m

Latissimus dorsi m

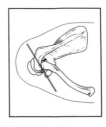

SHOULDER, SAGITTAL

Coracoacromial lig

Deltoid m

Biceps t, long head

Pectoralis major m

Coracobrachialis &
biceps (short head)
mm

Musculocutaneous
n

Subscapularis m
& t

Axillary a, v &
brachial plexus

Acromion

Supraspinatus m
& t

Infraspinatus m & t

Humerus, head

Deltoid m

Teres minor m

Triceps m, long
head

Axillary n

Teres major m

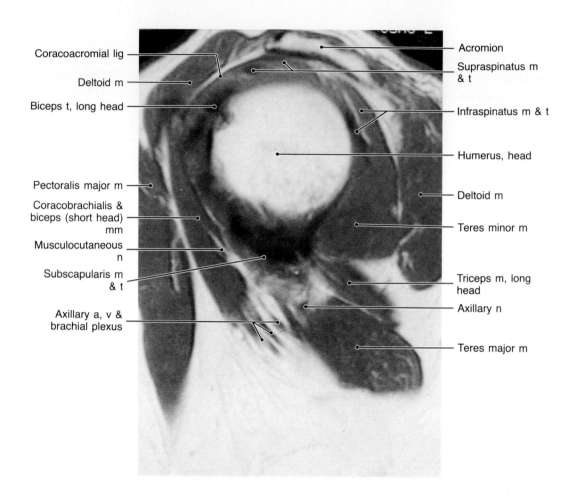

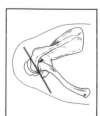

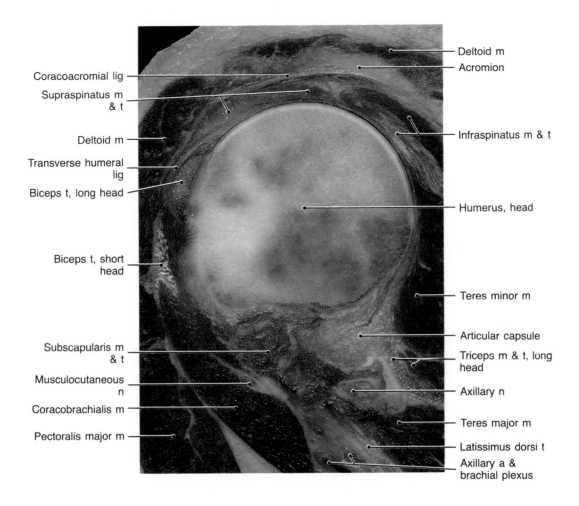

Coracoacromial lig

Supraspinatus m & t

Deltoid m

Transverse humeral lig

Biceps t, long head

Biceps t, short head

Subscapularis m & t

Musculocutaneous n

Coracobrachialis m

Pectoralis major m

Deltoid m

Acromion

Infraspinatus m & t

Humerus, head

Teres minor m

Articular capsule

Triceps m & t, long head

Axillary n

Teres major m

Latissimus dorsi t

Axillary a & brachial plexus

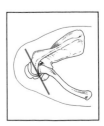

SHOULDER, SAGITTAL

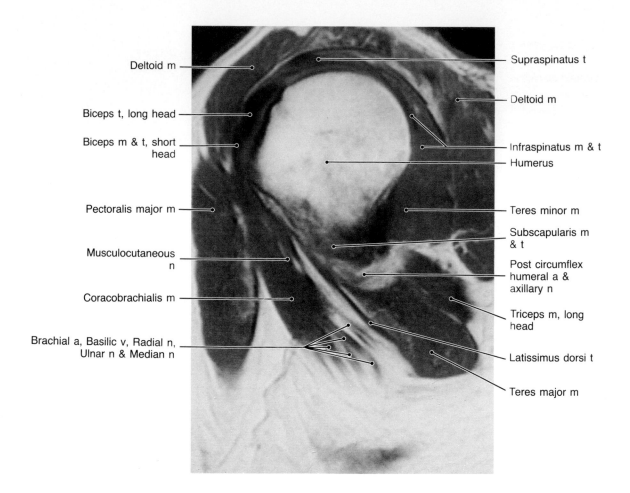

Deltoid m

Biceps t, long head

Biceps m & t, short head

Pectoralis major m

Musculocutaneous n

Coracobrachialis m

Brachial a, Basilic v, Radial n, Ulnar n & Median n

Supraspinatus t

Deltoid m

Infraspinatus m & t

Humerus

Teres minor m

Subscapularis m & t

Post circumflex humeral a & axillary n

Triceps m, long head

Latissimus dorsi t

Teres major m

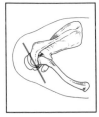

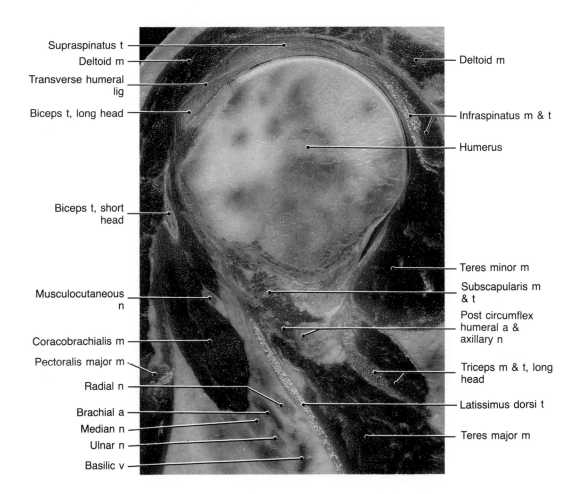

Supraspinatus t

Deltoid m

Transverse humeral lig

Biceps t, long head

Biceps t, short head

Musculocutaneous n

Coracobrachialis m

Pectoralis major m

Radial n

Brachial a

Median n

Ulnar n

Basilic v

Deltoid m

Infraspinatus m & t

Humerus

Teres minor m

Subscapularis m & t

Post circumflex humeral a & axillary n

Triceps m & t, long head

Latissimus dorsi t

Teres major m

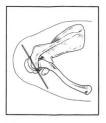

SHOULDER, SAGITTAL

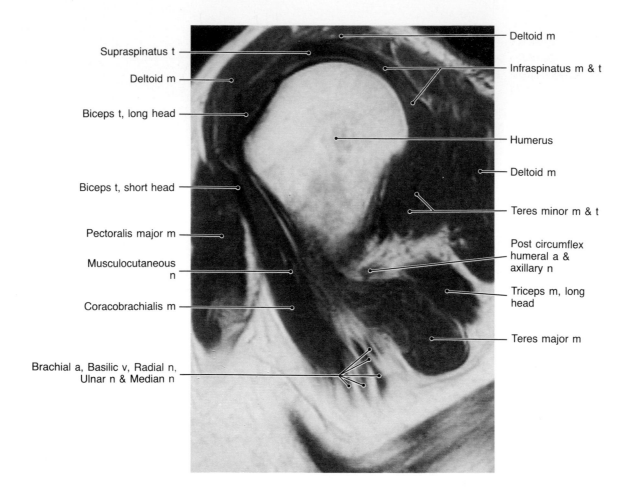

Supraspinatus t

Deltoid m

Biceps t, long head

Biceps t, short head

Pectoralis major m

Musculocutaneous n

Coracobrachialis m

Brachial a, Basilic v, Radial n, Ulnar n & Median n

Deltoid m

Infraspinatus m & t

Humerus

Deltoid m

Teres minor m & t

Post circumflex humeral a & axillary n

Triceps m, long head

Teres major m

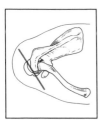

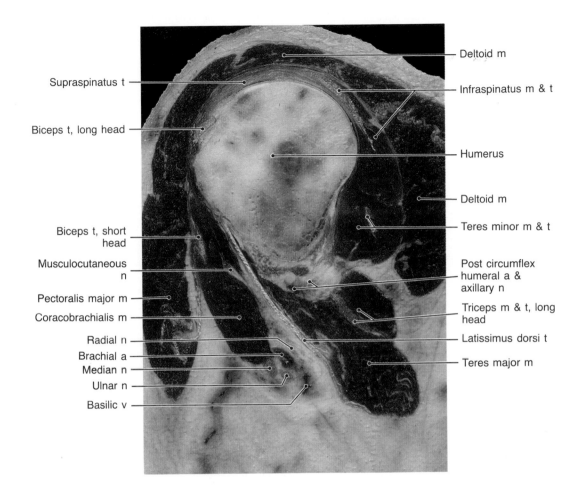

Supraspinatus t

Biceps t, long head

Biceps t, short head

Musculocutaneous n

Pectoralis major m

Coracobrachialis m

Radial n

Brachial a

Median n

Ulnar n

Basilic v

Deltoid m

Infraspinatus m & t

Humerus

Deltoid m

Teres minor m & t

Post circumflex humeral a & axillary n

Triceps m & t, long head

Latissimus dorsi t

Teres major m

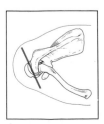

SHOULDER, SAGITTAL

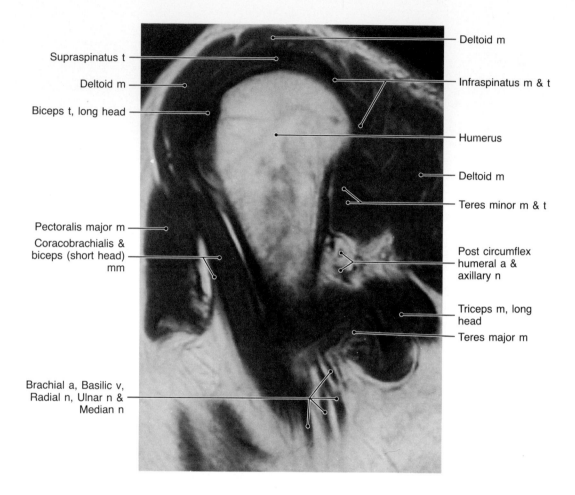

Supraspinatus t

Deltoid m

Biceps t, long head

Pectoralis major m

Coracobrachialis & biceps (short head) mm

Brachial a, Basilic v, Radial n, Ulnar n & Median n

Deltoid m

Infraspinatus m & t

Humerus

Deltoid m

Teres minor m & t

Post circumflex humeral a & axillary n

Triceps m, long head

Teres major m

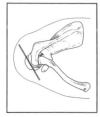

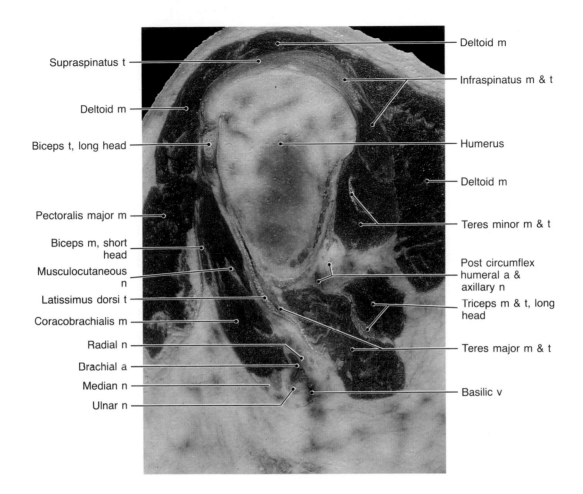

Supraspinatus t

Deltoid m

Biceps t, long head

Pectoralis major m

Biceps m, short head

Musculocutaneous n

Latissimus dorsi t

Coracobrachialis m

Radial n

Brachial a

Median n

Ulnar n

Deltoid m

Infraspinatus m & t

Humerus

Deltoid m

Teres minor m & t

Post circumflex humeral a & axillary n

Triceps m & t, long head

Teres major m & t

Basilic v

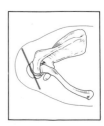

SHOULDER, SAGITTAL

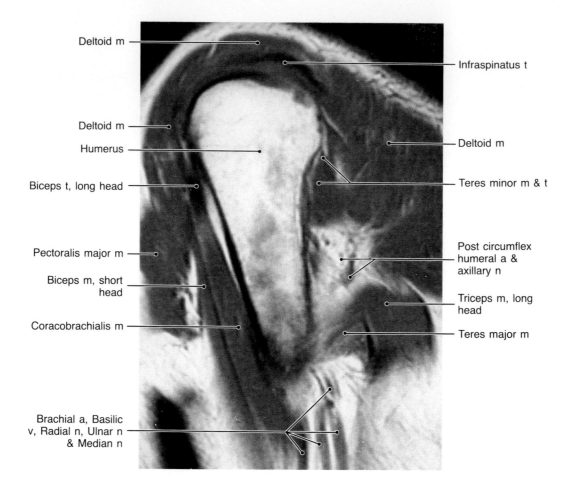

Deltoid m

Deltoid m

Humerus

Biceps t, long head

Pectoralis major m

Biceps m, short head

Coracobrachialis m

Brachial a, Basilic v, Radial n, Ulnar n & Median n

Infraspinatus t

Deltoid m

Teres minor m & t

Post circumflex humeral a & axillary n

Triceps m, long head

Teres major m

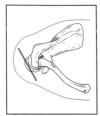

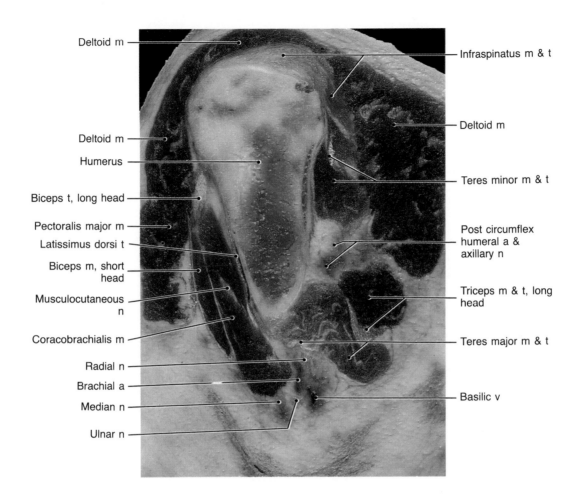

Deltoid m — Infraspinatus m & t

Deltoid m — Deltoid m

Humerus — Teres minor m & t

Biceps t, long head —

Pectoralis major m — Post circumflex humeral a & axillary n

Latissimus dorsi t —

Biceps m, short head —

Musculocutaneous n — Triceps m & t, long head

Coracobrachialis m — Teres major m & t

Radial n —

Brachial a — Basilic v

Median n —

Ulnar n —

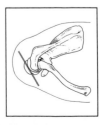

SHOULDER, SAGITTAL

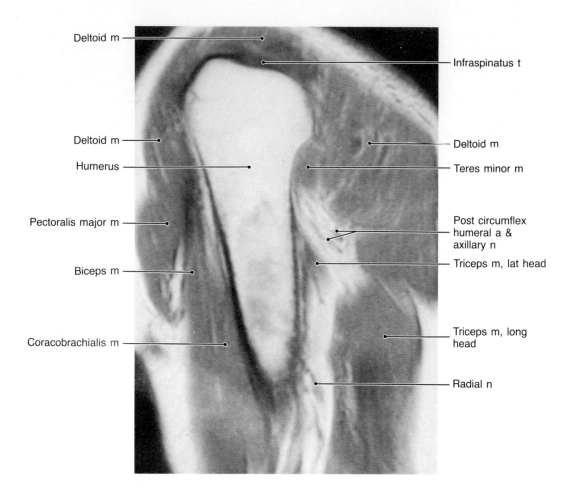

Deltoid m

Deltoid m

Humerus

Pectoralis major m

Biceps m

Coracobrachialis m

Infraspinatus t

Deltoid m

Teres minor m

Post circumflex humeral a & axillary n

Triceps m, lat head

Triceps m, long head

Radial n

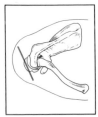

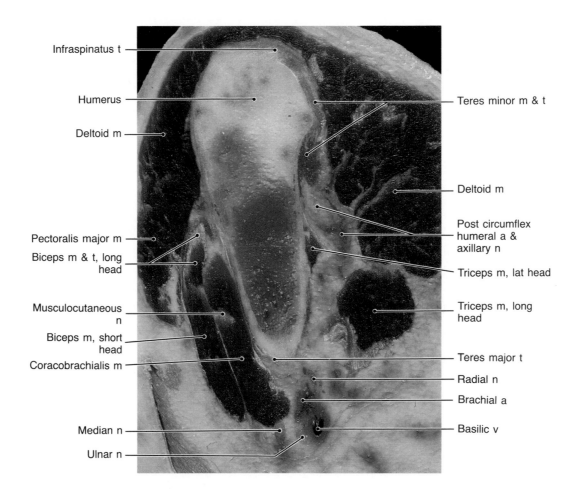

Infraspinatus t

Humerus

Deltoid m

Pectoralis major m

Biceps m & t, long head

Musculocutaneous n

Biceps m, short head

Coracobrachialis m

Median n

Ulnar n

Teres minor m & t

Deltoid m

Post circumflex humeral a & axillary n

Triceps m, lat head

Triceps m, long head

Teres major t

Radial n

Brachial a

Basilic v

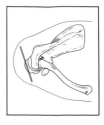

SHOULDER, SAGITTAL

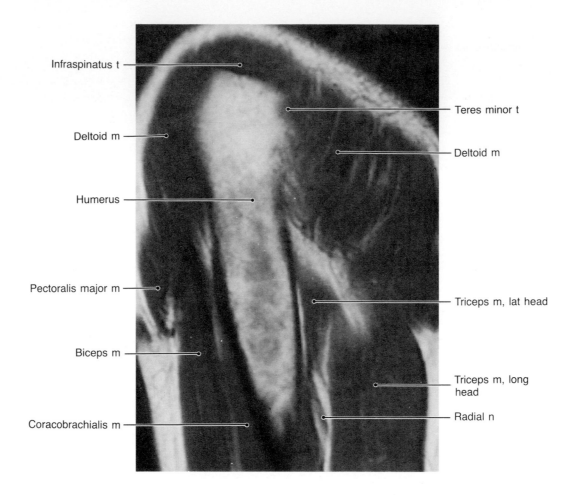

Infraspinatus t

Teres minor t

Deltoid m

Deltoid m

Humerus

Pectoralis major m

Triceps m, lat head

Biceps m

Triceps m, long head

Coracobrachialis m

Radial n

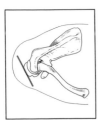

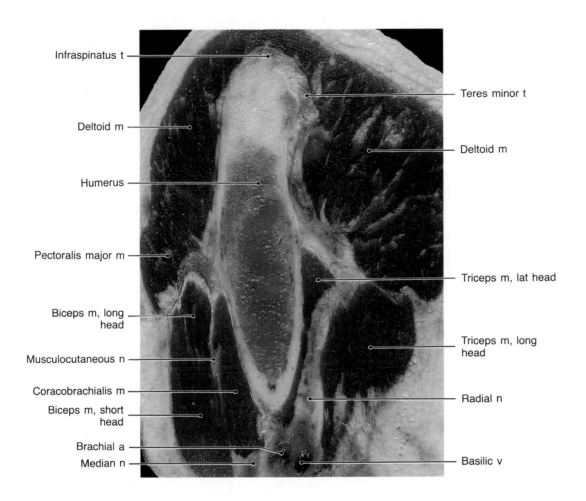

Infraspinatus t

Teres minor t

Deltoid m

Deltoid m

Humerus

Pectoralis major m

Triceps m, lat head

Biceps m, long head

Triceps m, long head

Musculocutaneous n

Coracobrachialis m

Radial n

Biceps m, short head

Brachial a

Median n

Basilic v

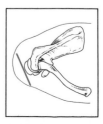

SHOULDER, SAGITTAL

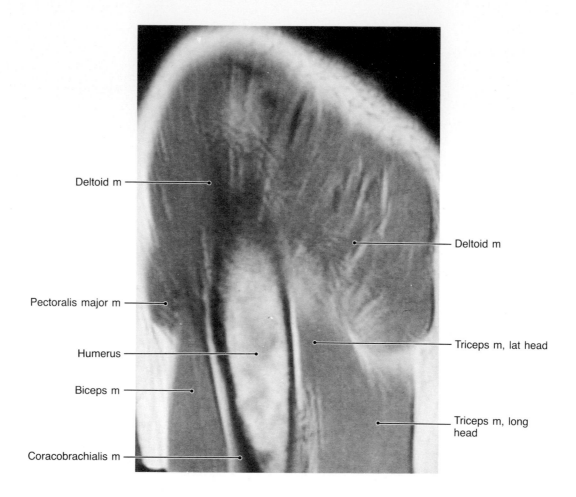

Deltoid m

Deltoid m

Pectoralis major m

Triceps m, lat head

Humerus

Biceps m

Triceps m, long head

Coracobrachialis m

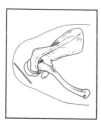

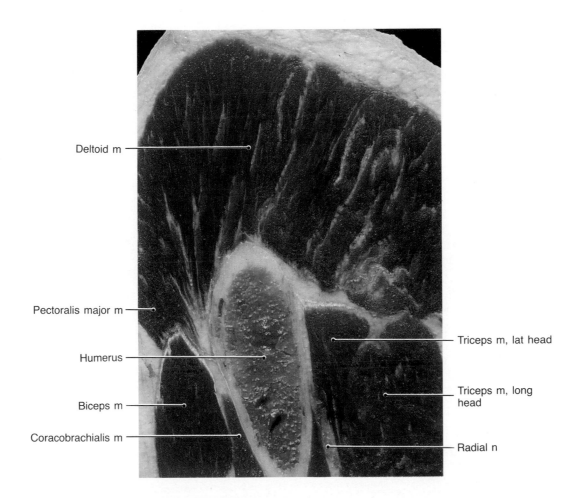

Deltoid m

Pectoralis major m

Humerus

Biceps m

Coracobrachialis m

Triceps m, lat head

Triceps m, long head

Radial n

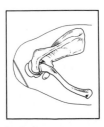

SHOULDER, CORONAL, INJECTED

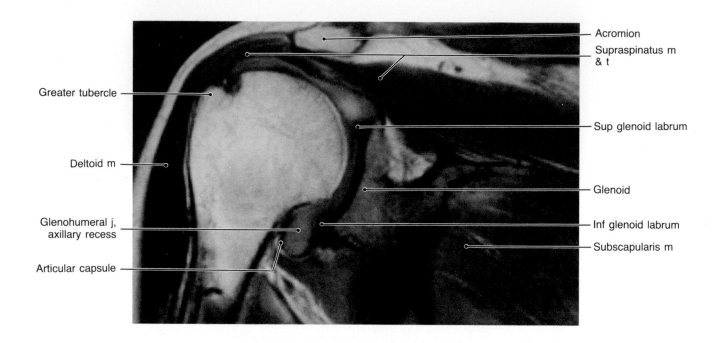

Acromion

Supraspinatus m & t

Greater tubercle

Sup glenoid labrum

Deltoid m

Glenoid

Glenohumeral j, axillary recess

Inf glenoid labrum

Subscapularis m

Articular capsule

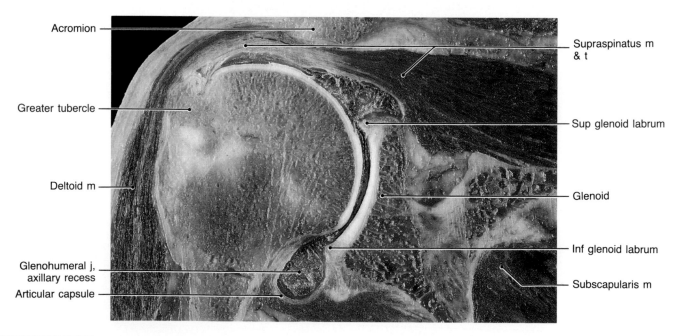

Acromion

Supraspinatus m & t

Greater tubercle

Sup glenoid labrum

Deltoid m

Glenoid

Glenohumeral j, axillary recess

Inf glenoid labrum

Subscapularis m

Articular capsule

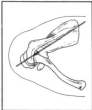

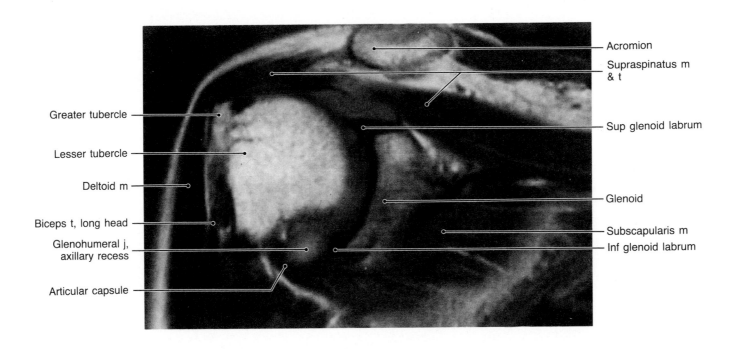

Acromion

Supraspinatus m & t

Greater tubercle

Sup glenoid labrum

Lesser tubercle

Deltoid m

Glenoid

Biceps t, long head

Subscapularis m

Glenohumeral j, axillary recess

Inf glenoid labrum

Articular capsule

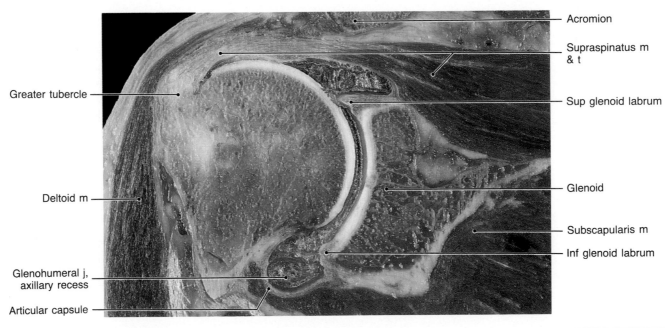

Acromion

Supraspinatus m & t

Greater tubercle

Sup glenoid labrum

Deltoid m

Glenoid

Subscapularis m

Inf glenoid labrum

Glenohumeral j, axillary recess

Articular capsule

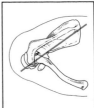

SHOULDER, CORONAL, INJECTED

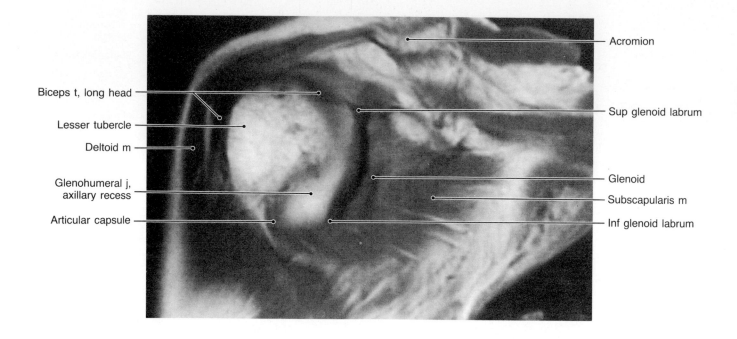

Biceps t, long head

Lesser tubercle

Deltoid m

Glenohumeral j, axillary recess

Articular capsule

Acromion

Sup glenoid labrum

Glenoid

Subscapularis m

Inf glenoid labrum

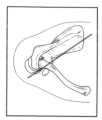

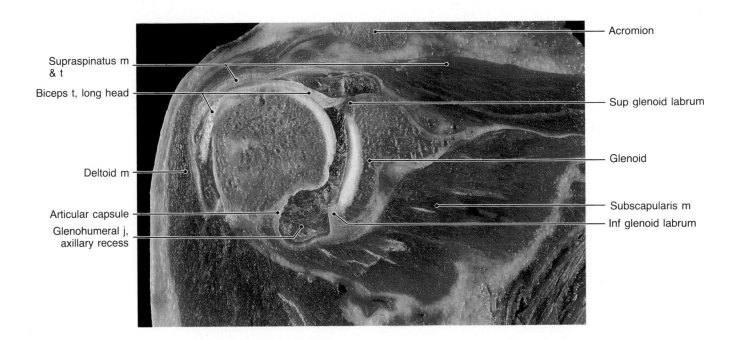

Acromion

Supraspinatus m & t

Biceps t, long head

Sup glenoid labrum

Deltoid m

Glenoid

Articular capsule

Subscapularis m

Glenohumeral j, axillary recess

Inf glenoid labrum

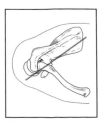

SHOULDER, TRANSVERSE, INJECTED

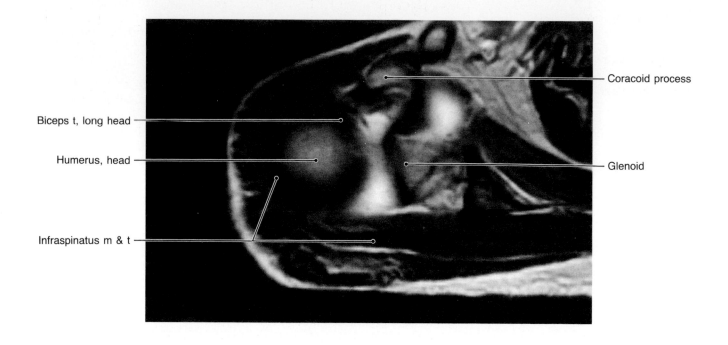

Biceps t, long head

Humerus, head

Infraspinatus m & t

Coracoid process

Glenoid

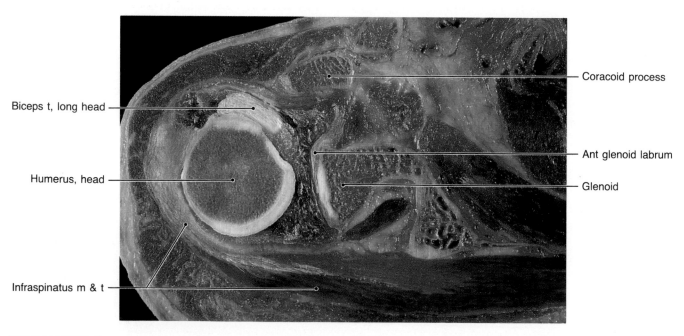

Biceps t, long head

Humerus, head

Infraspinatus m & t

Coracoid process

Ant glenoid labrum

Glenoid

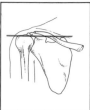

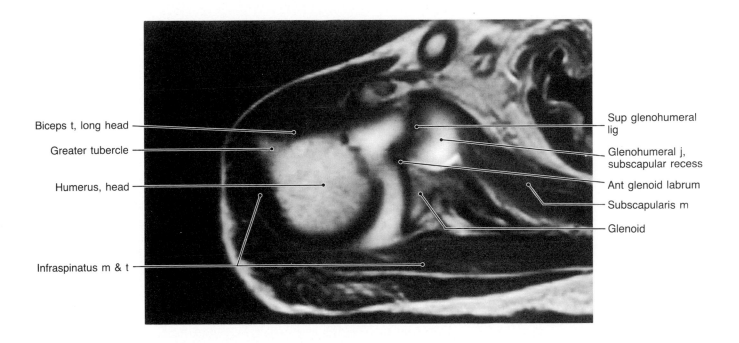

Biceps t, long head

Greater tubercle

Humerus, head

Infraspinatus m & t

Sup glenohumeral lig

Glenohumeral j, subscapular recess

Ant glenoid labrum

Subscapularis m

Glenoid

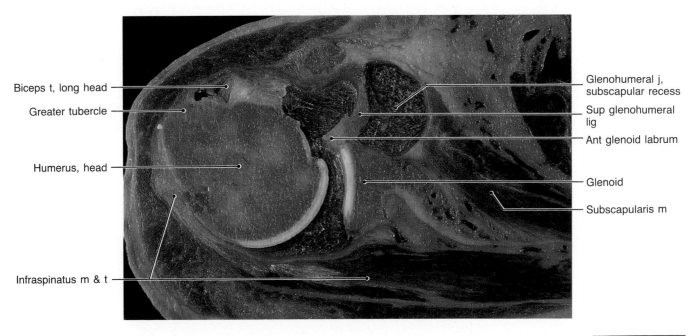

Biceps t, long head

Greater tubercle

Humerus, head

Infraspinatus m & t

Glenohumeral j, subscapular recess

Sup glenohumeral lig

Ant glenoid labrum

Glenoid

Subscapularis m

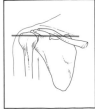

SHOULDER, TRANSVERSE, INJECTED

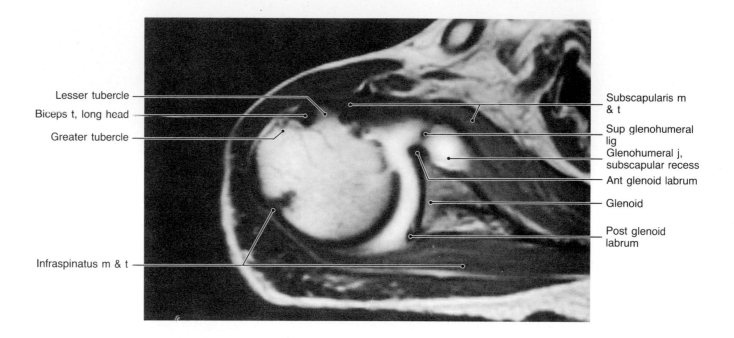

Lesser tubercle

Biceps t, long head

Greater tubercle

Infraspinatus m & t

Subscapularis m & t

Sup glenohumeral lig

Glenohumeral j, subscapular recess

Ant glenoid labrum

Glenoid

Post glenoid labrum

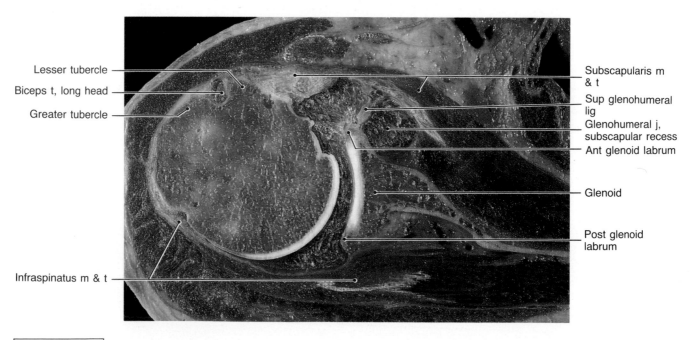

Lesser tubercle

Biceps t, long head

Greater tubercle

Infraspinatus m & t

Subscapularis m & t

Sup glenohumeral lig

Glenohumeral j, subscapular recess

Ant glenoid labrum

Glenoid

Post glenoid labrum

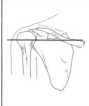

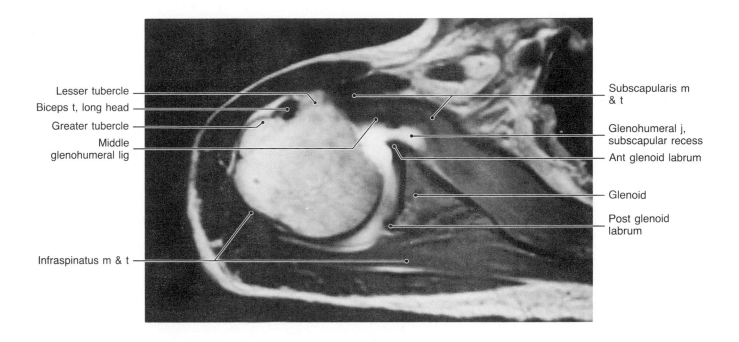

Lesser tubercle

Biceps t, long head

Greater tubercle

Middle
glenohumeral lig

Infraspinatus m & t

Subscapularis m
& t

Glenohumeral j,
subscapular recess

Ant glenoid labrum

Glenoid

Post glenoid
labrum

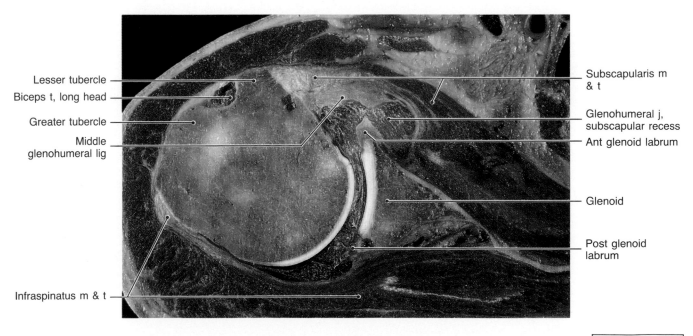

Lesser tubercle

Biceps t, long head

Greater tubercle

Middle
glenohumeral lig

Infraspinatus m & t

Subscapularis m
& t

Glenohumeral j,
subscapular recess

Ant glenoid labrum

Glenoid

Post glenoid
labrum

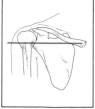

2 ELBOW

ELBOW, CORONAL

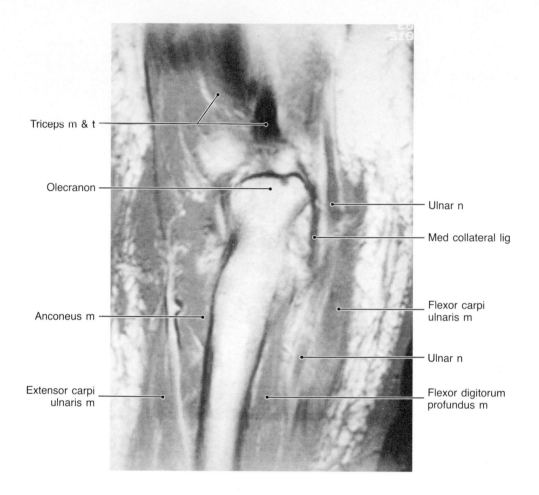

Triceps m & t

Olecranon

Ulnar n

Med collateral lig

Anconeus m

Flexor carpi
ulnaris m

Ulnar n

Extensor carpi
ulnaris m

Flexor digitorum
profundus m

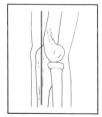

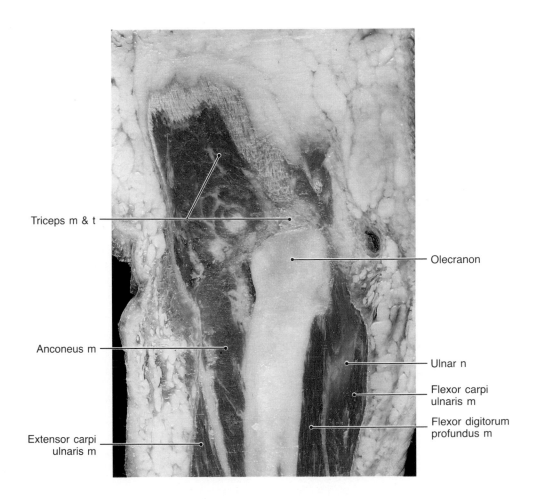

Triceps m & t

Olecranon

Anconeus m

Ulnar n

Flexor carpi
ulnaris m

Extensor carpi
ulnaris m

Flexor digitorum
profundus m

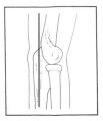

ELBOW, CORONAL

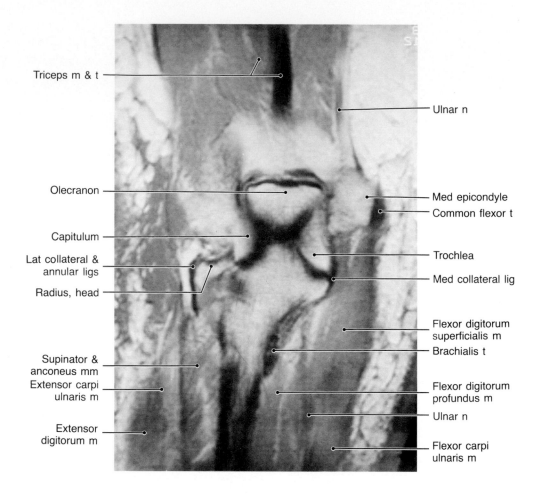

Triceps m & t

Ulnar n

Olecranon

Med epicondyle

Common flexor t

Capitulum

Trochlea

Lat collateral & annular ligs

Med collateral lig

Radius, head

Flexor digitorum superficialis m

Supinator & anconeus mm

Brachialis t

Extensor carpi ulnaris m

Flexor digitorum profundus m

Ulnar n

Extensor digitorum m

Flexor carpi ulnaris m

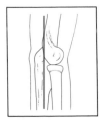

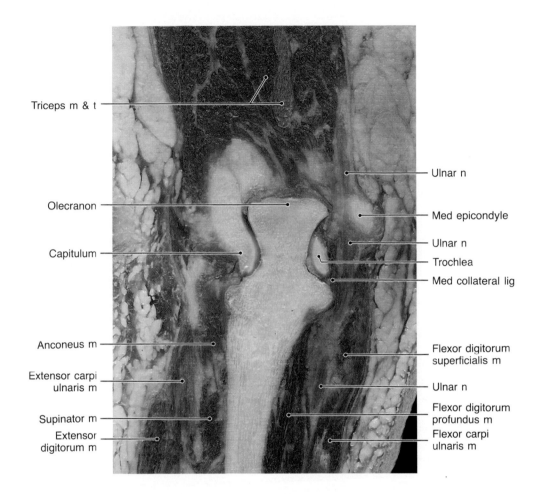

Triceps m & t

Olecranon

Capitulum

Anconeus m

Extensor carpi
ulnaris m

Supinator m

Extensor
digitorum m

Ulnar n

Med epicondyle

Ulnar n

Trochlea

Med collateral lig

Flexor digitorum
superficialis m

Ulnar n

Flexor digitorum
profundus m

Flexor carpi
ulnaris m

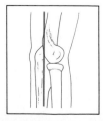

ELBOW, CORONAL

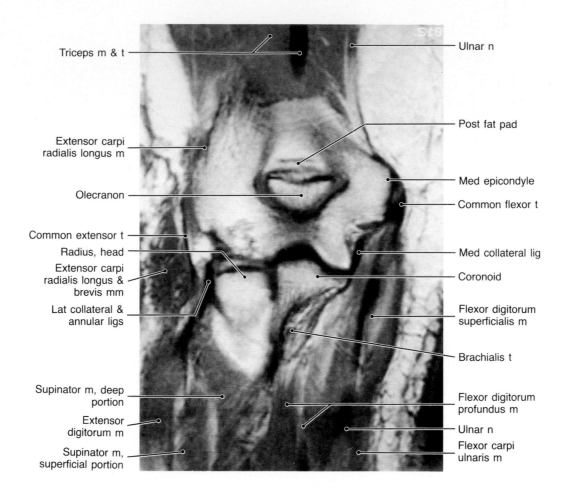

Triceps m & t

Ulnar n

Extensor carpi radialis longus m

Post fat pad

Olecranon

Med epicondyle

Common flexor t

Common extensor t

Radius, head

Med collateral lig

Extensor carpi radialis longus & brevis mm

Coronoid

Lat collateral & annular ligs

Flexor digitorum superficialis m

Brachialis t

Supinator m, deep portion

Flexor digitorum profundus m

Extensor digitorum m

Ulnar n

Supinator m, superficial portion

Flexor carpi ulnaris m

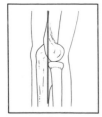

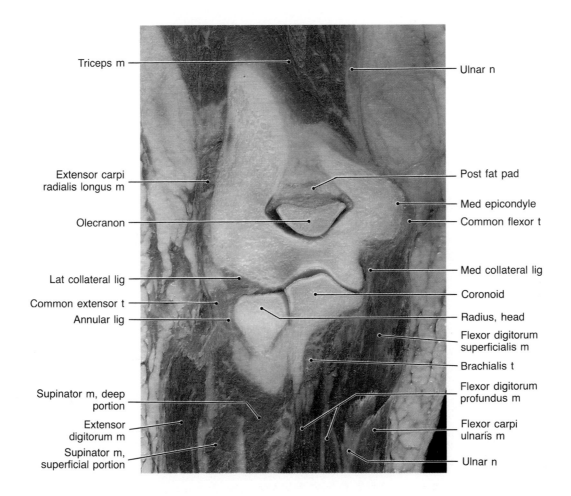

Triceps m

Ulnar n

Extensor carpi
radialis longus m

Post fat pad

Med epicondyle

Olecranon

Common flexor t

Lat collateral lig

Med collateral lig

Common extensor t

Coronoid

Annular lig

Radius, head

Flexor digitorum
superficialis m

Brachialis t

Supinator m, deep
portion

Flexor digitorum
profundus m

Extensor
digitorum m

Flexor carpi
ulnaris m

Supinator m,
superficial portion

Ulnar n

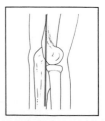

ELBOW, CORONAL

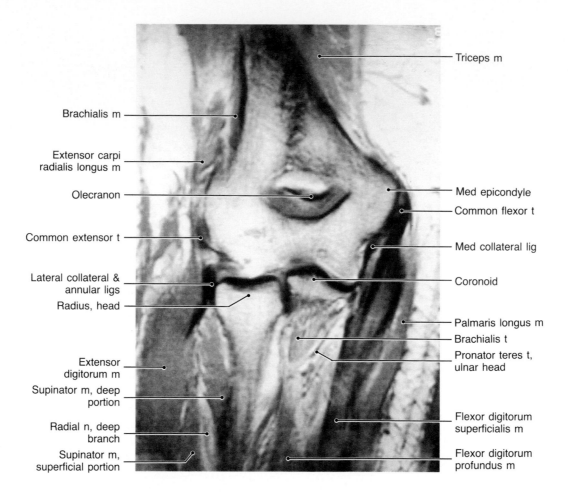

Triceps m

Brachialis m

Extensor carpi
radialis longus m

Olecranon

Med epicondyle

Common flexor t

Common extensor t

Med collateral lig

Lateral collateral &
annular ligs

Coronoid

Radius, head

Palmaris longus m

Brachialis t

Extensor
digitorum m

Pronator teres t,
ulnar head

Supinator m, deep
portion

Radial n, deep
branch

Flexor digitorum
superficialis m

Supinator m,
superficial portion

Flexor digitorum
profundus m

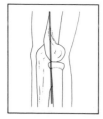

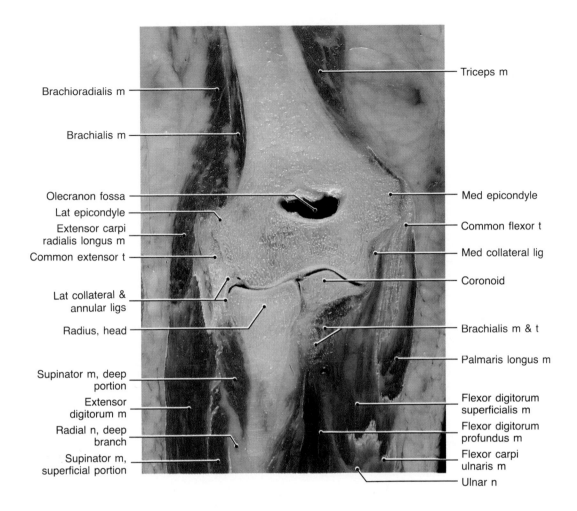

Brachioradialis m

Brachialis m

Olecranon fossa

Lat epicondyle

Extensor carpi radialis longus m

Common extensor t

Lat collateral & annular ligs

Radius, head

Supinator m, deep portion

Extensor digitorum m

Radial n, deep branch

Supinator m, superficial portion

Triceps m

Med epicondyle

Common flexor t

Med collateral lig

Coronoid

Brachialis m & t

Palmaris longus m

Flexor digitorum superficialis m

Flexor digitorum profundus m

Flexor carpi ulnaris m

Ulnar n

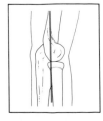

ELBOW, CORONAL

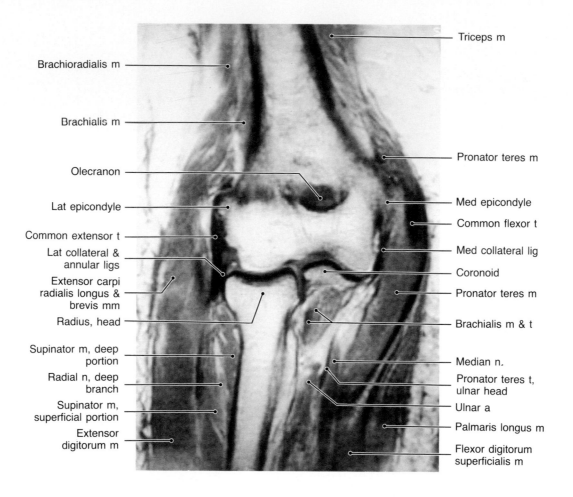

Brachioradialis m

Brachialis m

Olecranon

Lat epicondyle

Common extensor t

Lat collateral & annular ligs

Extensor carpi radialis longus & brevis mm

Radius, head

Supinator m, deep portion

Radial n, deep branch

Supinator m, superficial portion

Extensor digitorum m

Triceps m

Pronator teres m

Med epicondyle

Common flexor t

Med collateral lig

Coronoid

Pronator teres m

Brachialis m & t

Median n.

Pronator teres t, ulnar head

Ulnar a

Palmaris longus m

Flexor digitorum superficialis m

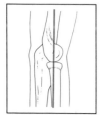

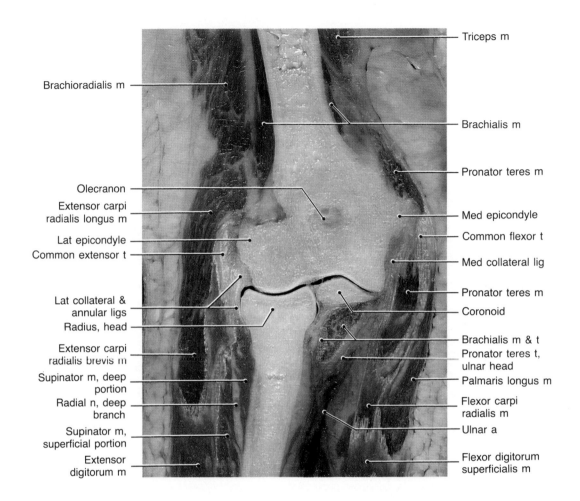

Triceps m

Brachioradialis m

Brachialis m

Pronator teres m

Olecranon

Extensor carpi
radialis longus m

Med epicondyle

Lat epicondyle

Common flexor t

Common extensor t

Med collateral lig

Lat collateral &
annular ligs

Pronator teres m

Coronoid

Radius, head

Extensor carpi
radialis brevis m

Brachialis m & t

Pronator teres t,
ulnar head

Supinator m, deep
portion

Palmaris longus m

Radial n, deep
branch

Flexor carpi
radialis m

Supinator m,
superficial portion

Ulnar a

Extensor
digitorum m

Flexor digitorum
superficialis m

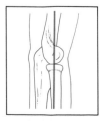

ELBOW, CORONAL

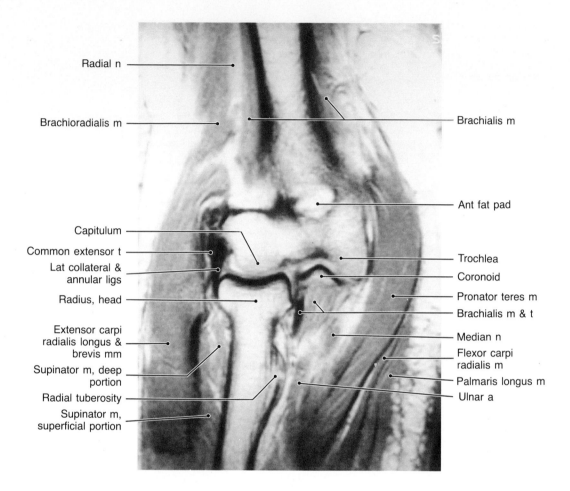

Radial n

Brachioradialis m — Brachialis m

Ant fat pad

Capitulum
Common extensor t — Trochlea
Lat collateral & annular ligs — Coronoid
Radius, head — Pronator teres m
Brachialis m & t
Extensor carpi radialis longus & brevis mm — Median n
Supinator m, deep portion — Flexor carpi radialis m
Radial tuberosity — Palmaris longus m
Supinator m, superficial portion — Ulnar a

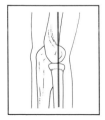

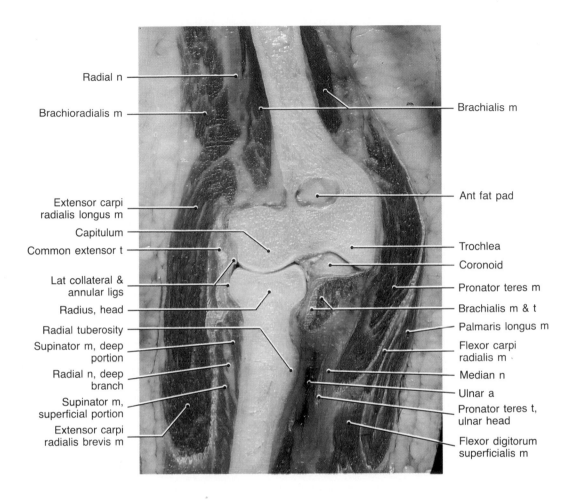

Radial n

Brachialis m

Brachioradialis m

Extensor carpi
radialis longus m

Ant fat pad

Capitulum

Trochlea

Common extensor t

Coronoid

Lat collateral &
annular ligs

Pronator teres m

Radius, head

Brachialis m & t

Radial tuberosity

Palmaris longus m

Supinator m, deep
portion

Flexor carpi
radialis m

Radial n, deep
branch

Median n

Supinator m,
superficial portion

Ulnar a

Pronator teres t,
ulnar head

Extensor carpi
radialis brevis m

Flexor digitorum
superficialis m

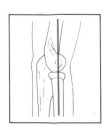

ELBOW, CORONAL

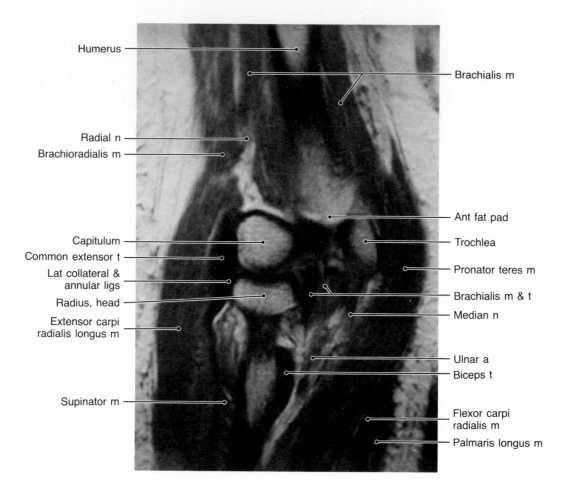

Humerus

Brachialis m

Radial n

Brachioradialis m

Ant fat pad

Capitulum

Trochlea

Common extensor t

Lat collateral &
annular ligs

Pronator teres m

Brachialis m & t

Radius, head

Median n

Extensor carpi
radialis longus m

Ulnar a

Biceps t

Supinator m

Flexor carpi
radialis m

Palmaris longus m

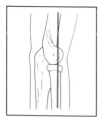

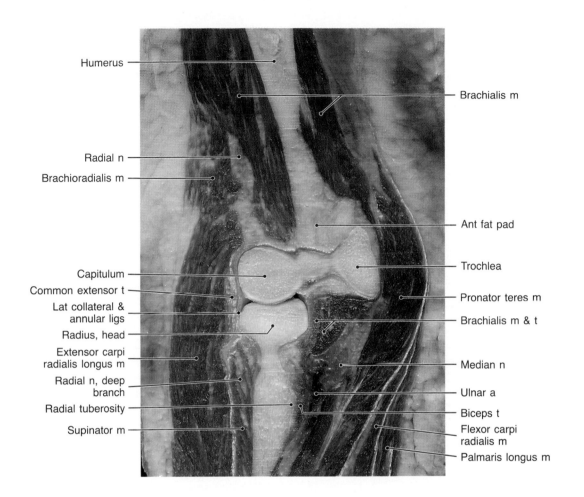

Humerus

Radial n

Brachioradialis m

Capitulum

Common extensor t

Lat collateral &
annular ligs

Radius, head

Extensor carpi
radialis longus m

Radial n, deep
branch

Radial tuberosity

Supinator m

Brachialis m

Ant fat pad

Trochlea

Pronator teres m

Brachialis m & t

Median n

Ulnar a

Biceps t

Flexor carpi
radialis m

Palmaris longus m

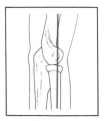

ELBOW, CORONAL

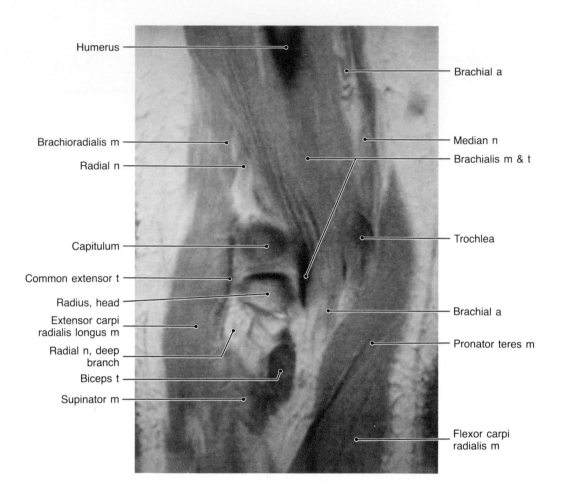

Humerus

Brachioradialis m

Radial n

Capitulum

Common extensor t

Radius, head

Extensor carpi radialis longus m

Radial n, deep branch

Biceps t

Supinator m

Brachial a

Median n

Brachialis m & t

Trochlea

Brachial a

Pronator teres m

Flexor carpi radialis m

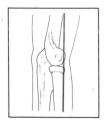

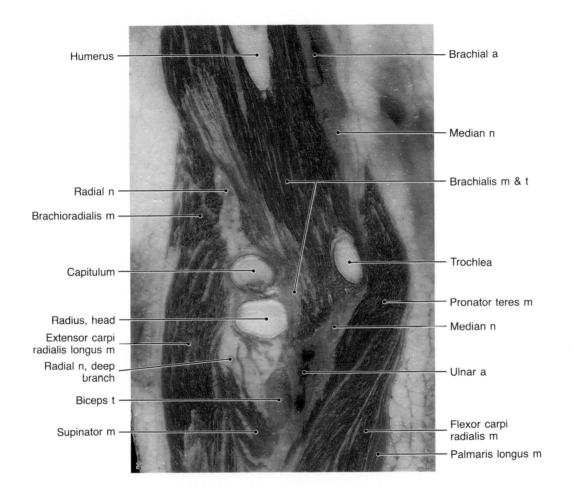

Humerus

Brachial a

Median n

Radial n

Brachialis m & t

Brachioradialis m

Capitulum

Trochlea

Radius, head

Pronator teres m

Extensor carpi
radialis longus m

Median n

Radial n, deep
branch

Ulnar a

Biceps t

Supinator m

Flexor carpi
radialis m

Palmaris longus m

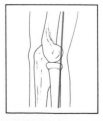

ELBOW, CORONAL

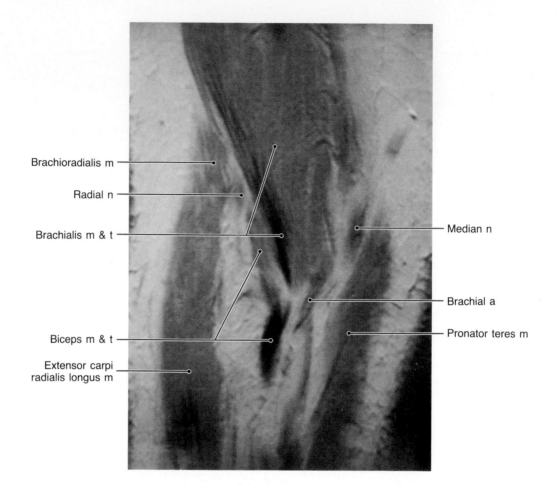

Brachioradialis m

Radial n

Brachialis m & t

Biceps m & t

Extensor carpi
radialis longus m

Median n

Brachial a

Pronator teres m

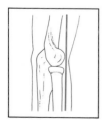

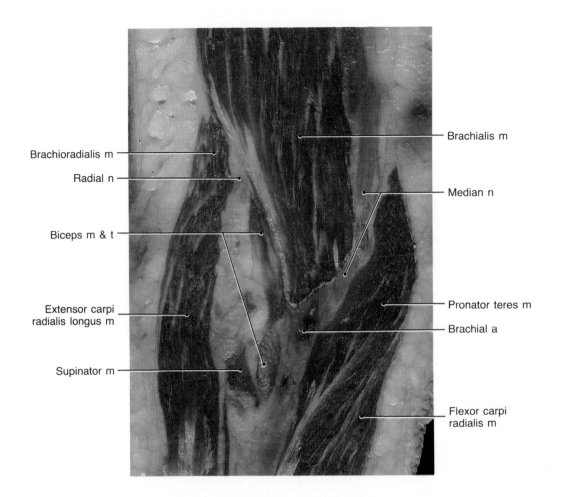

Brachioradialis m

Radial n

Biceps m & t

Extensor carpi
radialis longus m

Supinator m

Brachialis m

Median n

Pronator teres m

Brachial a

Flexor carpi
radialis m

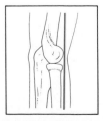

ELBOW, TRANSVERSE

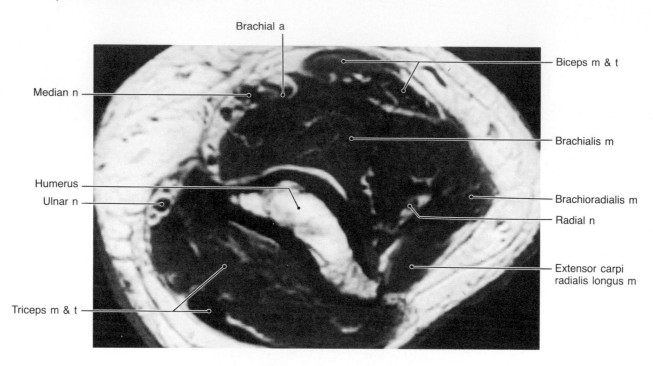

Brachial a

Median n

Humerus

Ulnar n

Triceps m & t

Biceps m & t

Brachialis m

Brachioradialis m

Radial n

Extensor carpi radialis longus m

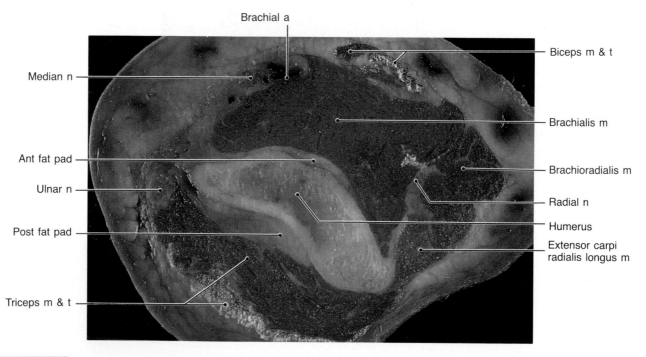

Brachial a

Median n

Ant fat pad

Ulnar n

Post fat pad

Triceps m & t

Biceps m & t

Brachialis m

Brachioradialis m

Radial n

Humerus

Extensor carpi radialis longus m

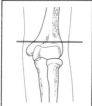

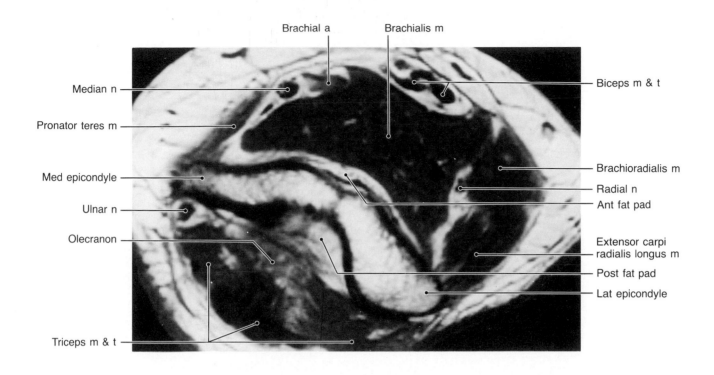

Brachial a

Brachialis m

Median n

Biceps m & t

Pronator teres m

Med epicondyle

Brachioradialis m

Ulnar n

Radial n

Ant fat pad

Olecranon

Extensor carpi
radialis longus m

Post fat pad

Lat epicondyle

Triceps m & t

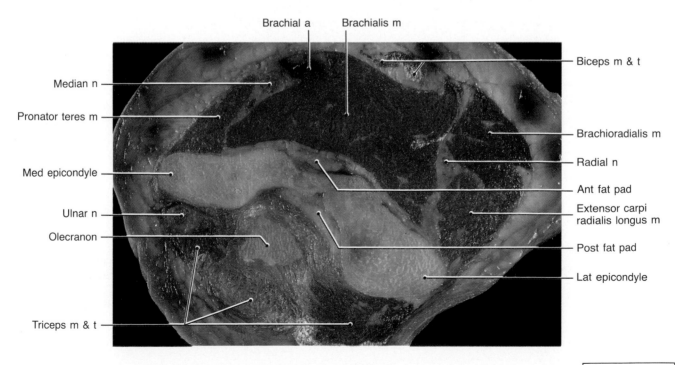

Brachial a

Brachialis m

Median n

Biceps m & t

Pronator teres m

Brachioradialis m

Med epicondyle

Radial n

Ulnar n

Ant fat pad

Olecranon

Extensor carpi
radialis longus m

Post fat pad

Lat epicondyle

Triceps m & t

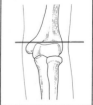

ELBOW, TRANSVERSE

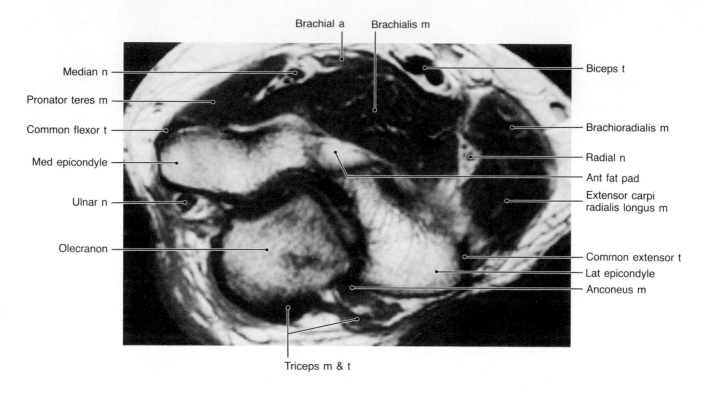

Brachial a
Brachialis m
Median n
Pronator teres m
Common flexor t
Med epicondyle
Ulnar n
Olecranon
Biceps t
Brachioradialis m
Radial n
Ant fat pad
Extensor carpi radialis longus m
Common extensor t
Lat epicondyle
Anconeus m
Triceps m & t

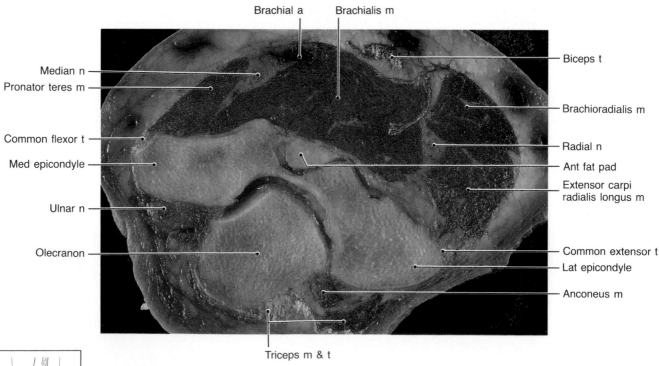

Brachial a
Brachialis m
Median n
Pronator teres m
Common flexor t
Med epicondyle
Ulnar n
Olecranon
Biceps t
Brachioradialis m
Radial n
Ant fat pad
Extensor carpi radialis longus m
Common extensor t
Lat epicondyle
Anconeus m
Triceps m & t

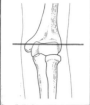

Brachial a   Brachialis m

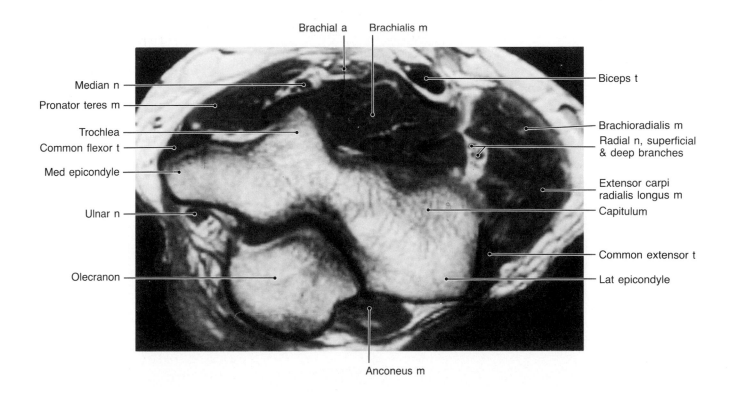

Median n
Pronator teres m
Trochlea
Common flexor t
Med epicondyle
Ulnar n
Olecranon

Biceps t
Brachioradialis m
Radial n, superficial & deep branches
Extensor carpi radialis longus m
Capitulum
Common extensor t
Lat epicondyle

Anconeus m

Brachial a   Brachialis m

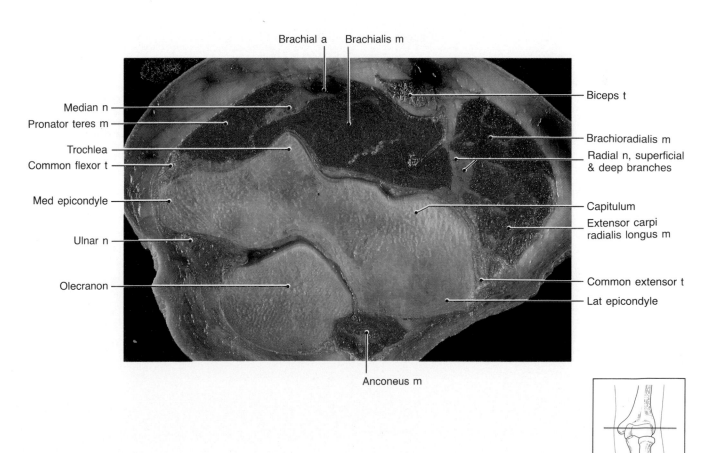

Median n
Pronator teres m
Trochlea
Common flexor t
Med epicondyle
Ulnar n
Olecranon

Biceps t
Brachioradialis m
Radial n, superficial & deep branches
Capitulum
Extensor carpi radialis longus m
Common extensor t
Lat epicondyle

Anconeus m

ELBOW, TRANSVERSE

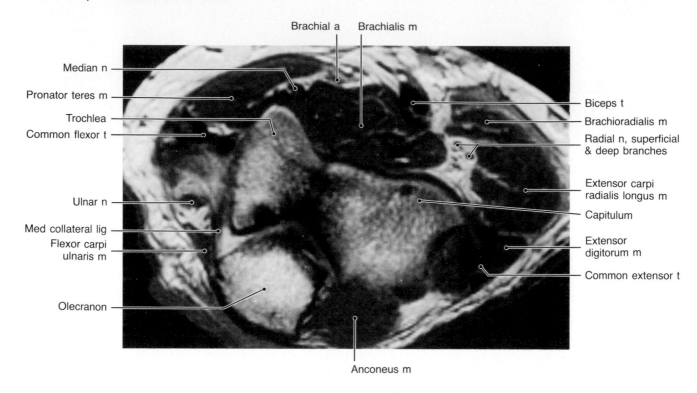

Brachial a   Brachialis m

Median n

Pronator teres m

Trochlea

Common flexor t

Ulnar n

Med collateral lig

Flexor carpi ulnaris m

Olecranon

Biceps t

Brachioradialis m

Radial n, superficial & deep branches

Extensor carpi radialis longus m

Capitulum

Extensor digitorum m

Common extensor t

Anconeus m

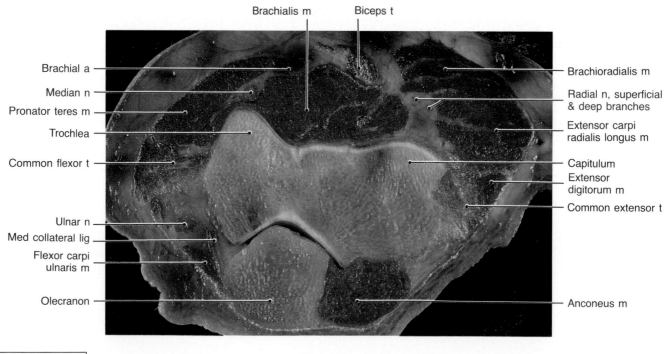

Brachialis m   Biceps t

Brachial a

Median n

Pronator teres m

Trochlea

Common flexor t

Ulnar n

Med collateral lig

Flexor carpi ulnaris m

Olecranon

Brachioradialis m

Radial n, superficial & deep branches

Extensor carpi radialis longus m

Capitulum

Extensor digitorum m

Common extensor t

Anconeus m

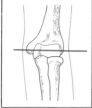

Brachial a   Biceps aponeurosis

Pronator teres m

Median n

Brachialis m

Flexor carpi
radialis m

Palmaris longus m

Flexor digitorum
superficialis m

Trochlea

Ulnar n

Med collateral lig

Flexor carpi
ulnaris m

Olecranon

Biceps t

Brachioradialis m

Radial n, superficial
& deep branches

Extensor carpi
radialis longus m

Lat collateral &
annular ligs

Capitulum

Extensor
digitorum m

Common extensor t

Anconeus m

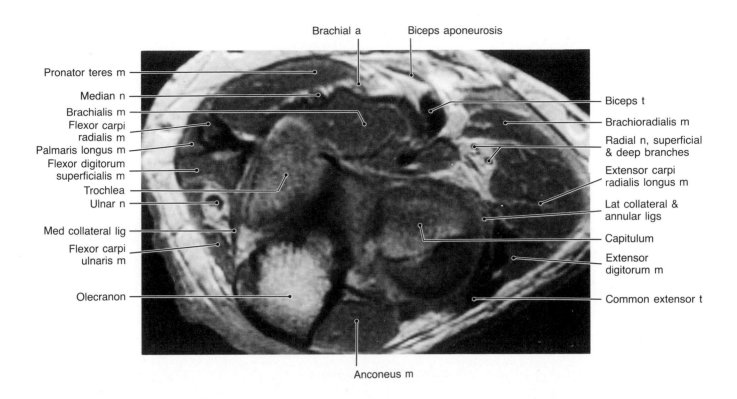

Brachial a   Biceps aponeurosis

Pronator teres m

Median n

Brachialis m

Coronoid

Flexor carpi
radialis m

Palmaris longus m

Flexor digitorum
superficialis m

Trochlea

Ulnar n

Med collateral lig

Flexor carpi
ulnaris m

Flexor digitorum
profundus m

Olecranon

Biceps t

Brachioradialis m

Radial n, superficial
& deep branches

Extensor carpi
radialis longus m

Lat collateral &
annular ligs

Capitulum

Extensor
digitorum m

Lat collateral lig

Common extensor t

Anconeus m

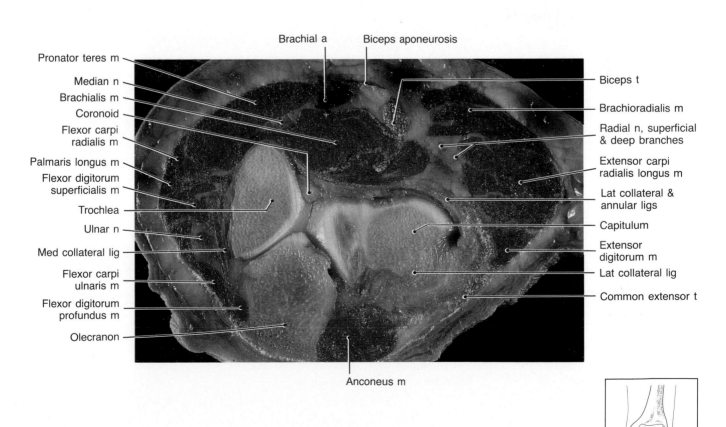

ELBOW, TRANSVERSE

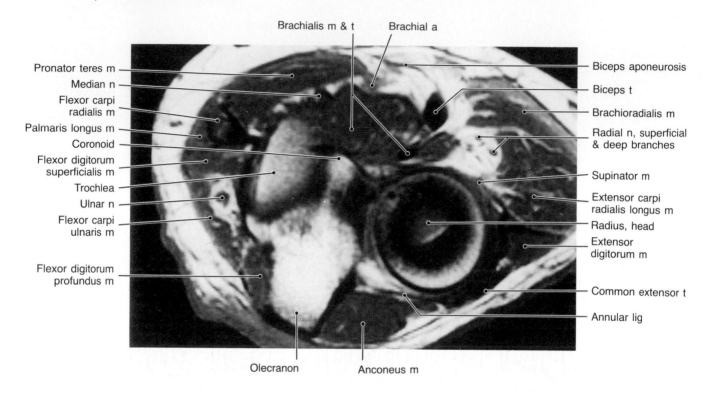

Brachialis m & t

Brachial a

Pronator teres m

Median n

Flexor carpi radialis m

Palmaris longus m

Coronoid

Flexor digitorum superficialis m

Trochlea

Ulnar n

Flexor carpi ulnaris m

Flexor digitorum profundus m

Biceps aponeurosis

Biceps t

Brachioradialis m

Radial n, superficial & deep branches

Supinator m

Extensor carpi radialis longus m

Radius, head

Extensor digitorum m

Common extensor t

Annular lig

Olecranon

Anconeus m

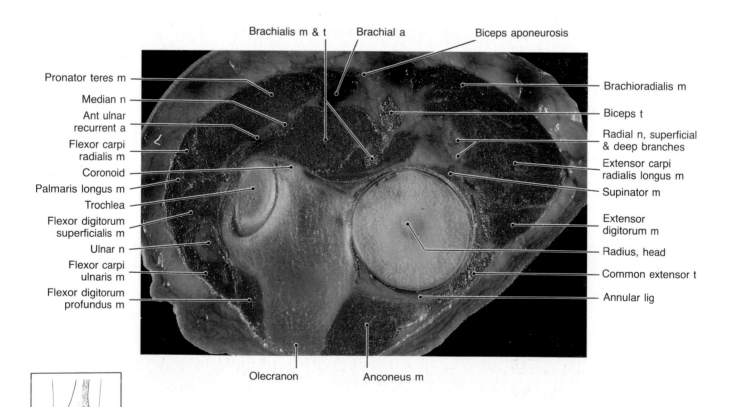

Brachialis m & t

Brachial a

Biceps aponeurosis

Pronator teres m

Median n

Ant ulnar recurrent a

Flexor carpi radialis m

Coronoid

Palmaris longus m

Trochlea

Flexor digitorum superficialis m

Ulnar n

Flexor carpi ulnaris m

Flexor digitorum profundus m

Brachioradialis m

Biceps t

Radial n, superficial & deep branches

Extensor carpi radialis longus m

Supinator m

Extensor digitorum m

Radius, head

Common extensor t

Annular lig

Olecranon

Anconeus m

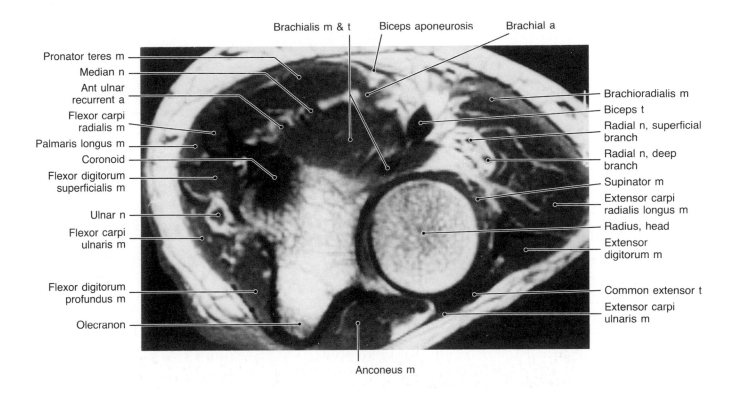

Brachialis m & t | Biceps aponeurosis | Brachial a

Pronator teres m
Median n
Ant ulnar recurrent a
Flexor carpi radialis m
Palmaris longus m
Coronoid
Flexor digitorum superficialis m
Ulnar n
Flexor carpi ulnaris m
Flexor digitorum profundus m
Olecranon

Brachioradialis m
Biceps t
Radial n, superficial branch
Radial n, deep branch
Supinator m
Extensor carpi radialis longus m
Radius, head
Extensor digitorum m
Common extensor t
Extensor carpi ulnaris m

Anconeus m

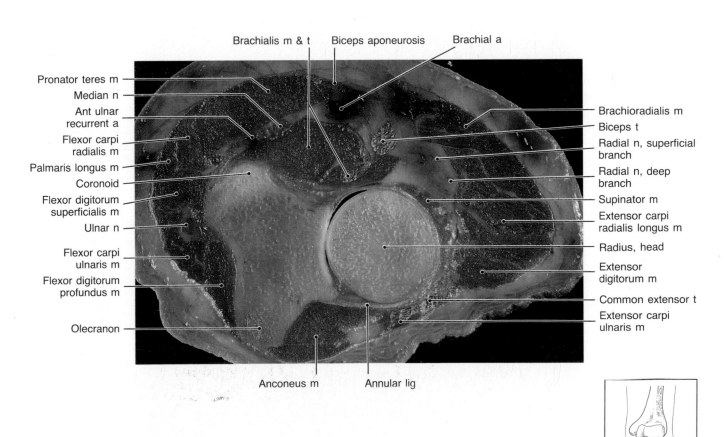

Brachialis m & t | Biceps aponeurosis | Brachial a

Pronator teres m
Median n
Ant ulnar recurrent a
Flexor carpi radialis m
Palmaris longus m
Coronoid
Flexor digitorum superficialis m
Ulnar n
Flexor carpi ulnaris m
Flexor digitorum profundus m
Olecranon

Brachioradialis m
Biceps t
Radial n, superficial branch
Radial n, deep branch
Supinator m
Extensor carpi radialis longus m
Radius, head
Extensor digitorum m
Common extensor t
Extensor carpi ulnaris m

Anconeus m | Annular lig

ELBOW, TRANSVERSE

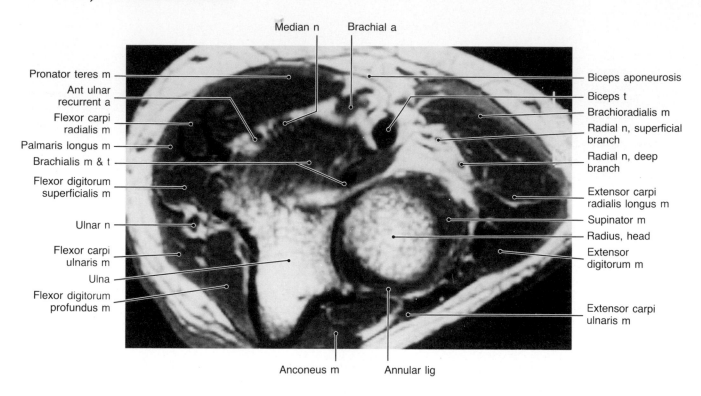

Median n

Brachial a

Pronator teres m

Ant ulnar recurrent a

Flexor carpi radialis m

Palmaris longus m

Brachialis m & t

Flexor digitorum superficialis m

Ulnar n

Flexor carpi ulnaris m

Ulna

Flexor digitorum profundus m

Biceps aponeurosis

Biceps t

Brachioradialis m

Radial n, superficial branch

Radial n, deep branch

Extensor carpi radialis longus m

Supinator m

Radius, head

Extensor digitorum m

Extensor carpi ulnaris m

Anconeus m

Annular lig

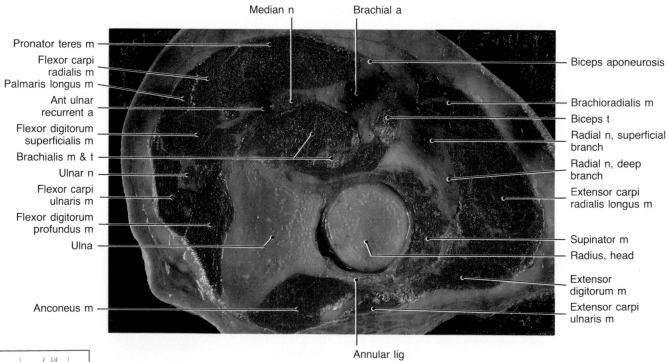

Median n

Brachial a

Pronator teres m

Flexor carpi radialis m

Palmaris longus m

Ant ulnar recurrent a

Flexor digitorum superficialis m

Brachialis m & t

Ulnar n

Flexor carpi ulnaris m

Flexor digitorum profundus m

Ulna

Anconeus m

Biceps aponeurosis

Brachioradialis m

Biceps t

Radial n, superficial branch

Radial n, deep branch

Extensor carpi radialis longus m

Supinator m

Radius, head

Extensor digitorum m

Extensor carpi ulnaris m

Annular lig

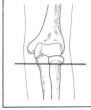

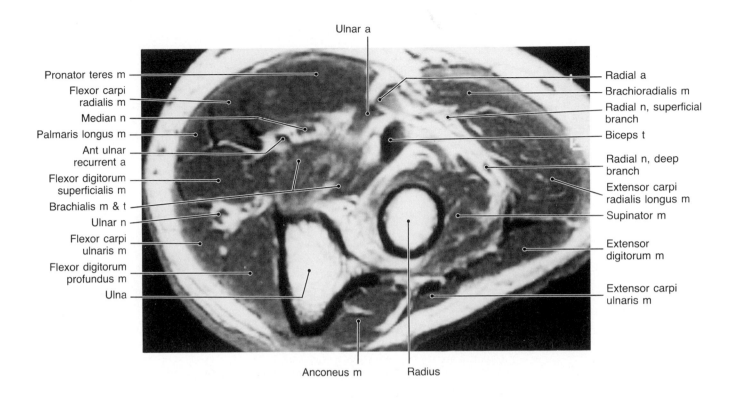

Ulnar a

Pronator teres m

Flexor carpi radialis m

Median n

Palmaris longus m

Ant ulnar recurrent a

Flexor digitorum superficialis m

Brachialis m & t

Ulnar n

Flexor carpi ulnaris m

Flexor digitorum profundus m

Ulna

Radial a

Brachioradialis m

Radial n, superficial branch

Biceps t

Radial n, deep branch

Extensor carpi radialis longus m

Supinator m

Extensor digitorum m

Extensor carpi ulnaris m

Anconeus m

Radius

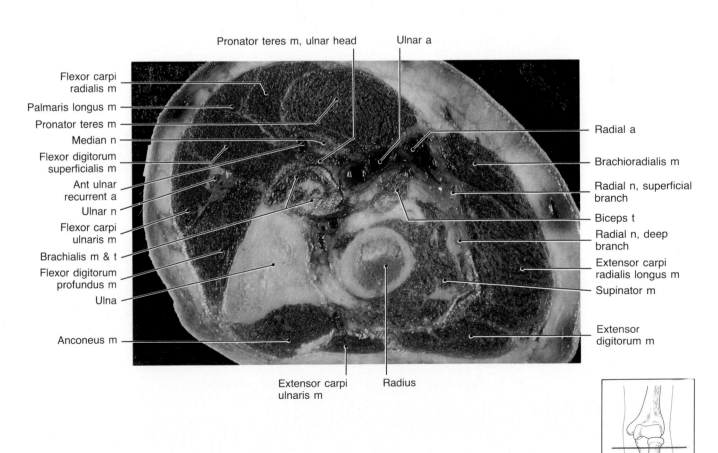

Pronator teres m, ulnar head

Ulnar a

Flexor carpi radialis m

Palmaris longus m

Pronator teres m

Median n

Flexor digitorum superficialis m

Ant ulnar recurrent a

Ulnar n

Flexor carpi ulnaris m

Brachialis m & t

Flexor digitorum profundus m

Ulna

Anconeus m

Radial a

Brachioradialis m

Radial n, superficial branch

Biceps t

Radial n, deep branch

Extensor carpi radialis longus m

Supinator m

Extensor digitorum m

Extensor carpi ulnaris m

Radius

ELBOW, TRANSVERSE

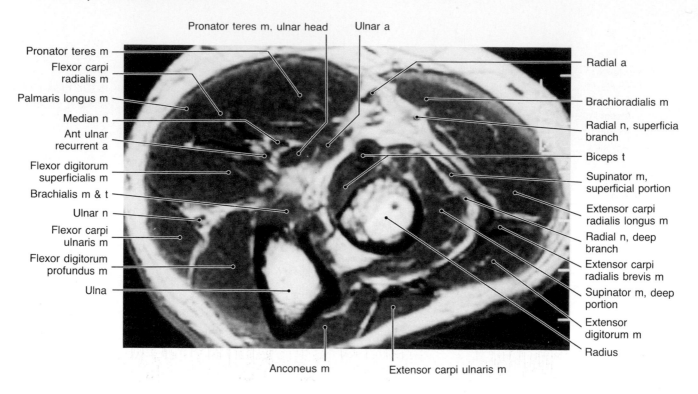

Pronator teres m, ulnar head
Ulnar a
Pronator teres m
Flexor carpi radialis m
Palmaris longus m
Median n
Ant ulnar recurrent a
Flexor digitorum superficialis m
Brachialis m & t
Ulnar n
Flexor carpi ulnaris m
Flexor digitorum profundus m
Ulna
Radial a
Brachioradialis m
Radial n, superficia branch
Biceps t
Supinator m, superficial portion
Extensor carpi radialis longus m
Radial n, deep branch
Extensor carpi radialis brevis m
Supinator m, deep portion
Extensor digitorum m
Radius
Anconeus m
Extensor carpi ulnaris m

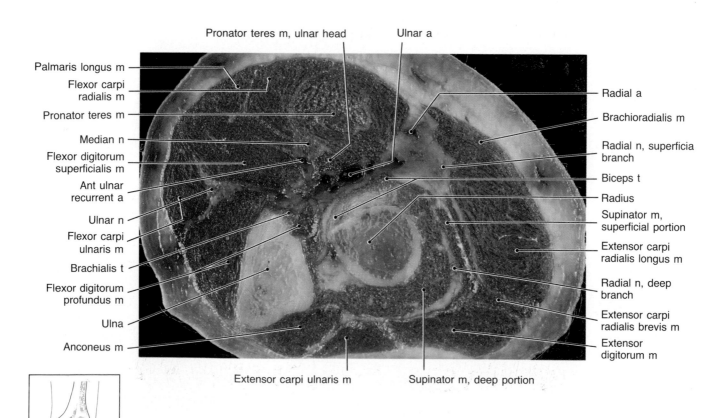

Pronator teres m, ulnar head
Ulnar a
Palmaris longus m
Flexor carpi radialis m
Pronator teres m
Median n
Flexor digitorum superficialis m
Ant ulnar recurrent a
Ulnar n
Flexor carpi ulnaris m
Brachialis t
Flexor digitorum profundus m
Ulna
Anconeus m
Radial a
Brachioradialis m
Radial n, superficia branch
Biceps t
Radius
Supinator m, superficial portion
Extensor carpi radialis longus m
Radial n, deep branch
Extensor carpi radialis brevis m
Extensor digitorum m
Extensor carpi ulnaris m
Supinator m, deep portion

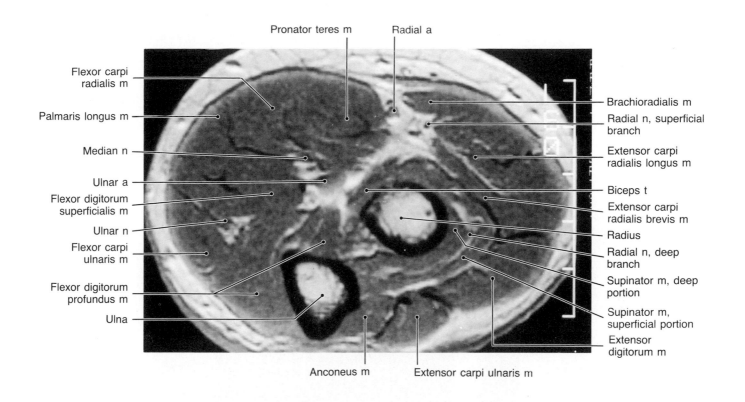

Pronator teres m — Radial a

Flexor carpi radialis m

Palmaris longus m

Median n

Ulnar a

Flexor digitorum superficialis m

Ulnar n

Flexor carpi ulnaris m

Flexor digitorum profundus m

Ulna

Brachioradialis m

Radial n, superficial branch

Extensor carpi radialis longus m

Biceps t

Extensor carpi radialis brevis m

Radius

Radial n, deep branch

Supinator m, deep portion

Supinator m, superficial portion

Extensor digitorum m

Anconeus m　Extensor carpi ulnaris m

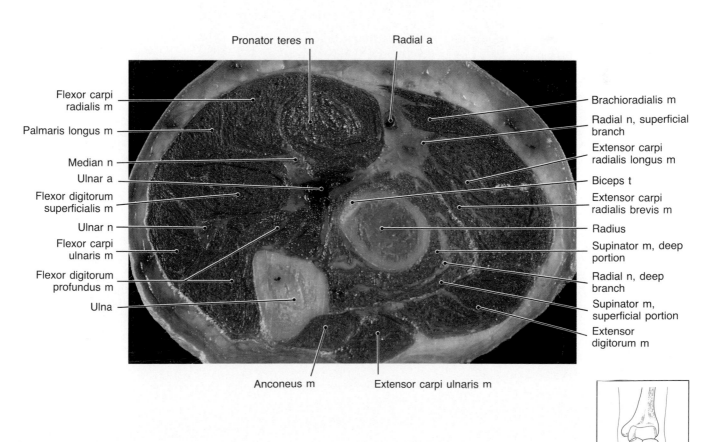

Pronator teres m — Radial a

Flexor carpi radialis m

Palmaris longus m

Median n

Ulnar a

Flexor digitorum superficialis m

Ulnar n

Flexor carpi ulnaris m

Flexor digitorum profundus m

Ulna

Brachioradialis m

Radial n, superficial branch

Extensor carpi radialis longus m

Biceps t

Extensor carpi radialis brevis m

Radius

Supinator m, deep portion

Radial n, deep branch

Supinator m, superficial portion

Extensor digitorum m

Anconeus m　Extensor carpi ulnaris m

ELBOW, SAGITTAL

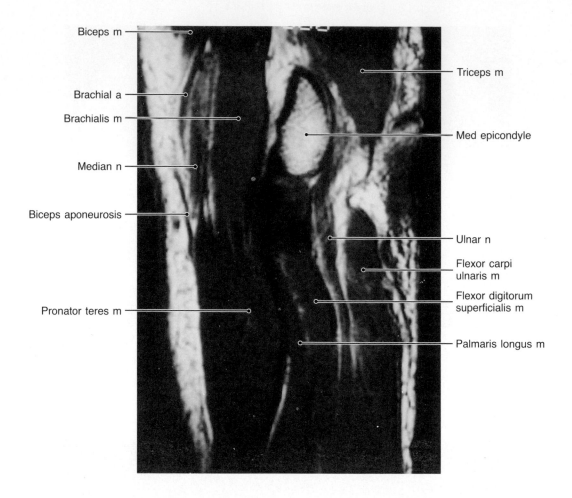

Biceps m

Brachial a

Brachialis m

Median n

Biceps aponeurosis

Pronator teres m

Triceps m

Med epicondyle

Ulnar n

Flexor carpi ulnaris m

Flexor digitorum superficialis m

Palmaris longus m

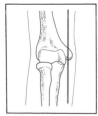

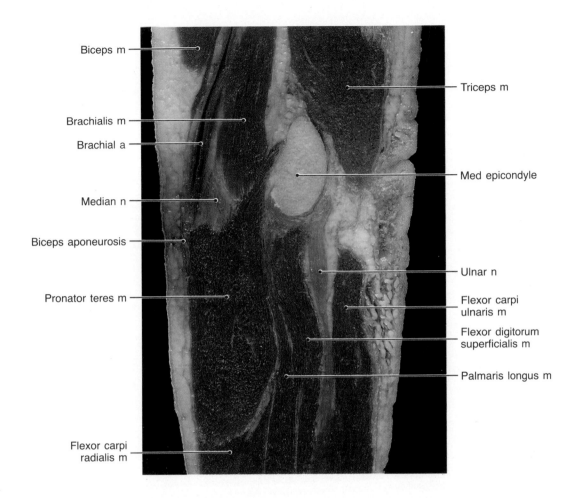

Biceps m

Brachialis m

Brachial a

Median n

Biceps aponeurosis

Pronator teres m

Flexor carpi
radialis m

Triceps m

Med epicondyle

Ulnar n

Flexor carpi
ulnaris m

Flexor digitorum
superficialis m

Palmaris longus m

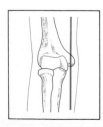

ELBOW, SAGITTAL

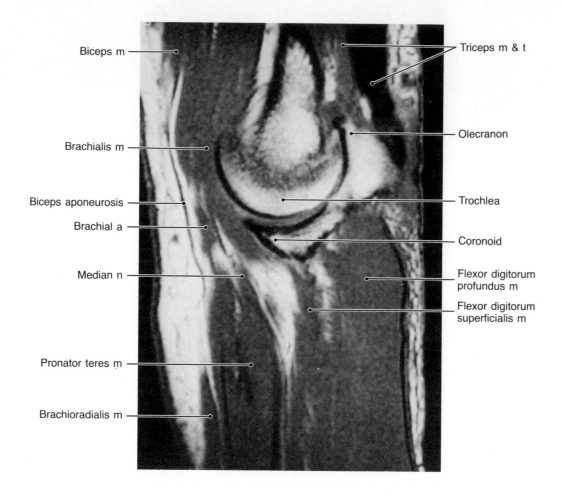

Biceps m

Brachialis m

Biceps aponeurosis

Brachial a

Median n

Pronator teres m

Brachioradialis m

Triceps m & t

Olecranon

Trochlea

Coronoid

Flexor digitorum profundus m

Flexor digitorum superficialis m

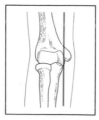

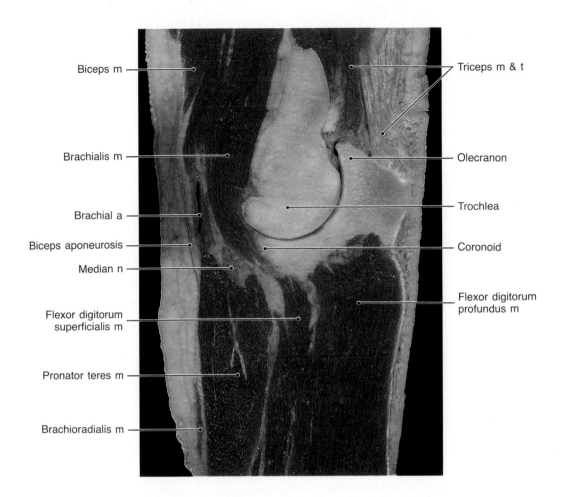

Biceps m

Brachialis m

Brachial a

Biceps aponeurosis

Median n

Flexor digitorum
superficialis m

Pronator teres m

Brachioradialis m

Triceps m & t

Olecranon

Trochlea

Coronoid

Flexor digitorum
profundus m

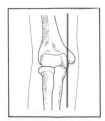

ELBOW, SAGITTAL

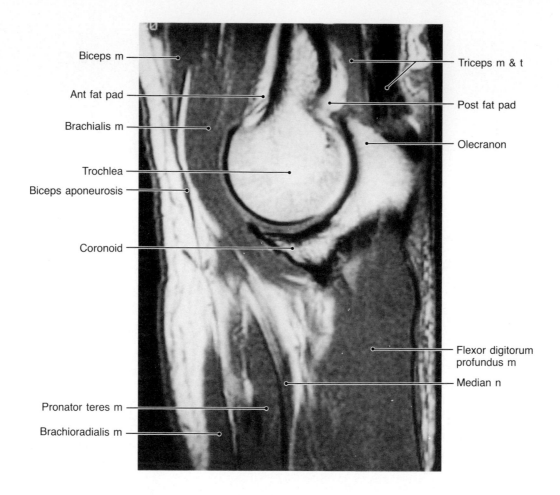

Biceps m

Ant fat pad

Brachialis m

Trochlea

Biceps aponeurosis

Coronoid

Pronator teres m

Brachioradialis m

Triceps m & t

Post fat pad

Olecranon

Flexor digitorum profundus m

Median n

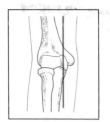

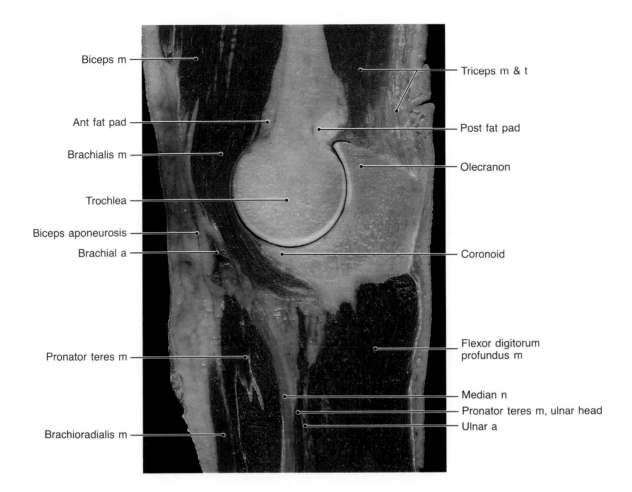

Biceps m

Ant fat pad

Brachialis m

Trochlea

Biceps aponeurosis

Brachial a

Pronator teres m

Brachioradialis m

Triceps m & t

Post fat pad

Olecranon

Coronoid

Flexor digitorum profundus m

Median n

Pronator teres m, ulnar head

Ulnar a

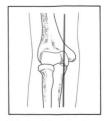

ELBOW, SAGITTAL

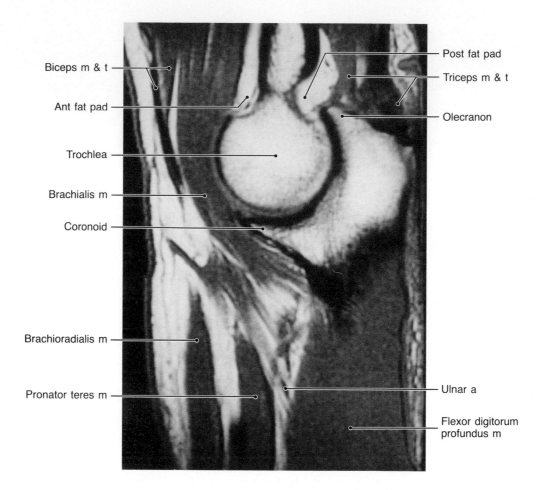

Biceps m & t

Ant fat pad

Trochlea

Brachialis m

Coronoid

Brachioradialis m

Pronator teres m

Post fat pad

Triceps m & t

Olecranon

Ulnar a

Flexor digitorum
profundus m

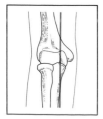

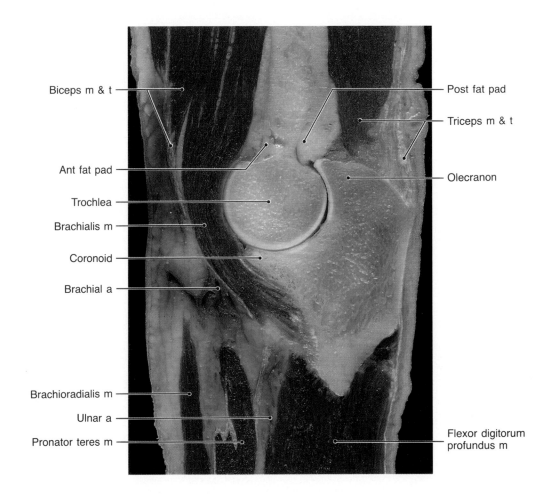

Biceps m & t

Ant fat pad

Trochlea

Brachialis m

Coronoid

Brachial a

Brachioradialis m

Ulnar a

Pronator teres m

Post fat pad

Triceps m & t

Olecranon

Flexor digitorum profundus m

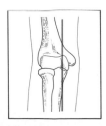

ELBOW, SAGITTAL

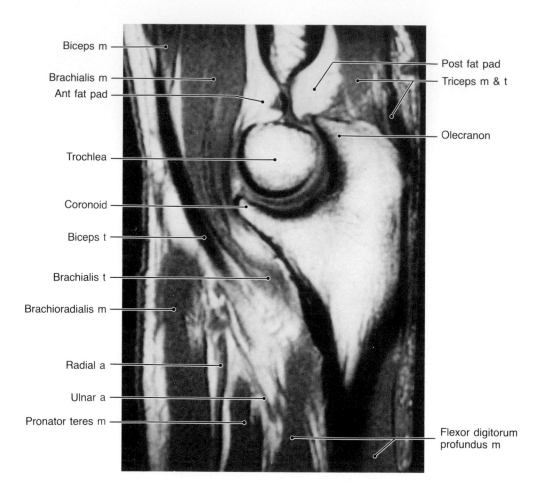

Biceps m

Brachialis m

Ant fat pad

Trochlea

Coronoid

Biceps t

Brachialis t

Brachioradialis m

Radial a

Ulnar a

Pronator teres m

Post fat pad

Triceps m & t

Olecranon

Flexor digitorum
profundus m

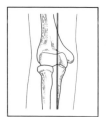

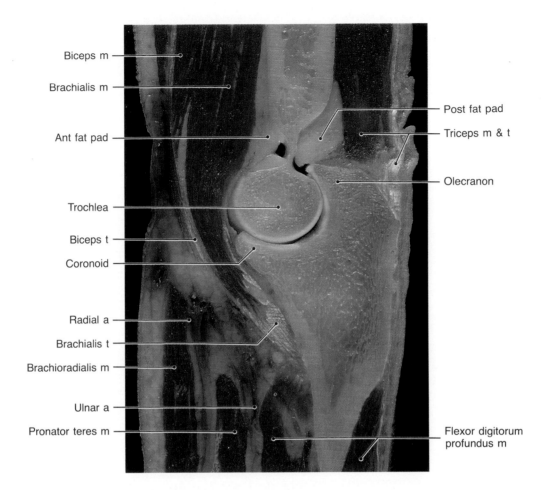

Biceps m

Brachialis m

Ant fat pad

Trochlea

Biceps t

Coronoid

Radial a

Brachialis t

Brachioradialis m

Ulnar a

Pronator teres m

Post fat pad

Triceps m & t

Olecranon

Flexor digitorum
profundus m

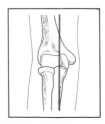

ELBOW, SAGITTAL

Biceps m

Ant fat pad

Brachialis m & t

Biceps t

Brachioradialis m

Supinator m

Radial a

Pronator teres m

Triceps m & t

Post fat pad

Olecranon

Trochlea

Coronoid

Anconeus m

Flexor digitorum
profundus m

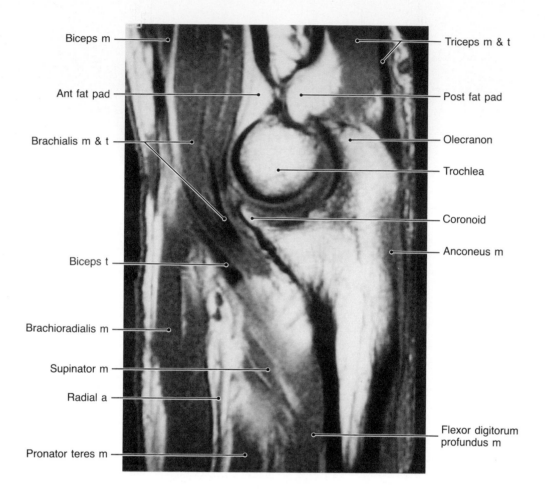

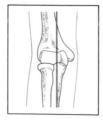

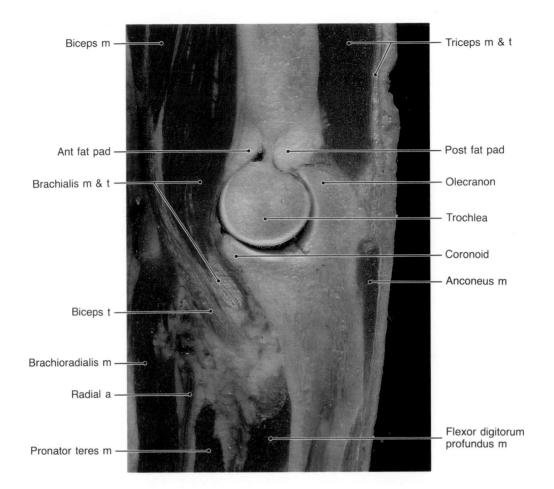

Biceps m

Triceps m & t

Ant fat pad

Post fat pad

Brachialis m & t

Olecranon

Trochlea

Coronoid

Anconeus m

Biceps t

Brachioradialis m

Radial a

Flexor digitorum
profundus m

Pronator teres m

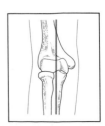

ELBOW, SAGITTAL

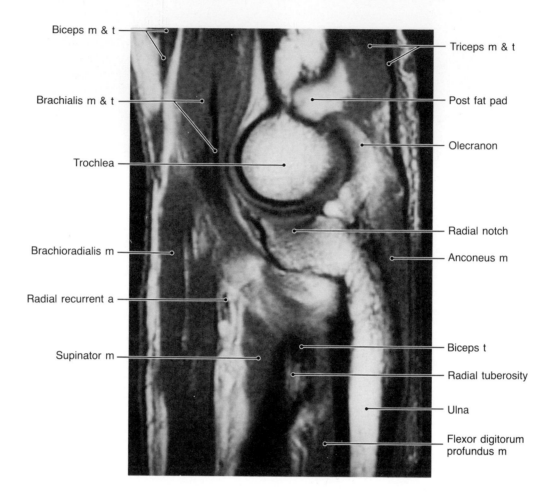

Biceps m & t

Brachialis m & t

Trochlea

Brachioradialis m

Radial recurrent a

Supinator m

Triceps m & t

Post fat pad

Olecranon

Radial notch

Anconeus m

Biceps t

Radial tuberosity

Ulna

Flexor digitorum
profundus m

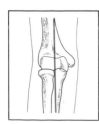

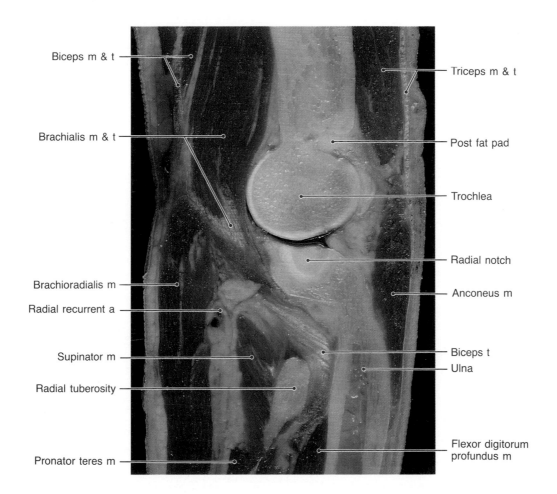

Biceps m & t

Brachialis m & t

Brachioradialis m

Radial recurrent a

Supinator m

Radial tuberosity

Pronator teres m

Triceps m & t

Post fat pad

Trochlea

Radial notch

Anconeus m

Biceps t
Ulna

Flexor digitorum
profundus m

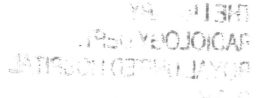

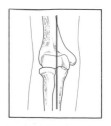

ELBOW, SAGITTAL

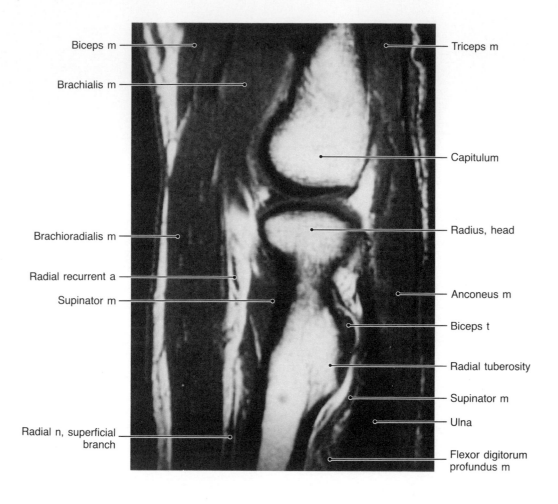

Biceps m

Brachialis m

Brachioradialis m

Radial recurrent a

Supinator m

Radial n, superficial branch

Triceps m

Capitulum

Radius, head

Anconeus m

Biceps t

Radial tuberosity

Supinator m

Ulna

Flexor digitorum profundus m

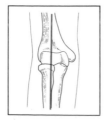

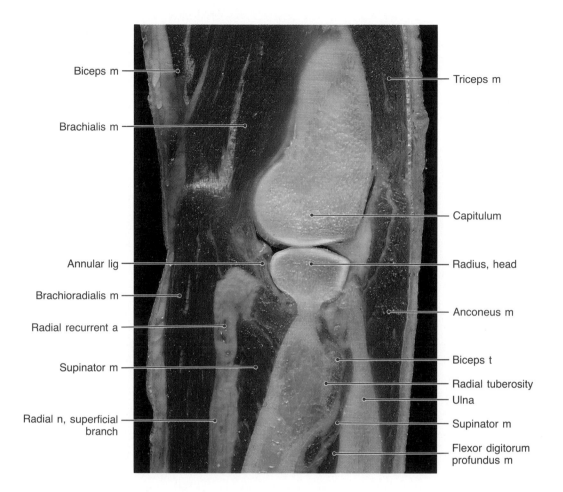

Biceps m

Brachialis m

Annular lig

Brachioradialis m

Radial recurrent a

Supinator m

Radial n, superficial branch

Triceps m

Capitulum

Radius, head

Anconeus m

Biceps t

Radial tuberosity

Ulna

Supinator m

Flexor digitorum profundus m

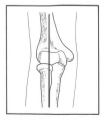

ELBOW, SAGITTAL

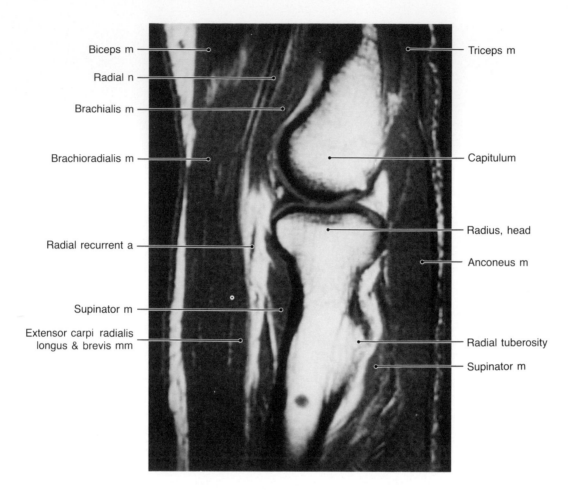

Biceps m

Radial n

Brachialis m

Brachioradialis m

Radial recurrent a

Supinator m

Extensor carpi radialis longus & brevis mm

Triceps m

Capitulum

Radius, head

Anconeus m

Radial tuberosity

Supinator m

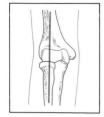

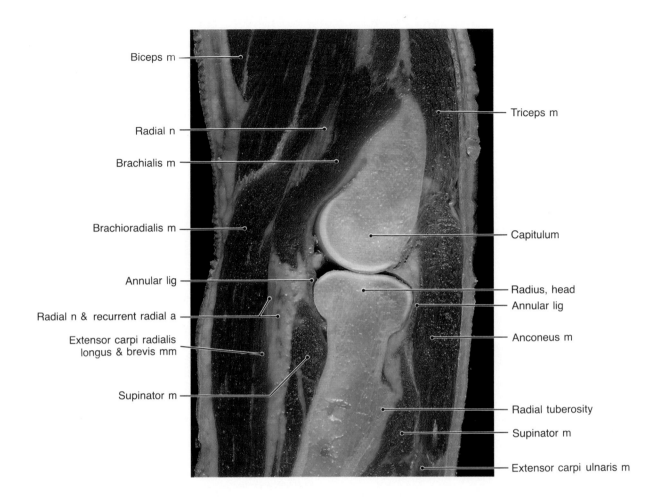

Biceps m

Radial n

Brachialis m

Brachioradialis m

Annular lig

Radial n & recurrent radial a

Extensor carpi radialis longus & brevis mm

Supinator m

Triceps m

Capitulum

Radius, head

Annular lig

Anconeus m

Radial tuberosity

Supinator m

Extensor carpi ulnaris m

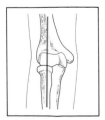

ELBOW, SAGITTAL

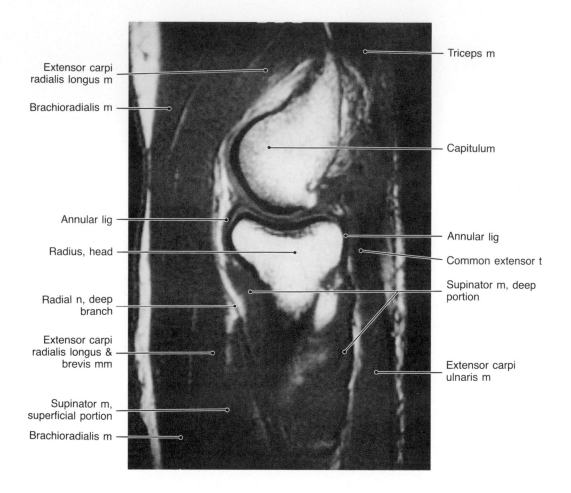

Extensor carpi radialis longus m

Brachioradialis m

Annular lig

Radius, head

Radial n, deep branch

Extensor carpi radialis longus & brevis mm

Supinator m, superficial portion

Brachioradialis m

Triceps m

Capitulum

Annular lig

Common extensor t

Supinator m, deep portion

Extensor carpi ulnaris m

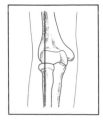

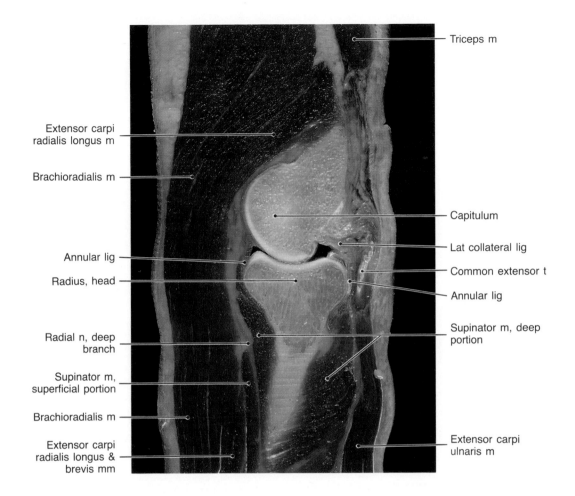

Triceps m

Extensor carpi
radialis longus m

Brachioradialis m

Capitulum

Lat collateral lig

Annular lig

Common extensor t

Radius, head

Annular lig

Radial n, deep
branch

Supinator m, deep
portion

Supinator m,
superficial portion

Brachioradialis m

Extensor carpi
radialis longus &
brevis mm

Extensor carpi
ulnaris m

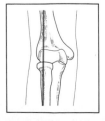

ELBOW, SAGITTAL

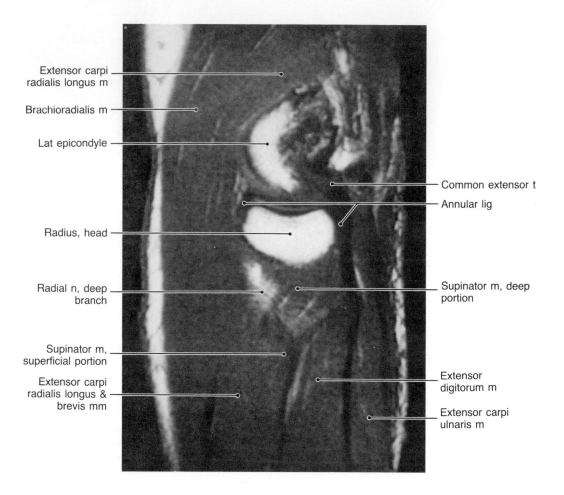

Extensor carpi radialis longus m

Brachioradialis m

Lat epicondyle

Radius, head

Radial n, deep branch

Supinator m, superficial portion

Extensor carpi radialis longus & brevis mm

Common extensor t

Annular lig

Supinator m, deep portion

Extensor digitorum m

Extensor carpi ulnaris m

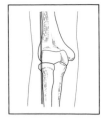

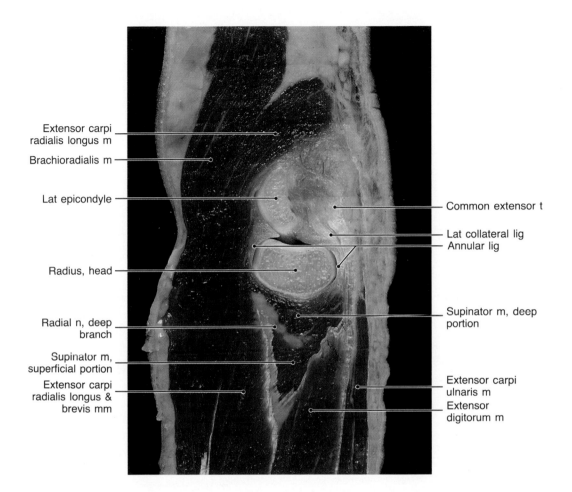

Extensor carpi radialis longus m

Brachioradialis m

Lat epicondyle

Radius, head

Radial n, deep branch

Supinator m, superficial portion

Extensor carpi radialis longus & brevis mm

Common extensor t

Lat collateral lig

Annular lig

Supinator m, deep portion

Extensor carpi ulnaris m

Extensor digitorum m

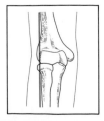

Elbow, Sagittal

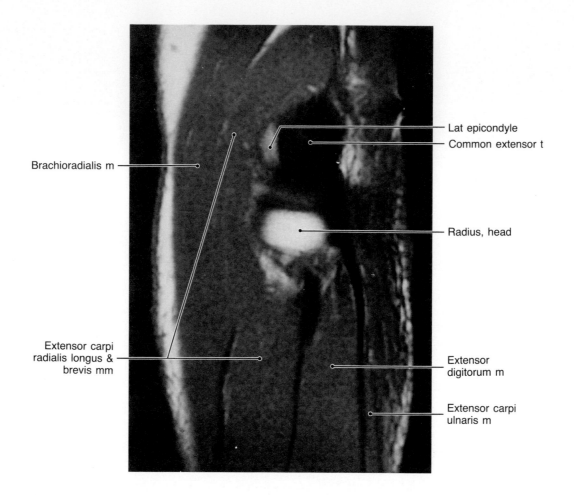

Brachioradialis m

Extensor carpi
radialis longus &
brevis mm

Lat epicondyle

Common extensor t

Radius, head

Extensor
digitorum m

Extensor carpi
ulnaris m

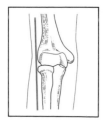

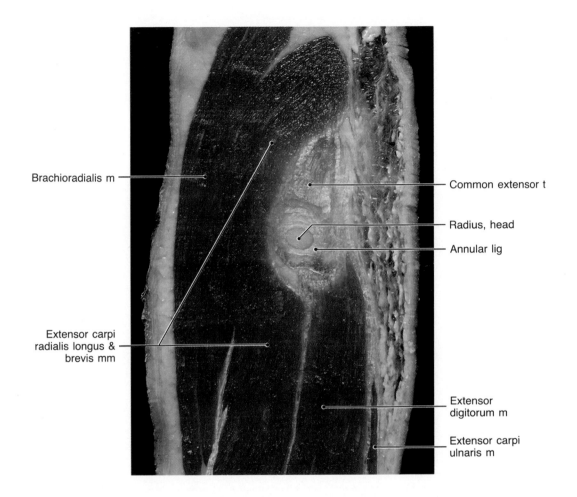

Brachioradialis m

Common extensor t

Radius, head

Annular lig

Extensor carpi
radialis longus &
brevis mm

Extensor
digitorum m

Extensor carpi
ulnaris m

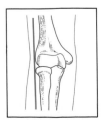

3 WRIST AND HAND

WRIST AND HAND, CORONAL

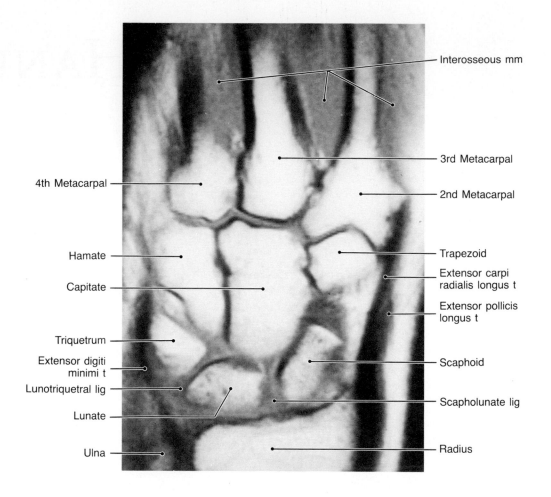

Interosseous mm

3rd Metacarpal

2nd Metacarpal

4th Metacarpal

Trapezoid

Hamate

Extensor carpi
radialis longus t

Capitate

Extensor pollicis
longus t

Triquetrum

Extensor digiti
minimi t

Scaphoid

Lunotriquetral lig

Lunate

Scapholunate lig

Ulna

Radius

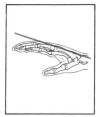

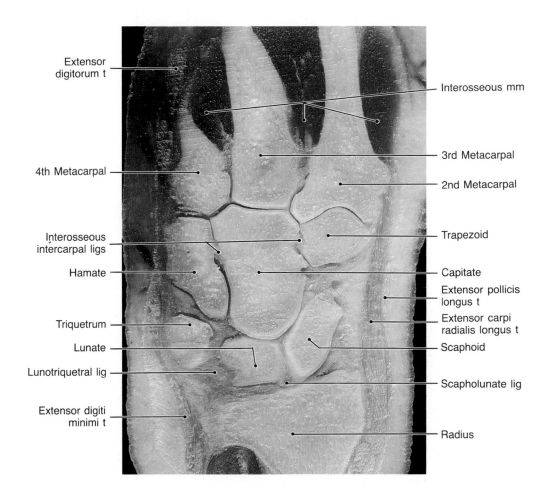

Extensor digitorum t

Interosseous mm

3rd Metacarpal

4th Metacarpal

2nd Metacarpal

Interosseous intercarpal ligs

Trapezoid

Hamate

Capitate

Extensor pollicis longus t

Triquetrum

Extensor carpi radialis longus t

Lunate

Scaphoid

Lunotriquetral lig

Scapholunate lig

Extensor digiti minimi t

Radius

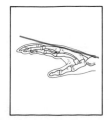

WRIST AND HAND, CORONAL

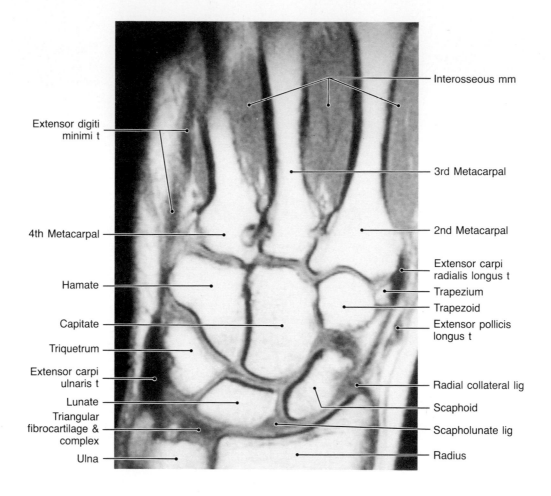

Extensor digiti minimi t

4th Metacarpal

Hamate

Capitate

Triquetrum

Extensor carpi ulnaris t

Lunate

Triangular fibrocartilage & complex

Ulna

Interosseous mm

3rd Metacarpal

2nd Metacarpal

Extensor carpi radialis longus t

Trapezium

Trapezoid

Extensor pollicis longus t

Radial collateral lig

Scaphoid

Scapholunate lig

Radius

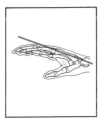

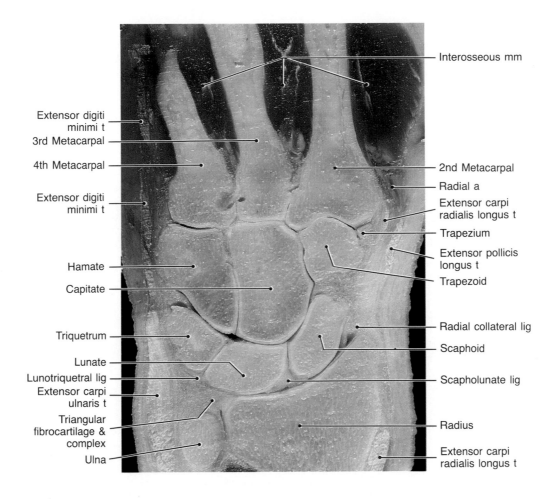

Interosseous mm

Extensor digiti minimi t

3rd Metacarpal

4th Metacarpal

Extensor digiti minimi t

Hamate

Capitate

Triquetrum

Lunate

Lunotriquetral lig

Extensor carpi ulnaris t

Triangular fibrocartilage & complex

Ulna

2nd Metacarpal

Radial a

Extensor carpi radialis longus t

Trapezium

Extensor pollicis longus t

Trapezoid

Radial collateral lig

Scaphoid

Scapholunate lig

Radius

Extensor carpi radialis longus t

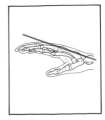

WRIST AND HAND, CORONAL

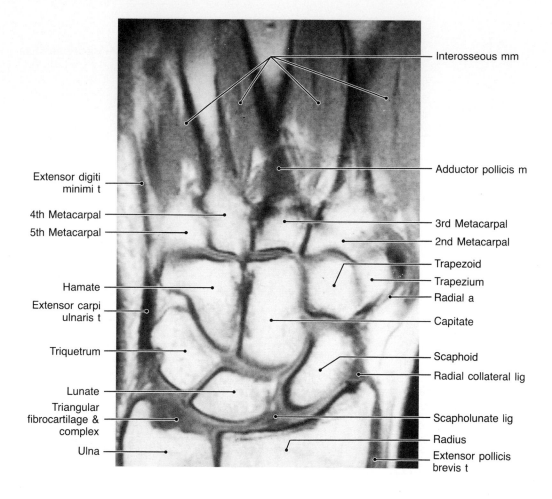

Interosseous mm

Extensor digiti minimi t

Adductor pollicis m

4th Metacarpal

3rd Metacarpal

5th Metacarpal

2nd Metacarpal

Trapezoid

Trapezium

Hamate

Radial a

Extensor carpi ulnaris t

Capitate

Triquetrum

Scaphoid

Radial collateral lig

Lunate

Triangular fibrocartilage & complex

Scapholunate lig

Radius

Ulna

Extensor pollicis brevis t

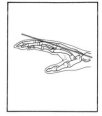

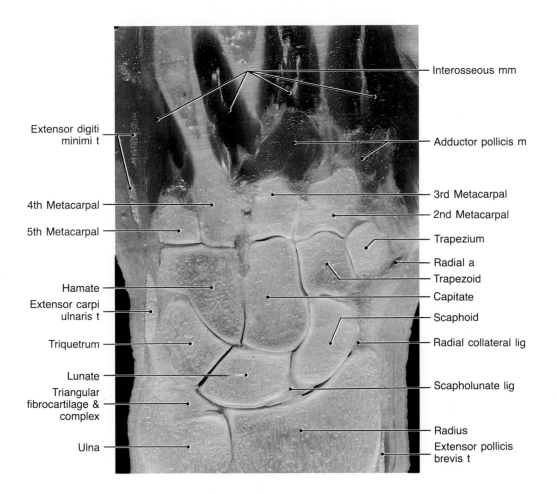

Interosseous mm

Extensor digiti
minimi t

Adductor pollicis m

4th Metacarpal

3rd Metacarpal

5th Metacarpal

2nd Metacarpal

Trapezium

Radial a

Hamate

Trapezoid

Extensor carpi
ulnaris t

Capitate

Triquetrum

Scaphoid

Radial collateral lig

Lunate

Triangular
fibrocartilage &
complex

Scapholunate lig

Ulna

Radius

Extensor pollicis
brevis t

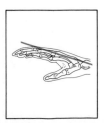

WRIST AND HAND, CORONAL

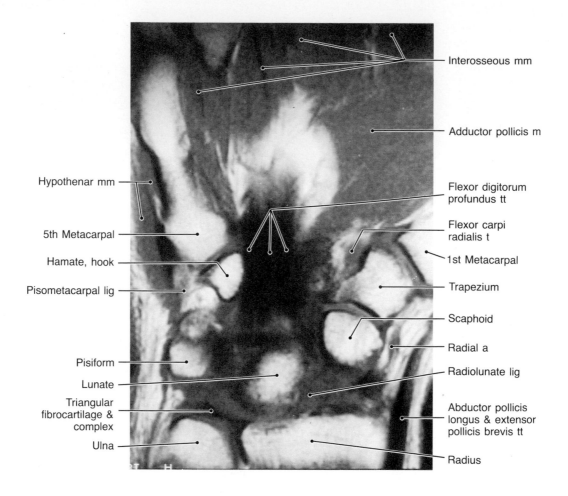

Interosseous mm

Adductor pollicis m

Hypothenar mm

Flexor digitorum profundus tt

5th Metacarpal

Flexor carpi radialis t

Hamate, hook

1st Metacarpal

Pisometacarpal lig

Trapezium

Scaphoid

Pisiform

Radial a

Lunate

Radiolunate lig

Triangular fibrocartilage & complex

Abductor pollicis longus & extensor pollicis brevis tt

Ulna

Radius

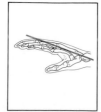

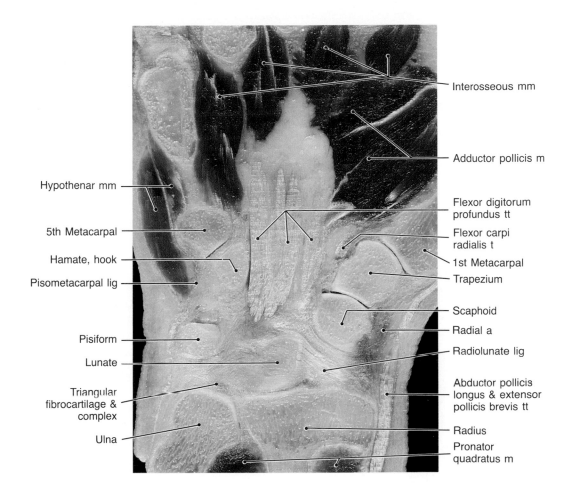

Interosseous mm

Adductor pollicis m

Hypothenar mm

Flexor digitorum profundus tt

5th Metacarpal

Flexor carpi radialis t

Hamate, hook

1st Metacarpal

Pisometacarpal lig

Trapezium

Scaphoid

Pisiform

Radial a

Lunate

Radiolunate lig

Triangular fibrocartilage & complex

Abductor pollicis longus & extensor pollicis brevis tt

Ulna

Radius

Pronator quadratus m

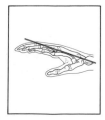

WRIST AND HAND, CORONAL

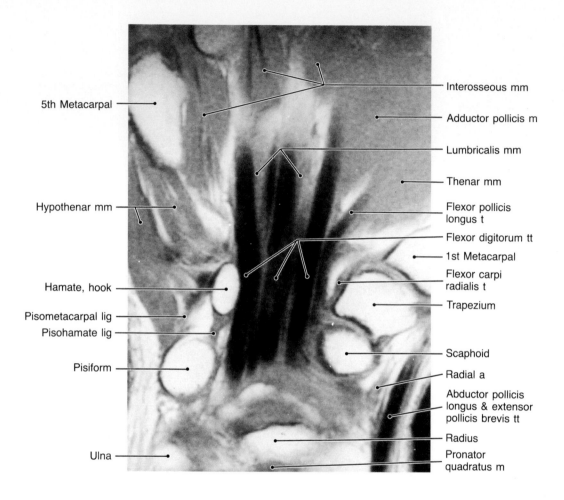

5th Metacarpal

Hypothenar mm

Hamate, hook

Pisometacarpal lig

Pisohamate lig

Pisiform

Ulna

Interosseous mm

Adductor pollicis m

Lumbricalis mm

Thenar mm

Flexor pollicis longus t

Flexor digitorum tt

1st Metacarpal

Flexor carpi radialis t

Trapezium

Scaphoid

Radial a

Abductor pollicis longus & extensor pollicis brevis tt

Radius

Pronator quadratus m

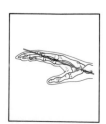

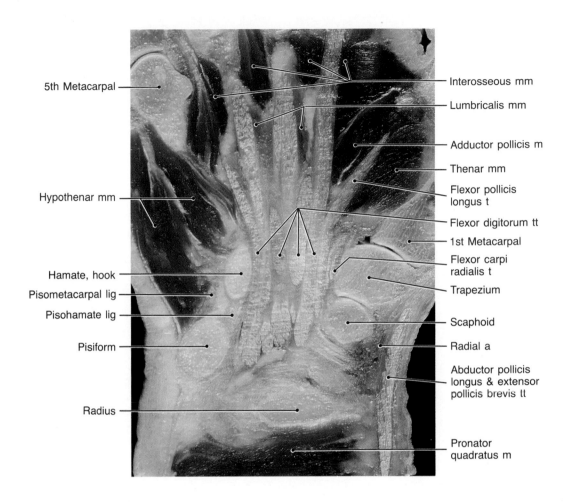

5th Metacarpal

Interosseous mm

Lumbricalis mm

Adductor pollicis m

Thenar mm

Hypothenar mm

Flexor pollicis longus t

Flexor digitorum tt

1st Metacarpal

Hamate, hook

Flexor carpi radialis t

Pisometacarpal lig

Trapezium

Pisohamate lig

Scaphoid

Pisiform

Radial a

Abductor pollicis longus & extensor pollicis brevis tt

Radius

Pronator quadratus m

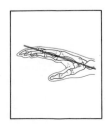

WRIST AND HAND, CORONAL

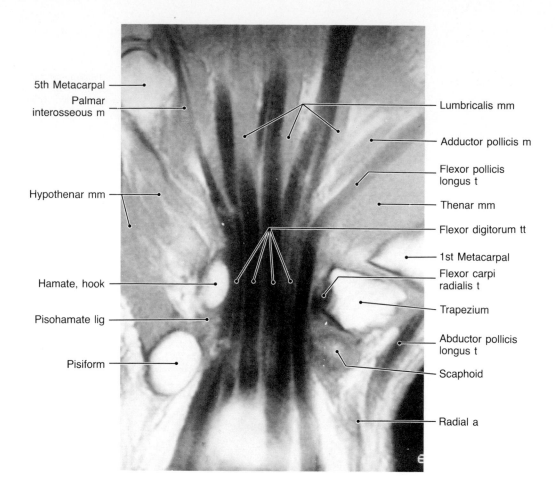

5th Metacarpal

Palmar interosseous m

Hypothenar mm

Hamate, hook

Pisohamate lig

Pisiform

Lumbricalis mm

Adductor pollicis m

Flexor pollicis longus t

Thenar mm

Flexor digitorum tt

1st Metacarpal

Flexor carpi radialis t

Trapezium

Abductor pollicis longus t

Scaphoid

Radial a

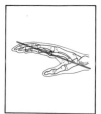

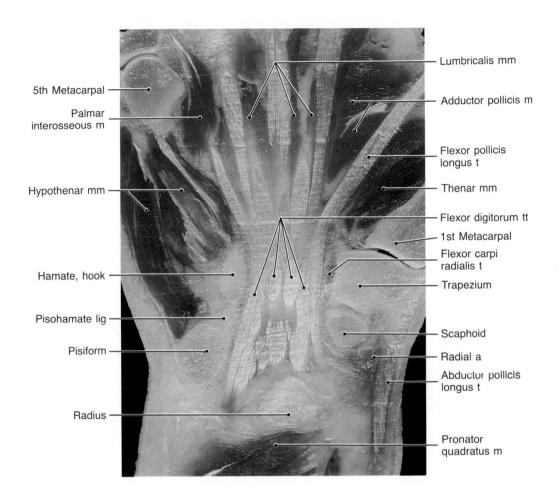

5th Metacarpal

Palmar
interosseous m

Hypothenar mm

Hamate, hook

Pisohamate lig

Pisiform

Radius

Lumbricalis mm

Adductor pollicis m

Flexor pollicis
longus t

Thenar mm

Flexor digitorum tt

1st Metacarpal

Flexor carpi
radialis t

Trapezium

Scaphoid

Radial a

Abductor pollicis
longus t

Pronator
quadratus m

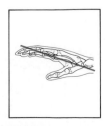

WRIST AND HAND, CORONAL

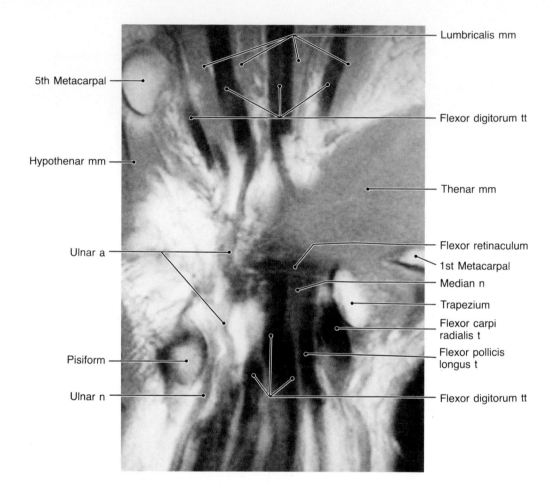

5th Metacarpal

Hypothenar mm

Ulnar a

Pisiform

Ulnar n

Lumbricalis mm

Flexor digitorum tt

Thenar mm

Flexor retinaculum

1st Metacarpal

Median n

Trapezium

Flexor carpi radialis t

Flexor pollicis longus t

Flexor digitorum tt

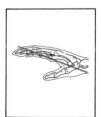

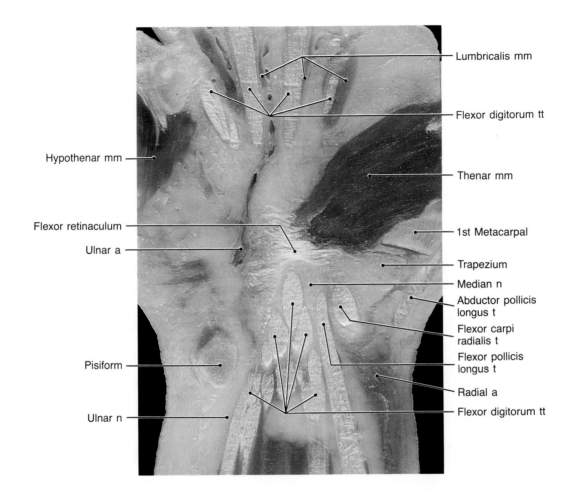

Lumbricalis mm

Flexor digitorum tt

Hypothenar mm

Thenar mm

Flexor retinaculum

1st Metacarpal

Ulnar a

Trapezium

Median n

Abductor pollicis longus t

Flexor carpi radialis t

Pisiform

Flexor pollicis longus t

Radial a

Ulnar n

Flexor digitorum tt

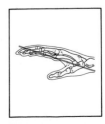

WRIST AND HAND, TRANSVERSE

Extensor digiti minimi t   Extensor digitorum & indicis tt

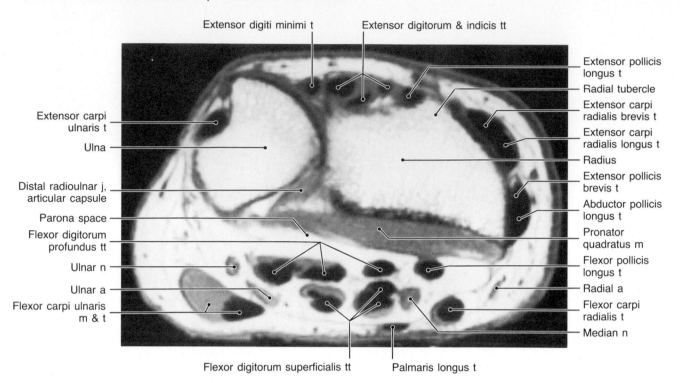

Extensor carpi ulnaris t

Ulna

Distal radioulnar j, articular capsule

Parona space

Flexor digitorum profundus tt

Ulnar n

Ulnar a

Flexor carpi ulnaris m & t

Extensor pollicis longus t

Radial tubercle

Extensor carpi radialis brevis t

Extensor carpi radialis longus t

Radius

Extensor pollicis brevis t

Abductor pollicis longus t

Pronator quadratus m

Flexor pollicis longus t

Radial a

Flexor carpi radialis t

Median n

Flexor digitorum superficialis tt   Palmaris longus t

Extensor digiti minimi t   Extensor digitorum & indicis tt

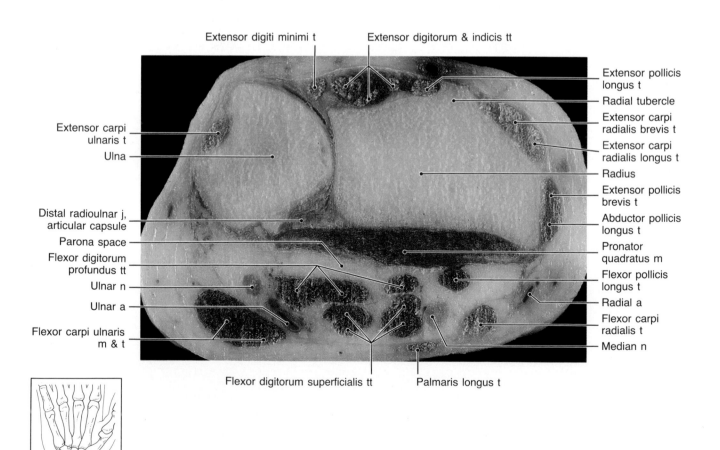

Extensor carpi ulnaris t

Ulna

Distal radioulnar j, articular capsule

Parona space

Flexor digitorum profundus tt

Ulnar n

Ulnar a

Flexor carpi ulnaris m & t

Extensor pollicis longus t

Radial tubercle

Extensor carpi radialis brevis t

Extensor carpi radialis longus t

Radius

Extensor pollicis brevis t

Abductor pollicis longus t

Pronator quadratus m

Flexor pollicis longus t

Radial a

Flexor carpi radialis t

Median n

Flexor digitorum superficialis tt   Palmaris longus t

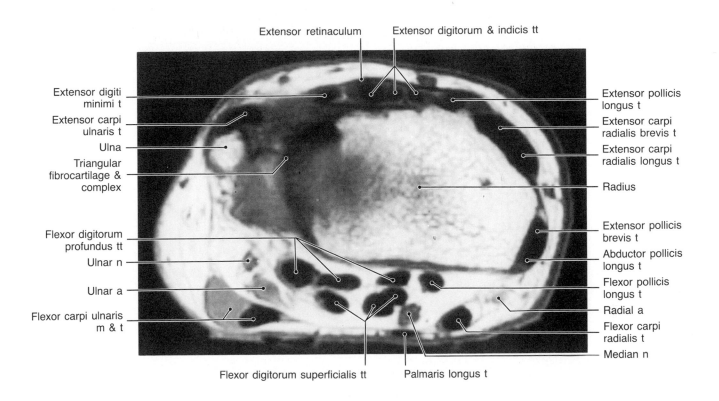

Extensor retinaculum

Extensor digitorum & indicis tt

Extensor digiti minimi t

Extensor carpi ulnaris t

Ulna

Triangular fibrocartilage & complex

Flexor digitorum profundus tt

Ulnar n

Ulnar a

Flexor carpi ulnaris m & t

Extensor pollicis longus t

Extensor carpi radialis brevis t

Extensor carpi radialis longus t

Radius

Extensor pollicis brevis t

Abductor pollicis longus t

Flexor pollicis longus t

Radial a

Flexor carpi radialis t

Median n

Flexor digitorum superficialis tt

Palmaris longus t

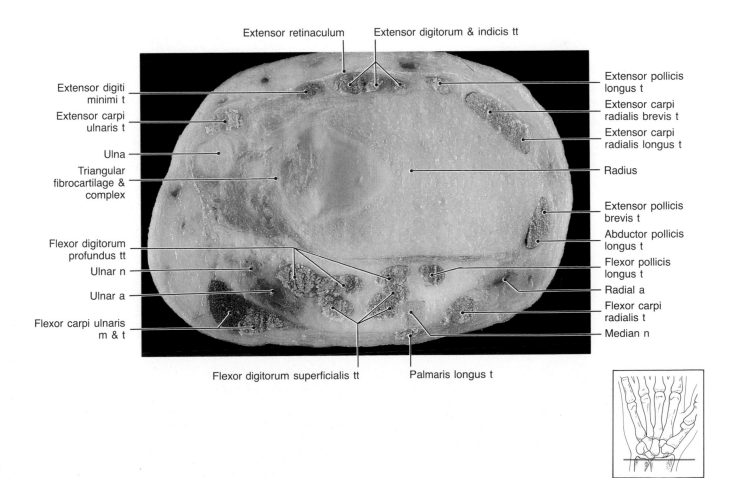

Extensor retinaculum

Extensor digitorum & indicis tt

Extensor digiti minimi t

Extensor carpi ulnaris t

Ulna

Triangular fibrocartilage & complex

Flexor digitorum profundus tt

Ulnar n

Ulnar a

Flexor carpi ulnaris m & t

Extensor pollicis longus t

Extensor carpi radialis brevis t

Extensor carpi radialis longus t

Radius

Extensor pollicis brevis t

Abductor pollicis longus t

Flexor pollicis longus t

Radial a

Flexor carpi radialis t

Median n

Flexor digitorum superficialis tt

Palmaris longus t

WRIST AND HAND, TRANSVERSE

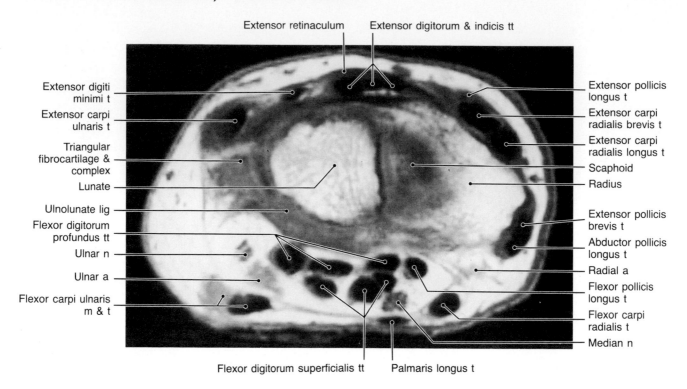

Extensor retinaculum · Extensor digitorum & indicis tt

Extensor digiti minimi t
Extensor carpi ulnaris t
Triangular fibrocartilage & complex
Lunate
Ulnolunate lig
Flexor digitorum profundus tt
Ulnar n
Ulnar a
Flexor carpi ulnaris m & t

Extensor pollicis longus t
Extensor carpi radialis brevis t
Extensor carpi radialis longus t
Scaphoid
Radius
Extensor pollicis brevis t
Abductor pollicis longus t
Radial a
Flexor pollicis longus t
Flexor carpi radialis t
Median n

Flexor digitorum superficialis tt · Palmaris longus t

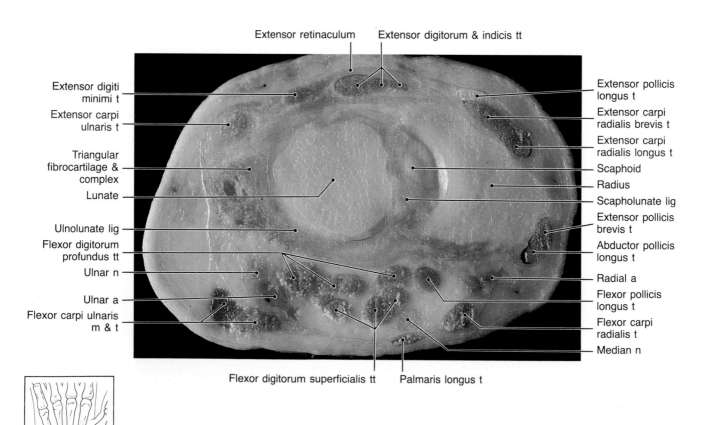

Extensor retinaculum · Extensor digitorum & indicis tt

Extensor digiti minimi t
Extensor carpi ulnaris t
Triangular fibrocartilage & complex
Lunate
Ulnolunate lig
Flexor digitorum profundus tt
Ulnar n
Ulnar a
Flexor carpi ulnaris m & t

Extensor pollicis longus t
Extensor carpi radialis brevis t
Extensor carpi radialis longus t
Scaphoid
Radius
Scapholunate lig
Extensor pollicis brevis t
Abductor pollicis longus t
Radial a
Flexor pollicis longus t
Flexor carpi radialis t
Median n

Flexor digitorum superficialis tt · Palmaris longus t

Extensor retinaculum   Extensor digitorum & indicis tt

Extensor digiti minimi t

Dorsal radiocarpal lig

Extensor carpi ulnaris t

Triquetrum

Lunate

Lunotriquetral lig

Flexor digitorum profundus tt

Ulnar n

Ulnar a

Flexor carpi ulnaris t

Scapholunate lig

Extensor pollicis longus t

Extensor carpi radialis brevis t

Extensor carpi radialis longus t

Scaphoid

Radius

Scapholunate lig

Radiolunate lig

Extensor pollicis brevis t

Abductor pollicis longus t

Radial a

Flexor pollicis longus t

Flexor carpi radialis t

Median n

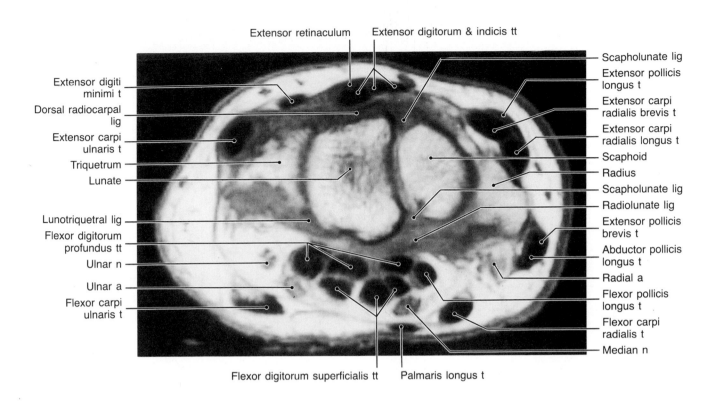

Flexor digitorum superficialis tt   Palmaris longus t

Extensor retinaculum   Extensor digitorum & indicis tt

Extensor digiti minimi t

Dorsal radiocarpal lig

Extensor carpi ulnaris t

Triquetrum

Lunate

Lunotriquetral lig

Flexor digitorum profundus tt

Ulnar n

Ulnar a

Flexor carpi ulnaris t

Scapholunate lig

Extensor pollicis longus t

Extensor carpi radialis brevis t

Extensor carpi radialis longus t

Scaphoid

Radius

Scapholunate lig

Radiolunate lig

Extensor pollicis brevis t

Abductor pollicis longus t

Radial a

Flexor pollicis longus t

Flexor carpi radialis t

Median n

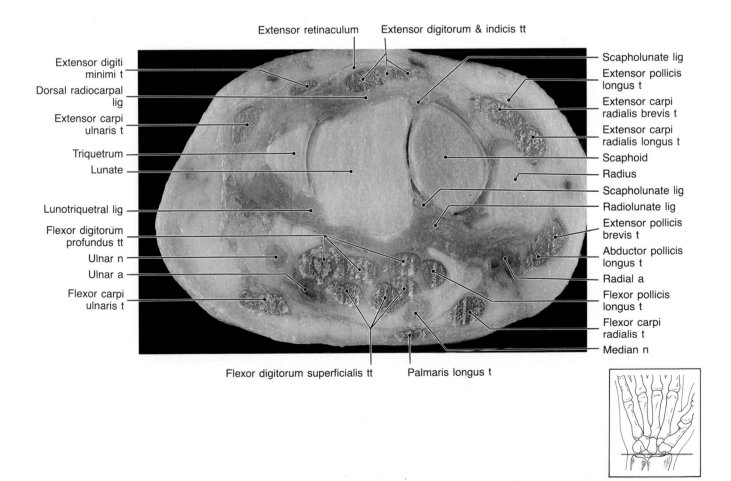

Flexor digitorum superficialis tt   Palmaris longus t

WRIST AND HAND, TRANSVERSE

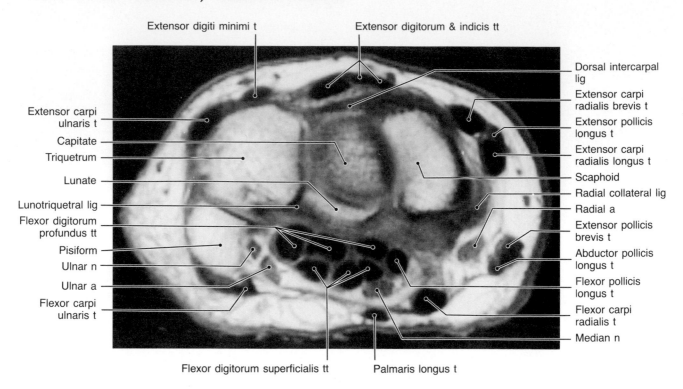

Extensor digiti minimi t

Extensor digitorum & indicis tt

Dorsal intercarpal lig

Extensor carpi radialis brevis t

Extensor pollicis longus t

Extensor carpi radialis longus t

Scaphoid

Radial collateral lig

Radial a

Extensor pollicis brevis t

Abductor pollicis longus t

Flexor pollicis longus t

Flexor carpi radialis t

Median n

Extensor carpi ulnaris t

Capitate

Triquetrum

Lunate

Lunotriquetral lig

Flexor digitorum profundus tt

Pisiform

Ulnar n

Ulnar a

Flexor carpi ulnaris t

Flexor digitorum superficialis tt

Palmaris longus t

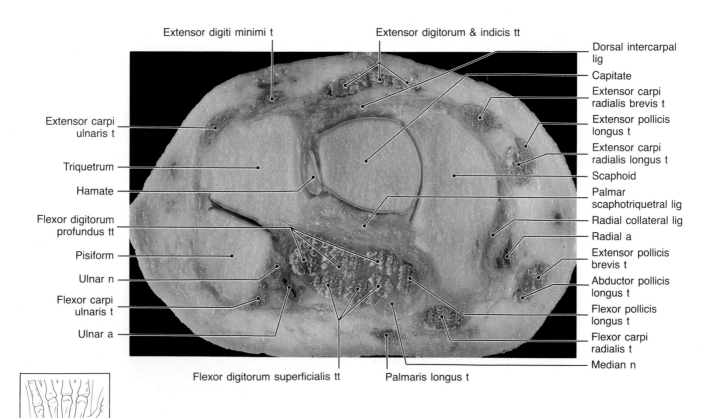

Extensor digiti minimi t

Extensor digitorum & indicis tt

Dorsal intercarpal lig

Capitate

Extensor carpi radialis brevis t

Extensor pollicis longus t

Extensor carpi radialis longus t

Scaphoid

Palmar scaphotriquetral lig

Radial collateral lig

Radial a

Extensor pollicis brevis t

Abductor pollicis longus t

Flexor pollicis longus t

Flexor carpi radialis t

Median n

Extensor carpi ulnaris t

Triquetrum

Hamate

Flexor digitorum profundus tt

Pisiform

Ulnar n

Flexor carpi ulnaris t

Ulnar a

Flexor digitorum superficialis tt

Palmaris longus t

Extensor digitorum & indicis tt

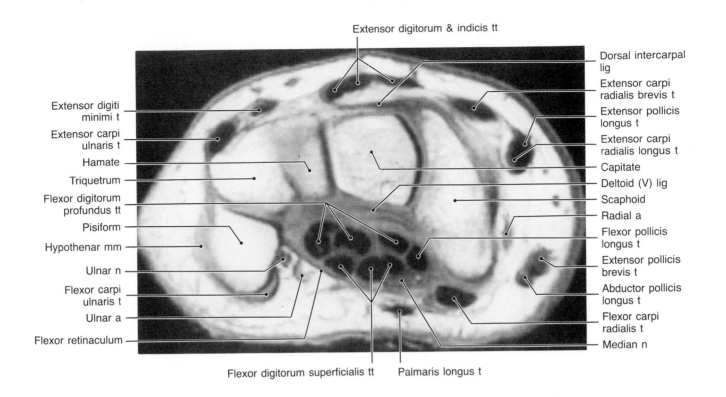

Extensor digiti minimi t

Extensor carpi ulnaris t

Hamate

Triquetrum

Flexor digitorum profundus tt

Pisiform

Hypothenar mm

Ulnar n

Flexor carpi ulnaris t

Ulnar a

Flexor retinaculum

Dorsal intercarpal lig

Extensor carpi radialis brevis t

Extensor pollicis longus t

Extensor carpi radialis longus t

Capitate

Deltoid (V) lig

Scaphoid

Radial a

Flexor pollicis longus t

Extensor pollicis brevis t

Abductor pollicis longus t

Flexor carpi radialis t

Median n

Flexor digitorum superficialis tt

Palmaris longus t

Extensor digiti minimi t

Extensor digitorum & indicis tt

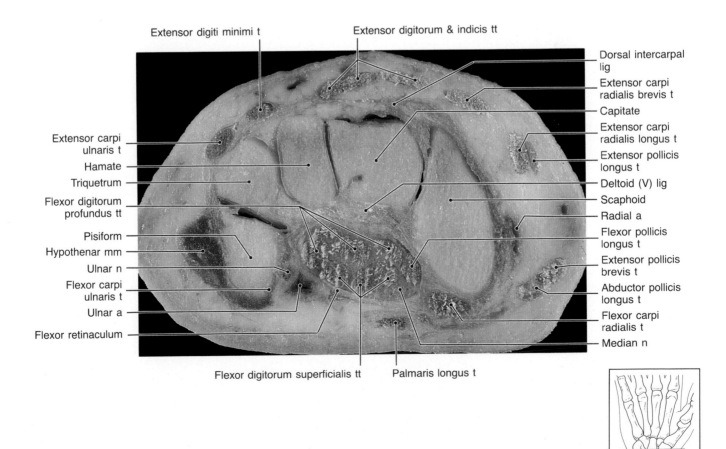

Dorsal intercarpal lig

Extensor carpi radialis brevis t

Capitate

Extensor carpi radialis longus t

Extensor pollicis longus t

Deltoid (V) lig

Scaphoid

Radial a

Flexor pollicis longus t

Extensor pollicis brevis t

Abductor pollicis longus t

Flexor carpi radialis t

Median n

Extensor carpi ulnaris t

Hamate

Triquetrum

Flexor digitorum profundus tt

Pisiform

Hypothenar mm

Ulnar n

Flexor carpi ulnaris t

Ulnar a

Flexor retinaculum

Flexor digitorum superficialis tt

Palmaris longus t

WRIST AND HAND, TRANSVERSE

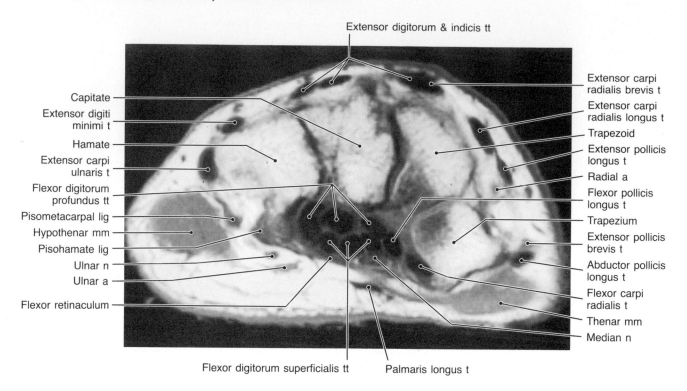

Extensor digitorum & indicis tt

Capitate

Extensor digiti minimi t

Hamate

Extensor carpi ulnaris t

Flexor digitorum profundus tt

Pisometacarpal lig

Hypothenar mm

Pisohamate lig

Ulnar n

Ulnar a

Flexor retinaculum

Extensor carpi radialis brevis t

Extensor carpi radialis longus t

Trapezoid

Extensor pollicis longus t

Radial a

Flexor pollicis longus t

Trapezium

Extensor pollicis brevis t

Abductor pollicis longus t

Flexor carpi radialis t

Thenar mm

Median n

Flexor digitorum superficialis tt

Palmaris longus t

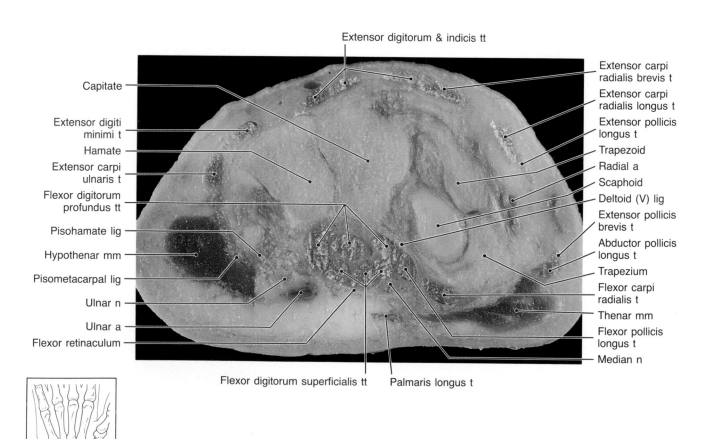

Extensor digitorum & indicis tt

Capitate

Extensor digiti minimi t

Hamate

Extensor carpi ulnaris t

Flexor digitorum profundus tt

Pisohamate lig

Hypothenar mm

Pisometacarpal lig

Ulnar n

Ulnar a

Flexor retinaculum

Extensor carpi radialis brevis t

Extensor carpi radialis longus t

Extensor pollicis longus t

Trapezoid

Radial a

Scaphoid

Deltoid (V) lig

Extensor pollicis brevis t

Abductor pollicis longus t

Trapezium

Flexor carpi radialis t

Thenar mm

Flexor pollicis longus t

Median n

Flexor digitorum superficialis tt

Palmaris longus t

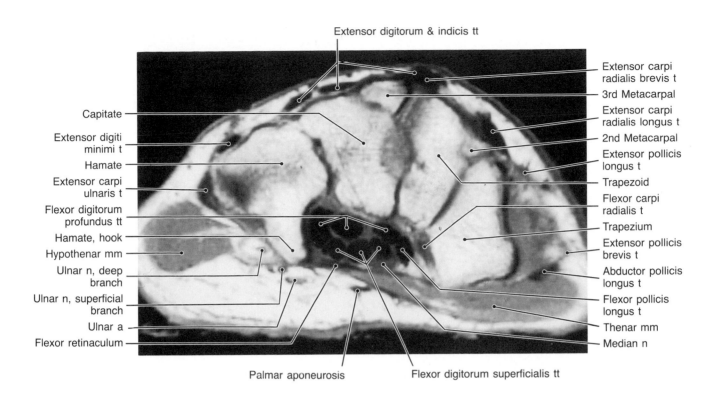

Extensor digitorum & indicis tt

Capitate

Extensor digiti minimi t

Hamate

Extensor carpi ulnaris t

Flexor digitorum profundus tt

Hamate, hook

Hypothenar mm

Ulnar n, deep branch

Ulnar n, superficial branch

Ulnar a

Flexor retinaculum

Extensor carpi radialis brevis t

3rd Metacarpal

Extensor carpi radialis longus t

2nd Metacarpal

Extensor pollicis longus t

Trapezoid

Flexor carpi radialis t

Trapezium

Extensor pollicis brevis t

Abductor pollicis longus t

Flexor pollicis longus t

Thenar mm

Median n

Palmar aponeurosis   Flexor digitorum superficialis tt

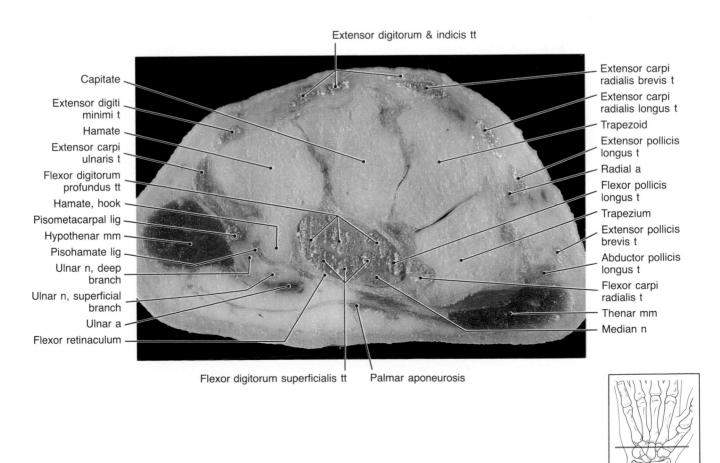

Extensor digitorum & indicis tt

Capitate

Extensor digiti minimi t

Hamate

Extensor carpi ulnaris t

Flexor digitorum profundus tt

Hamate, hook

Pisometacarpal lig

Hypothenar mm

Pisohamate lig

Ulnar n, deep branch

Ulnar n, superficial branch

Ulnar a

Flexor retinaculum

Extensor carpi radialis brevis t

Extensor carpi radialis longus t

Trapezoid

Extensor pollicis longus t

Radial a

Flexor pollicis longus t

Trapezium

Extensor pollicis brevis t

Abductor pollicis longus t

Flexor carpi radialis t

Thenar mm

Median n

Flexor digitorum superficialis tt   Palmar aponeurosis

WRIST AND HAND, TRANSVERSE

Extensor digitorum & indicis tt

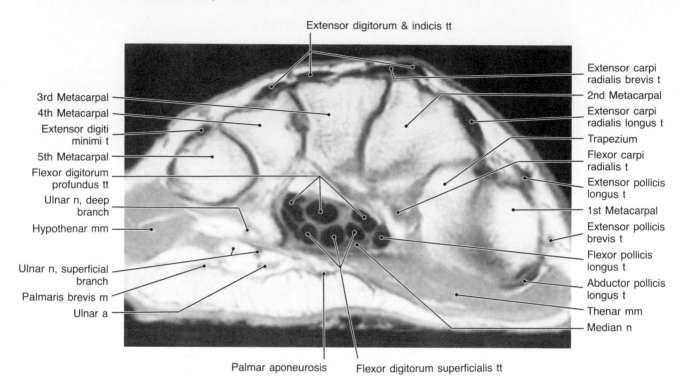

3rd Metacarpal
4th Metacarpal
Extensor digiti minimi t
5th Metacarpal
Flexor digitorum profundus tt
Ulnar n, deep branch
Hypothenar mm
Ulnar n, superficial branch
Palmaris brevis m
Ulnar a

Extensor carpi radialis brevis t
2nd Metacarpal
Extensor carpi radialis longus t
Trapezium
Flexor carpi radialis t
Extensor pollicis longus t
1st Metacarpal
Extensor pollicis brevis t
Flexor pollicis longus t
Abductor pollicis longus t
Thenar mm
Median n

Palmar aponeurosis   Flexor digitorum superficialis tt

Extensor digitorum & indicis tt

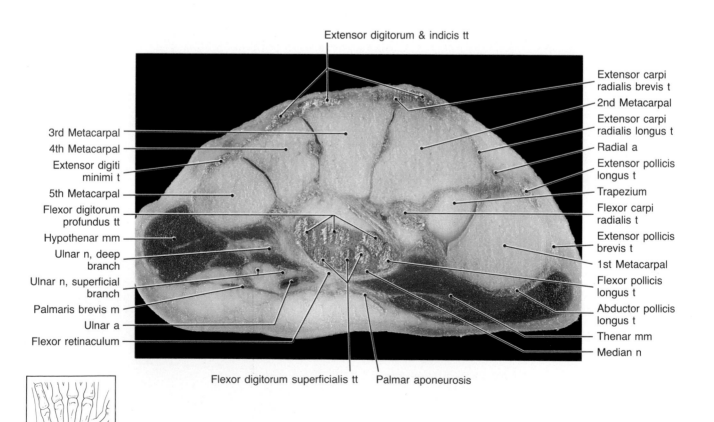

3rd Metacarpal
4th Metacarpal
Extensor digiti minimi t
5th Metacarpal
Flexor digitorum profundus tt
Hypothenar mm
Ulnar n, deep branch
Ulnar n, superficial branch
Palmaris brevis m
Ulnar a
Flexor retinaculum

Extensor carpi radialis brevis t
2nd Metacarpal
Extensor carpi radialis longus t
Radial a
Extensor pollicis longus t
Trapezium
Flexor carpi radialis t
Extensor pollicis brevis t
1st Metacarpal
Flexor pollicis longus t
Abductor pollicis longus t
Thenar mm
Median n

Flexor digitorum superficialis tt   Palmar aponeurosis

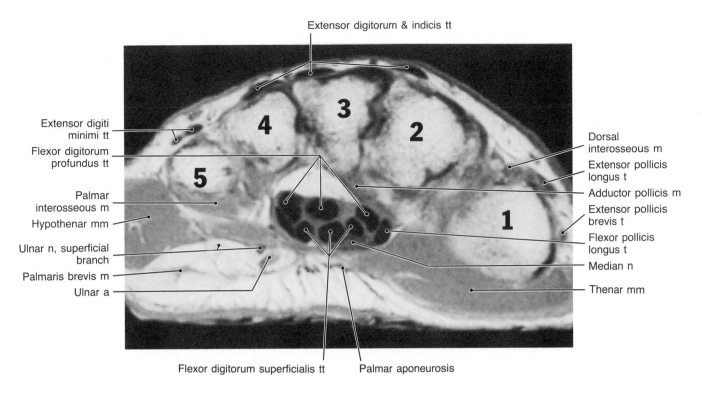

Extensor digitorum & indicis tt

Extensor digiti minimi tt

Flexor digitorum profundus tt

Palmar interosseous m

Hypothenar mm

Ulnar n, superficial branch

Palmaris brevis m

Ulnar a

Dorsal interosseous m

Extensor pollicis longus t

Adductor pollicis m

Extensor pollicis brevis t

Flexor pollicis longus t

Median n

Thenar mm

Flexor digitorum superficialis tt

Palmar aponeurosis

1, 2, 3, 4, 5: Metacarpals

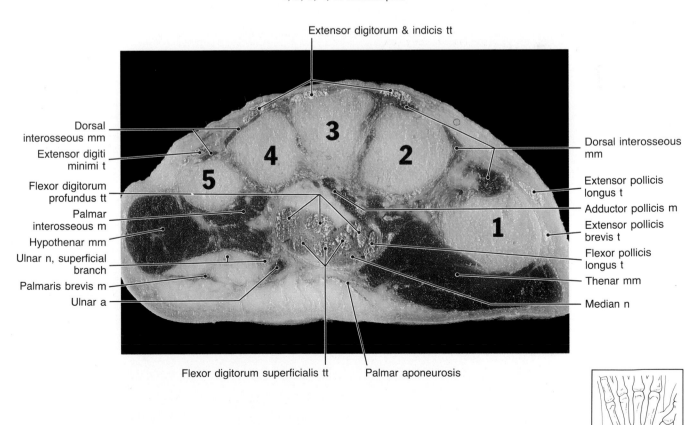

Extensor digitorum & indicis tt

Dorsal interosseous mm

Extensor digiti minimi t

Flexor digitorum profundus tt

Palmar interosseous m

Hypothenar mm

Ulnar n, superficial branch

Palmaris brevis m

Ulnar a

Dorsal interosseous mm

Extensor pollicis longus t

Adductor pollicis m

Extensor pollicis brevis t

Flexor pollicis longus t

Thenar mm

Median n

Flexor digitorum superficialis tt

Palmar aponeurosis

WRIST AND HAND, TRANSVERSE

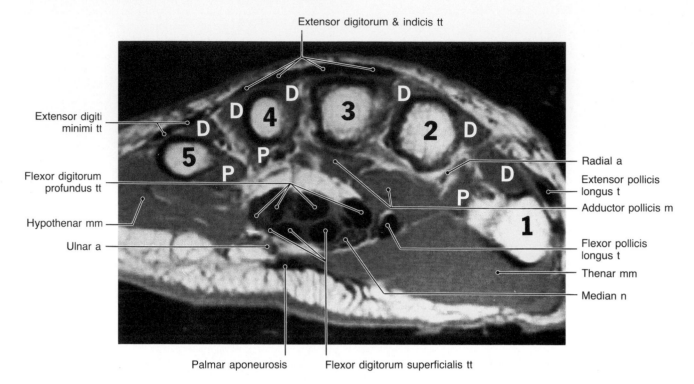

Extensor digitorum & indicis tt

Extensor digiti minimi tt

Flexor digitorum profundus tt

Hypothenar mm

Ulnar a

Radial a

Extensor pollicis longus t

Adductor pollicis m

Flexor pollicis longus t

Thenar mm

Median n

Palmar aponeurosis

Flexor digitorum superficialis tt

D: Dorsal interosseous m

P: Palmar interosseous m

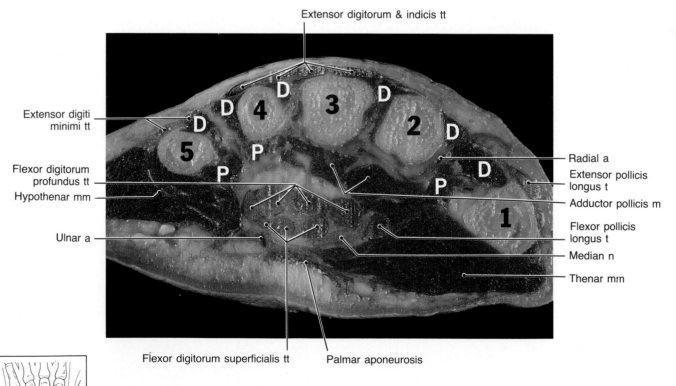

Extensor digitorum & indicis tt

Extensor digiti minimi tt

Flexor digitorum profundus tt

Hypothenar mm

Ulnar a

Radial a

Extensor pollicis longus t

Adductor pollicis m

Flexor pollicis longus t

Median n

Thenar mm

Flexor digitorum superficialis tt

Palmar aponeurosis

Extensor digitorum indicis tt

Extensor digiti minimi tt

Flexor digitorum profundus tt

Hypothenar mm

Flexor digitorum superficialis tt

Adductor pollicis m

Extensor pollicis longus t

Flexor pollicis longus t

Thenar mm

Common palmar digital aa & nn

Palmar aponeurosis

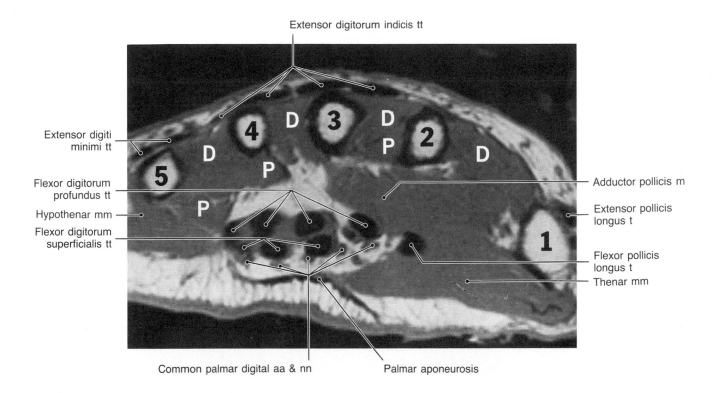

Extensor digitorum & indicis tt

Extensor digiti minimi tt

Flexor digitorum profundus tt

Hypothenar mm

Flexor digitorum superficialis tt

Adductor pollicis m

Extensor pollicis longus t

Flexor pollicis longus t

Thenar mm

Common palmar digital aa & nn

Palmar aponeurosis

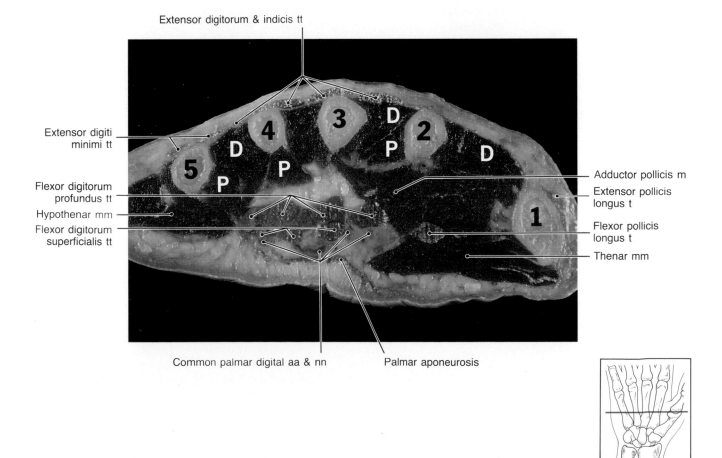

WRIST AND HAND, SAGITTAL

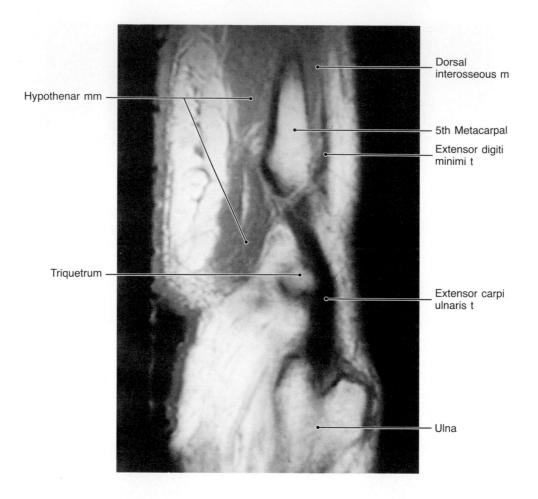

Hypothenar mm

Triquetrum

Dorsal interosseous m

5th Metacarpal

Extensor digiti minimi t

Extensor carpi ulnaris t

Ulna

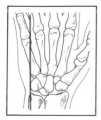

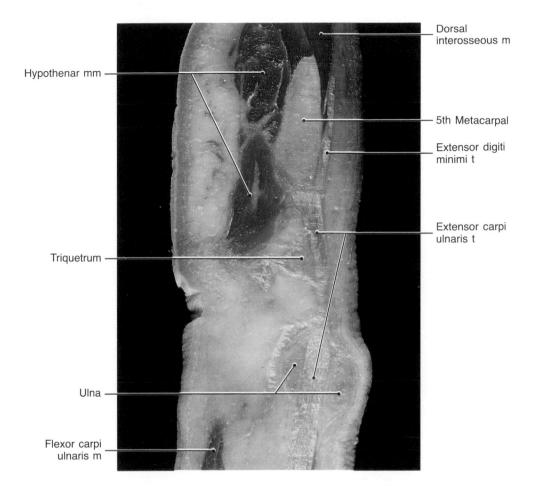

Hypothenar mm

Triquetrum

Ulna

Flexor carpi
ulnaris m

Dorsal
interosseous m

5th Metacarpal

Extensor digiti
minimi t

Extensor carpi
ulnaris t

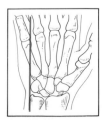

WRIST AND HAND, SAGITTAL

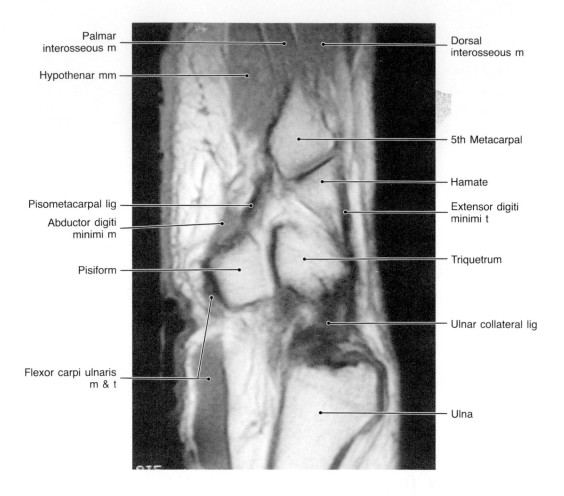

Palmar interosseous m

Hypothenar mm

Pisometacarpal lig

Abductor digiti minimi m

Pisiform

Flexor carpi ulnaris m & t

Dorsal interosseous m

5th Metacarpal

Hamate

Extensor digiti minimi t

Triquetrum

Ulnar collateral lig

Ulna

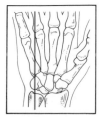

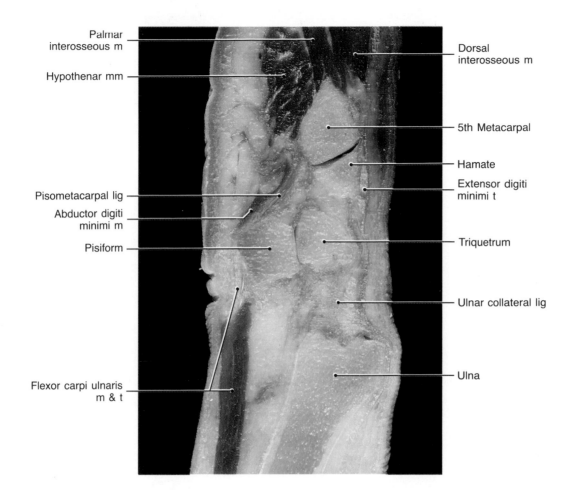

Palmar interosseous m

Hypothenar mm

Pisometacarpal lig

Abductor digiti minimi m

Pisiform

Flexor carpi ulnaris m & t

Dorsal interosseous m

5th Metacarpal

Hamate

Extensor digiti minimi t

Triquetrum

Ulnar collateral lig

Ulna

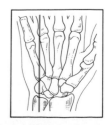

WRIST AND HAND, SAGITTAL

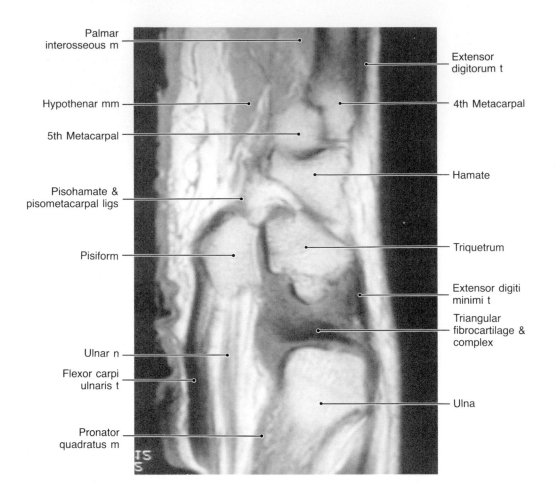

Palmar interosseous m

Hypothenar mm

5th Metacarpal

Pisohamate & pisometacarpal ligs

Pisiform

Ulnar n

Flexor carpi ulnaris t

Pronator quadratus m

Extensor digitorum t

4th Metacarpal

Hamate

Triquetrum

Extensor digiti minimi t

Triangular fibrocartilage & complex

Ulna

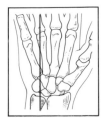

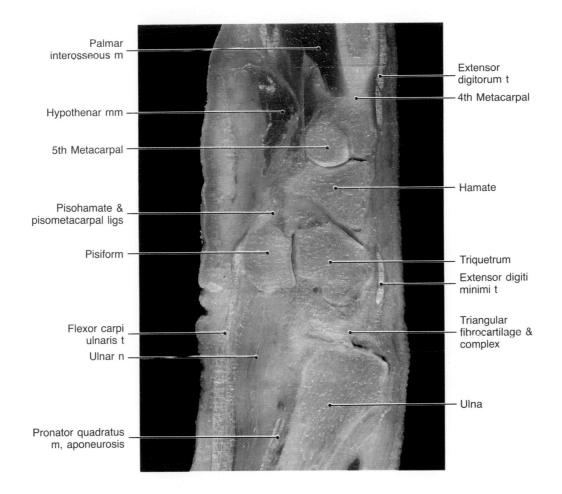

Palmar interosseous m

Hypothenar mm

5th Metacarpal

Pisohamate & pisometacarpal ligs

Pisiform

Flexor carpi ulnaris t

Ulnar n

Pronator quadratus m, aponeurosis

Extensor digitorum t

4th Metacarpal

Hamate

Triquetrum

Extensor digiti minimi t

Triangular fibrocartilage & complex

Ulna

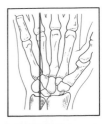

WRIST AND HAND, SAGITTAL

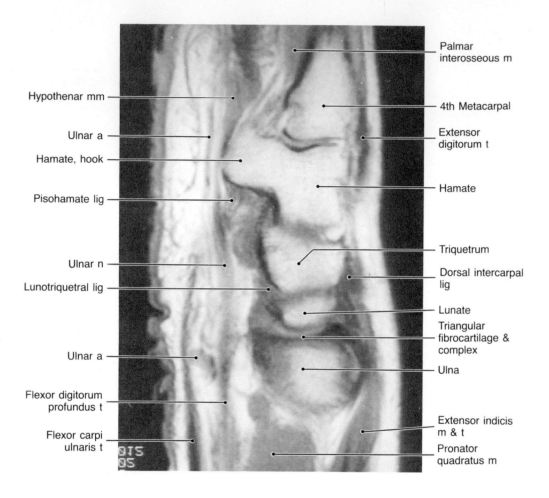

Hypothenar mm

Ulnar a

Hamate, hook

Pisohamate lig

Ulnar n

Lunotriquetral lig

Ulnar a

Flexor digitorum profundus t

Flexor carpi ulnaris t

Palmar interosseous m

4th Metacarpal

Extensor digitorum t

Hamate

Triquetrum

Dorsal intercarpal lig

Lunate

Triangular fibrocartilage & complex

Ulna

Extensor indicis m & t

Pronator quadratus m

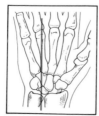

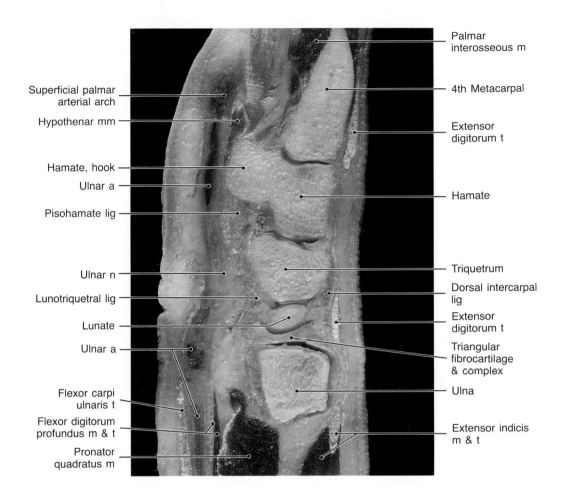

Superficial palmar arterial arch

Hypothenar mm

Hamate, hook

Ulnar a

Pisohamate lig

Ulnar n

Lunotriquetral lig

Lunate

Ulnar a

Flexor carpi ulnaris t

Flexor digitorum profundus m & t

Pronator quadratus m

Palmar interosseous m

4th Metacarpal

Extensor digitorum t

Hamate

Triquetrum

Dorsal intercarpal lig

Extensor digitorum t

Triangular fibrocartilage & complex

Ulna

Extensor indicis m & t

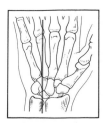

WRIST AND HAND, SAGITTAL

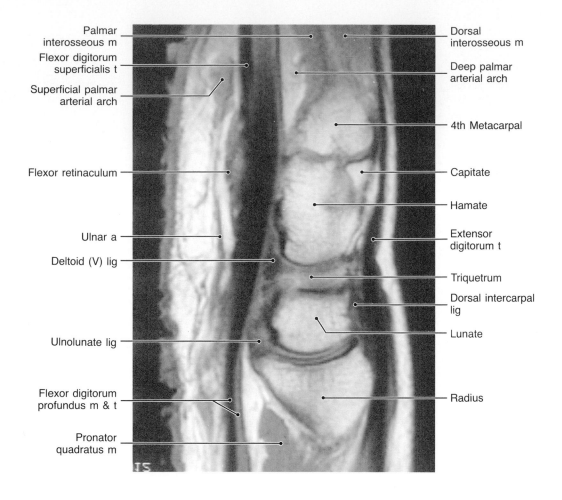

Palmar interosseous m

Flexor digitorum superficialis t

Superficial palmar arterial arch

Flexor retinaculum

Ulnar a

Deltoid (V) lig

Ulnolunate lig

Flexor digitorum profundus m & t

Pronator quadratus m

Dorsal interosseous m

Deep palmar arterial arch

4th Metacarpal

Capitate

Hamate

Extensor digitorum t

Triquetrum

Dorsal intercarpal lig

Lunate

Radius

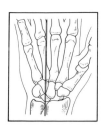

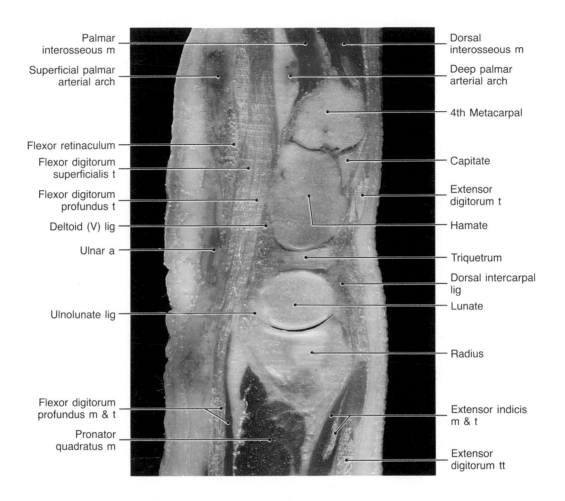

Palmar interosseous m

Superficial palmar arterial arch

Flexor retinaculum

Flexor digitorum superficialis t

Flexor digitorum profundus t

Deltoid (V) lig

Ulnar a

Ulnolunate lig

Flexor digitorum profundus m & t

Pronator quadratus m

Dorsal interosseous m

Deep palmar arterial arch

4th Metacarpal

Capitate

Extensor digitorum t

Hamate

Triquetrum

Dorsal intercarpal lig

Lunate

Radius

Extensor indicis m & t

Extensor digitorum tt

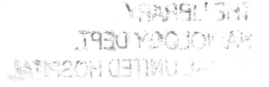

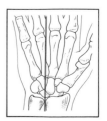

WRIST AND HAND, SAGITTAL

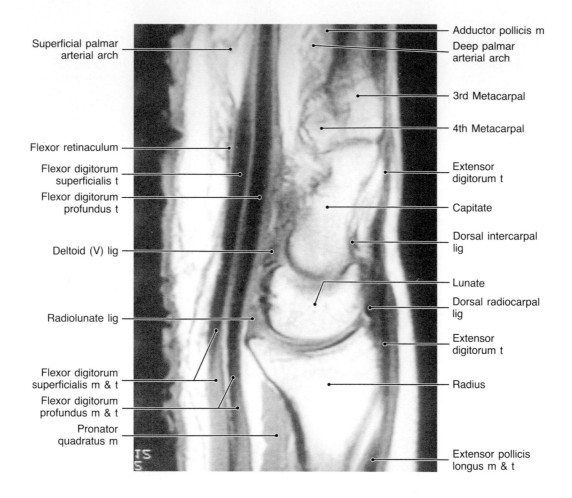

Superficial palmar arterial arch

Flexor retinaculum

Flexor digitorum superficialis t

Flexor digitorum profundus t

Deltoid (V) lig

Radiolunate lig

Flexor digitorum superficialis m & t

Flexor digitorum profundus m & t

Pronator quadratus m

Adductor pollicis m

Deep palmar arterial arch

3rd Metacarpal

4th Metacarpal

Extensor digitorum t

Capitate

Dorsal intercarpal lig

Lunate

Dorsal radiocarpal lig

Extensor digitorum t

Radius

Extensor pollicis longus m & t

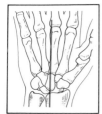

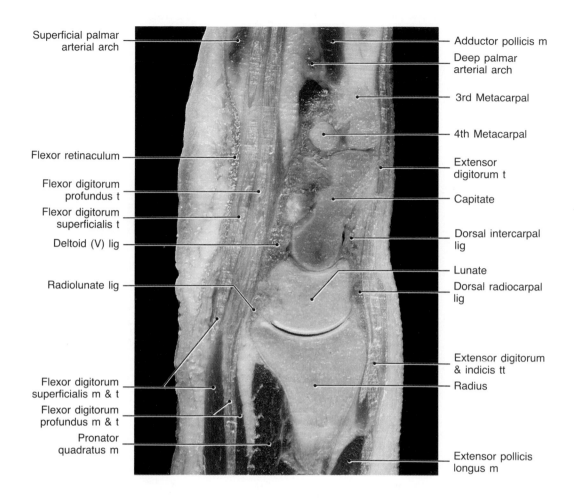

Superficial palmar arterial arch

Flexor retinaculum

Flexor digitorum profundus t

Flexor digitorum superficialis t

Deltoid (V) lig

Radiolunate lig

Flexor digitorum superficialis m & t

Flexor digitorum profundus m & t

Pronator quadratus m

Adductor pollicis m

Deep palmar arterial arch

3rd Metacarpal

4th Metacarpal

Extensor digitorum t

Capitate

Dorsal intercarpal lig

Lunate

Dorsal radiocarpal lig

Extensor digitorum & indicis tt

Radius

Extensor pollicis longus m

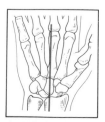

WRIST AND HAND, SAGITTAL

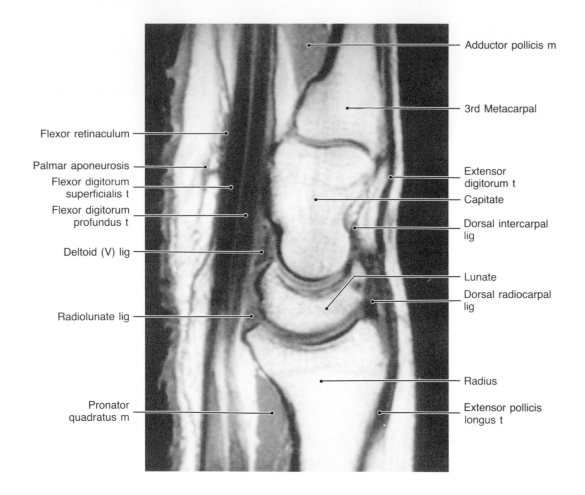

Flexor retinaculum

Palmar aponeurosis

Flexor digitorum
superficialis t

Flexor digitorum
profundus t

Deltoid (V) lig

Radiolunate lig

Pronator
quadratus m

Adductor pollicis m

3rd Metacarpal

Extensor
digitorum t

Capitate

Dorsal intercarpal
lig

Lunate

Dorsal radiocarpal
lig

Radius

Extensor pollicis
longus t

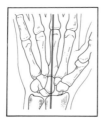

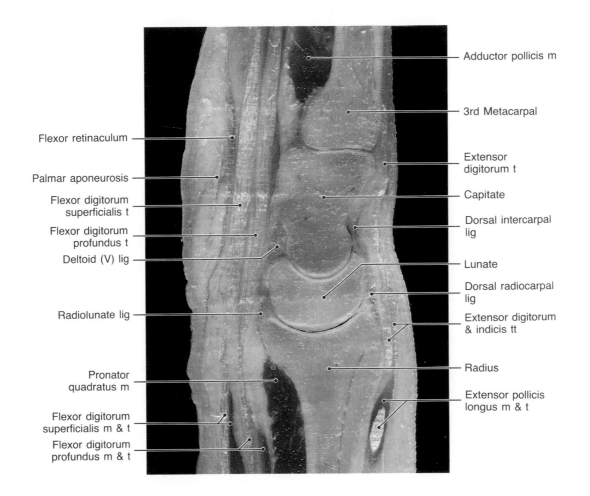

Adductor pollicis m

3rd Metacarpal

Extensor digitorum t

Capitate

Dorsal intercarpal lig

Lunate

Dorsal radiocarpal lig

Extensor digitorum & indicis tt

Radius

Extensor pollicis longus m & t

Flexor retinaculum

Palmar aponeurosis

Flexor digitorum superficialis t

Flexor digitorum profundus t

Deltoid (V) lig

Radiolunate lig

Pronator quadratus m

Flexor digitorum superficialis m & t

Flexor digitorum profundus m & t

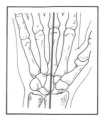

WRIST AND HAND, SAGITTAL

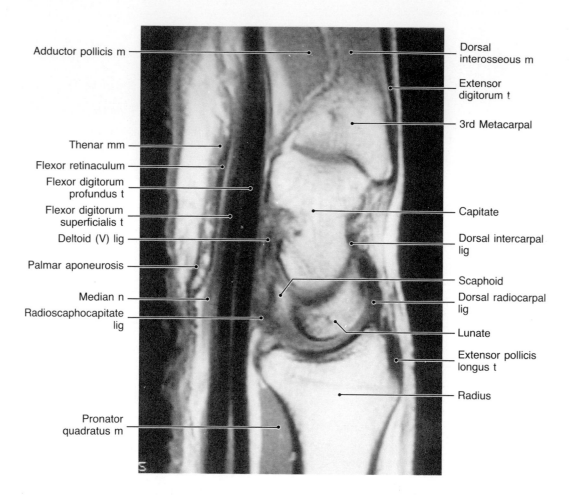

Adductor pollicis m

Dorsal
interosseous m

Extensor
digitorum t

3rd Metacarpal

Thenar mm

Flexor retinaculum

Flexor digitorum
profundus t

Flexor digitorum
superficialis t

Capitate

Deltoid (V) lig

Dorsal intercarpal
lig

Palmar aponeurosis

Scaphoid

Median n

Dorsal radiocarpal
lig

Radioscaphocapitate
lig

Lunate

Extensor pollicis
longus t

Radius

Pronator
quadratus m

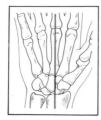

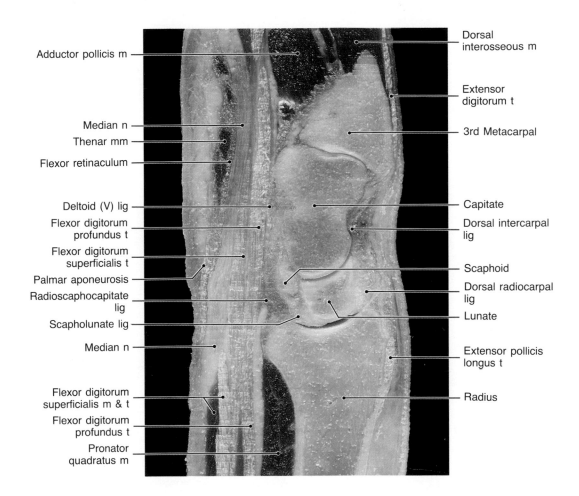

Adductor pollicis m

Median n
Thenar mm
Flexor retinaculum

Deltoid (V) lig
Flexor digitorum
profundus t
Flexor digitorum
superficialis t
Palmar aponeurosis
Radioscaphocapitate
lig
Scapholunate lig

Median n

Flexor digitorum
superficialis m & t
Flexor digitorum
profundus t
Pronator
quadratus m

Dorsal
interosseous m

Extensor
digitorum t

3rd Metacarpal

Capitate
Dorsal intercarpal
lig

Scaphoid
Dorsal radiocarpal
lig
Lunate

Extensor pollicis
longus t

Radius

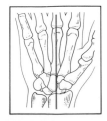

WRIST AND HAND, SAGITTAL

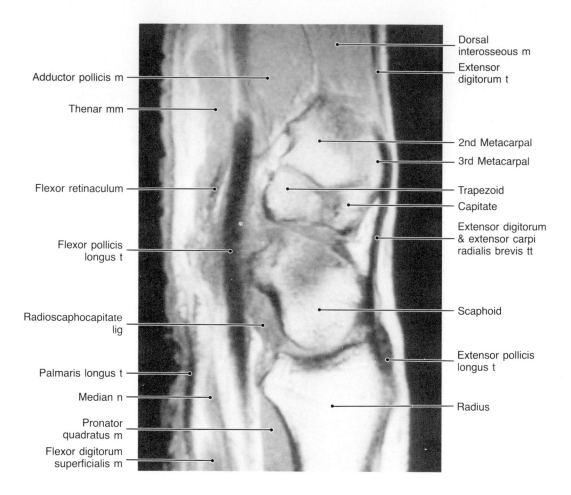

Adductor pollicis m

Thenar mm

Flexor retinaculum

Flexor pollicis longus t

Radioscaphocapitate lig

Palmaris longus t

Median n

Pronator quadratus m

Flexor digitorum superficialis m

Dorsal interosseous m

Extensor digitorum t

2nd Metacarpal

3rd Metacarpal

Trapezoid

Capitate

Extensor digitorum & extensor carpi radialis brevis tt

Scaphoid

Extensor pollicis longus t

Radius

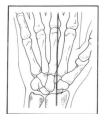

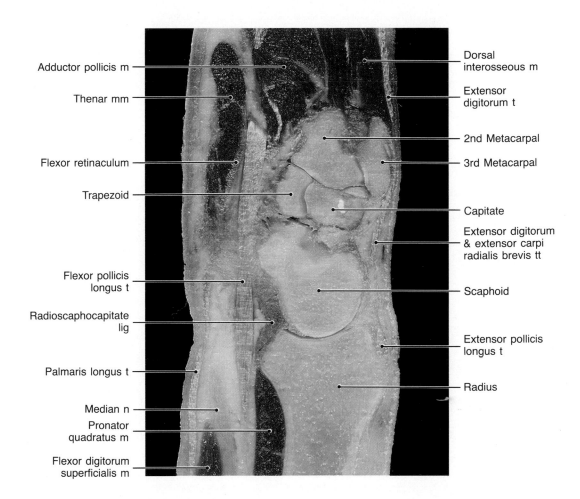

Adductor pollicis m

Thenar mm

Flexor retinaculum

Trapezoid

Flexor pollicis longus t

Radioscaphocapitate lig

Palmaris longus t

Median n

Pronator quadratus m

Flexor digitorum superficialis m

Dorsal interosseous m

Extensor digitorum t

2nd Metacarpal

3rd Metacarpal

Capitate

Extensor digitorum & extensor carpi radialis brevis tt

Scaphoid

Extensor pollicis longus t

Radius

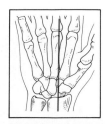

WRIST AND HAND, SAGITTAL

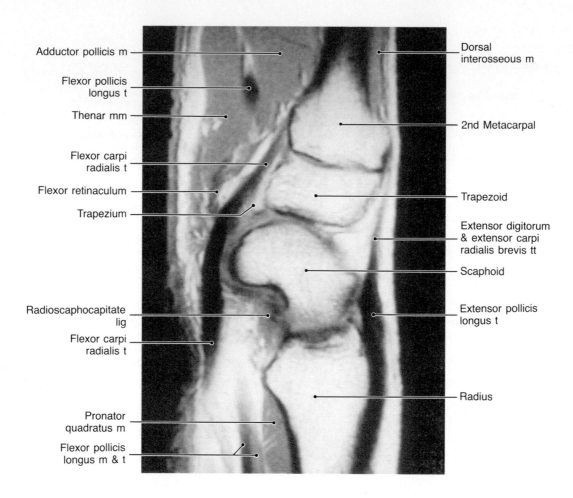

Adductor pollicis m

Flexor pollicis longus t

Thenar mm

Flexor carpi radialis t

Flexor retinaculum

Trapezium

Radioscaphocapitate lig

Flexor carpi radialis t

Pronator quadratus m

Flexor pollicis longus m & t

Dorsal interosseous m

2nd Metacarpal

Trapezoid

Extensor digitorum & extensor carpi radialis brevis tt

Scaphoid

Extensor pollicis longus t

Radius

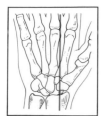

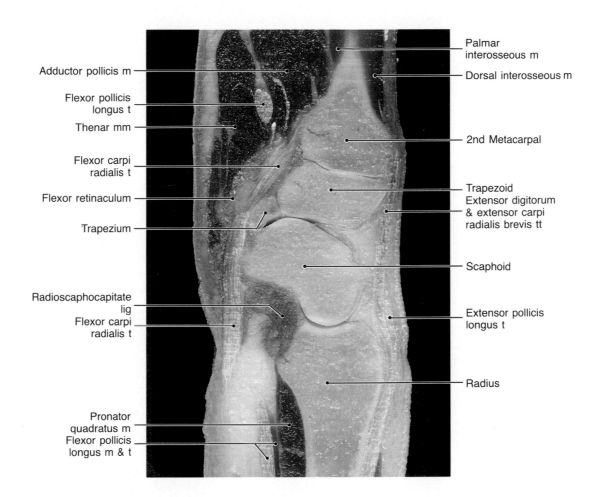

Adductor pollicis m

Flexor pollicis longus t

Thenar mm

Flexor carpi radialis t

Flexor retinaculum

Trapezium

Radioscaphocapitate lig

Flexor carpi radialis t

Pronator quadratus m

Flexor pollicis longus m & t

Palmar interosseous m

Dorsal interosseous m

2nd Metacarpal

Trapezoid

Extensor digitorum & extensor carpi radialis brevis tt

Scaphoid

Extensor pollicis longus t

Radius

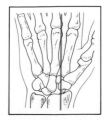

WRIST AND HAND, SAGITTAL

Adductor pollicis m

Flexor pollicis
longus t

Thenar mm

Trapezium

Scaphoid

Radioscaphocapitate
lig

Radial a

Flexor carpi
radialis t

Pronator
quadratus m

Dorsal
interosseous m

2nd Metacarpal

Trapezoid

Extensor pollicis
longus t

Extensor carpi
radialis longus t

Radius

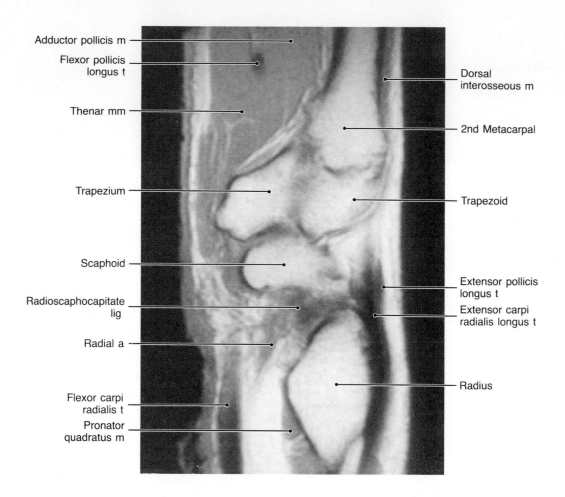

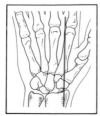

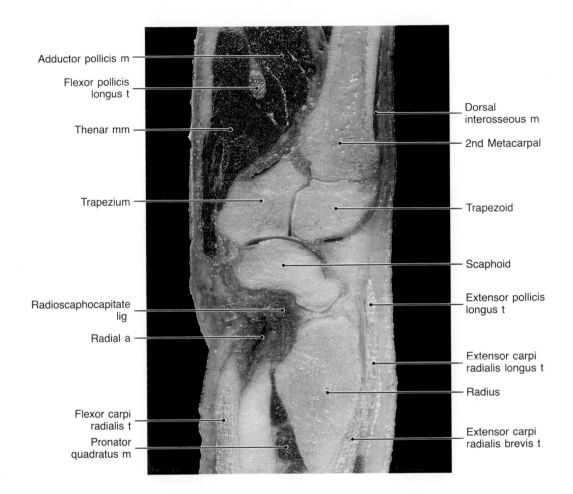

Adductor pollicis m

Flexor pollicis longus t

Thenar mm

Trapezium

Radioscaphocapitate lig

Radial a

Flexor carpi radialis t

Pronator quadratus m

Dorsal interosseous m

2nd Metacarpal

Trapezoid

Scaphoid

Extensor pollicis longus t

Extensor carpi radialis longus t

Radius

Extensor carpi radialis brevis t

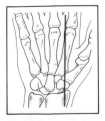

WRIST AND HAND, SAGITTAL

Flexor pollicis
longus t

Adductor pollicis m

Thenar mm

Carpometacarpal
lig

Trapezium

Radial a

Palmar
interosseous m

2nd Metacarpal

Extensor carpi
radialis longus t

Abductor pollicis
longus & extensor
pollicis brevis tt

Radius

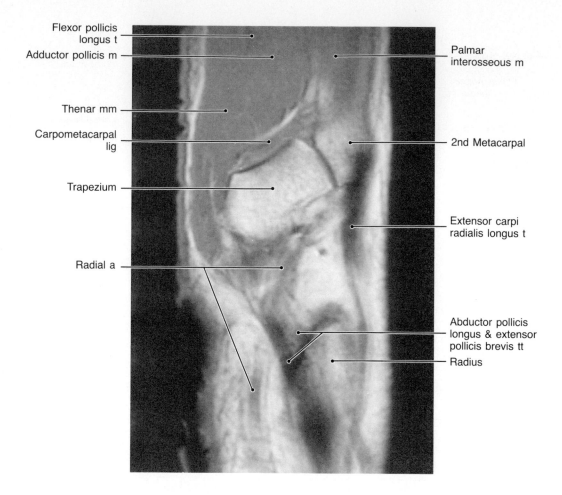

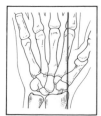

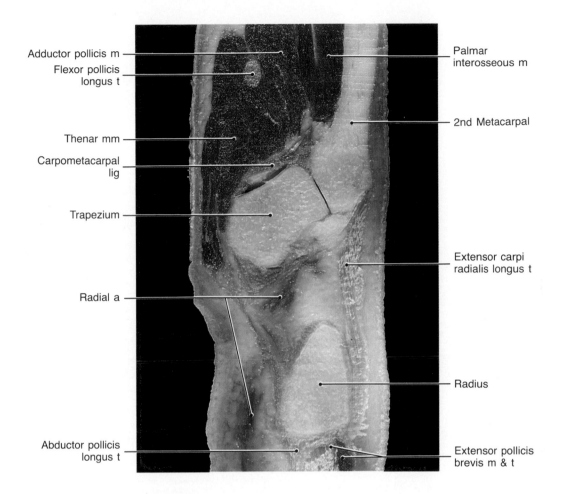

Adductor pollicis m

Flexor pollicis longus t

Thenar mm

Carpometacarpal lig

Trapezium

Radial a

Abductor pollicis longus t

Palmar interosseous m

2nd Metacarpal

Extensor carpi radialis longus t

Radius

Extensor pollicis brevis m & t

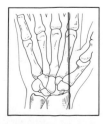

WRIST, CORONAL, INJECTED

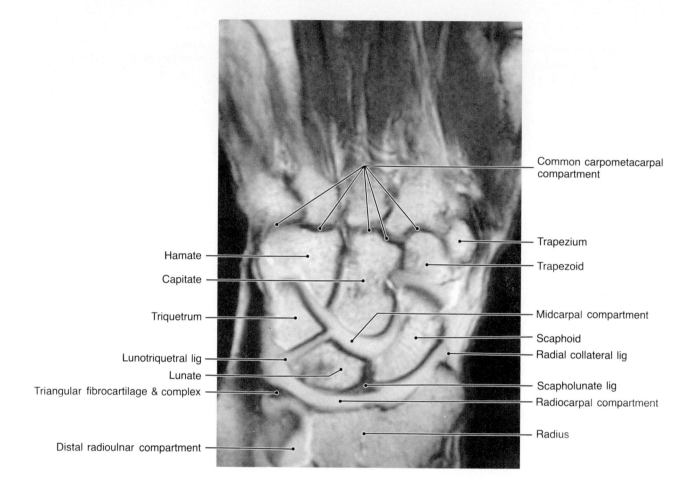

Common carpometacarpal compartment

Trapezium

Trapezoid

Hamate

Capitate

Triquetrum

Midcarpal compartment

Scaphoid

Lunotriquetral lig

Radial collateral lig

Lunate

Triangular fibrocartilage & complex

Scapholunate lig

Radiocarpal compartment

Radius

Distal radioulnar compartment

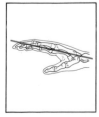

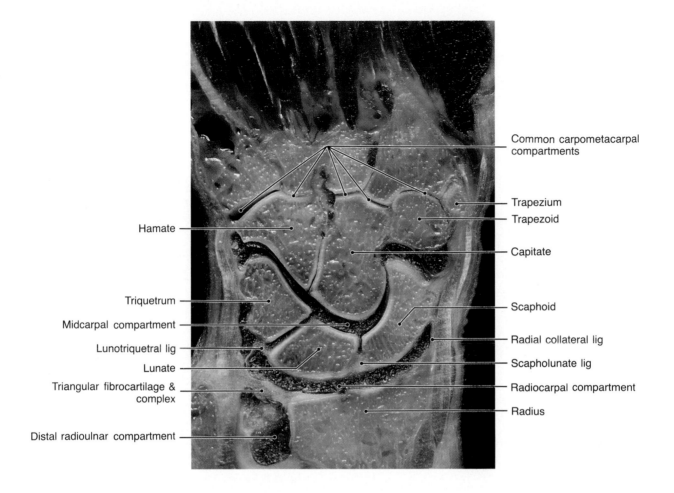

Common carpometacarpal compartments

Trapezium

Trapezoid

Capitate

Scaphoid

Radial collateral lig

Scapholunate lig

Radiocarpal compartment

Radius

Hamate

Triquetrum

Midcarpal compartment

Lunotriquetral lig

Lunate

Triangular fibrocartilage & complex

Distal radioulnar compartment

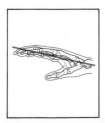

WRIST, SAGITTAL, INJECTED

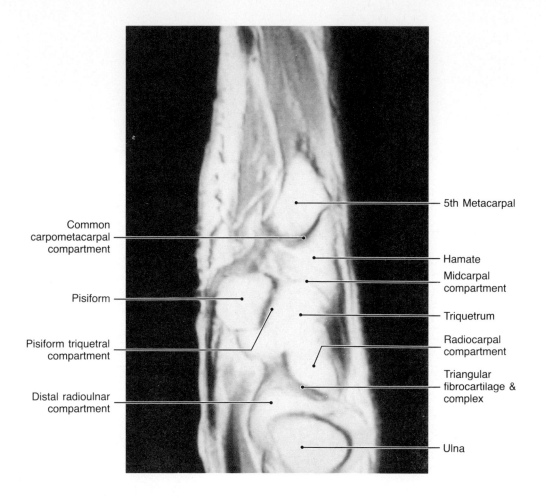

Common carpometacarpal compartment

Pisiform

Pisiform triquetral compartment

Distal radioulnar compartment

5th Metacarpal

Hamate

Midcarpal compartment

Triquetrum

Radiocarpal compartment

Triangular fibrocartilage & complex

Ulna

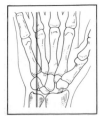

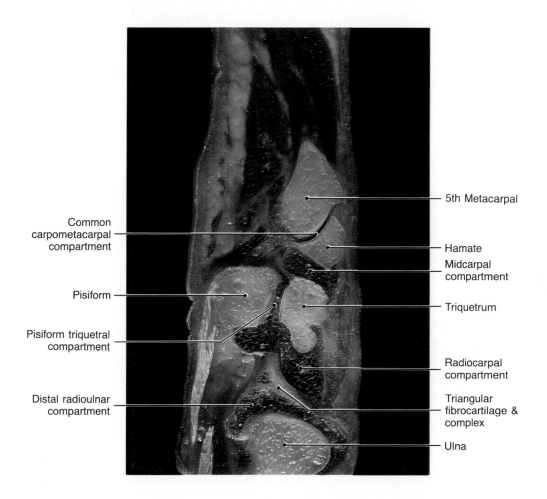

Common carpometacarpal compartment

5th Metacarpal

Hamate

Midcarpal compartment

Pisiform

Triquetrum

Pisiform triquetral compartment

Radiocarpal compartment

Distal radioulnar compartment

Triangular fibrocartilage & complex

Ulna

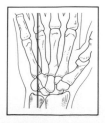

WRIST, SAGITTAL, INJECTED

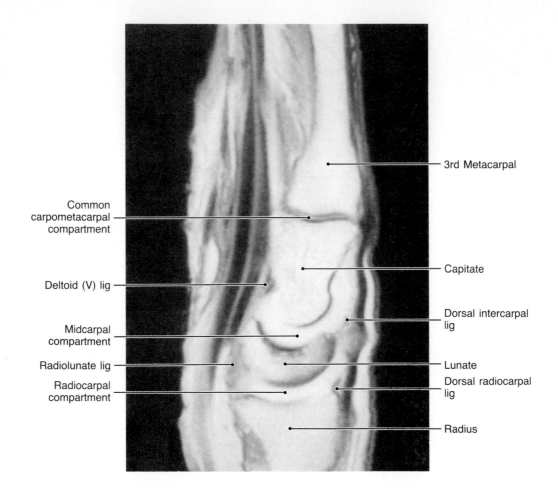

3rd Metacarpal

Common carpometacarpal compartment

Capitate

Deltoid (V) lig

Dorsal intercarpal lig

Midcarpal compartment

Radiolunate lig

Lunate

Dorsal radiocarpal lig

Radiocarpal compartment

Radius

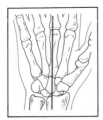

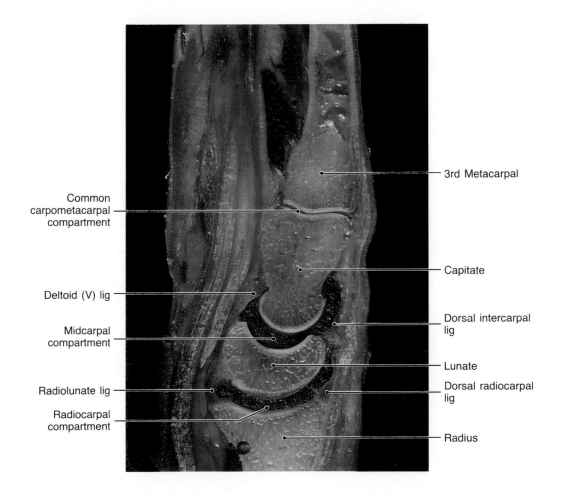

Common carpometacarpal compartment

Deltoid (V) lig

Midcarpal compartment

Radiolunate lig

Radiocarpal compartment

3rd Metacarpal

Capitate

Dorsal intercarpal lig

Lunate

Dorsal radiocarpal lig

Radius

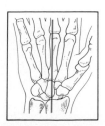

WRIST, SAGITTAL, INJECTED

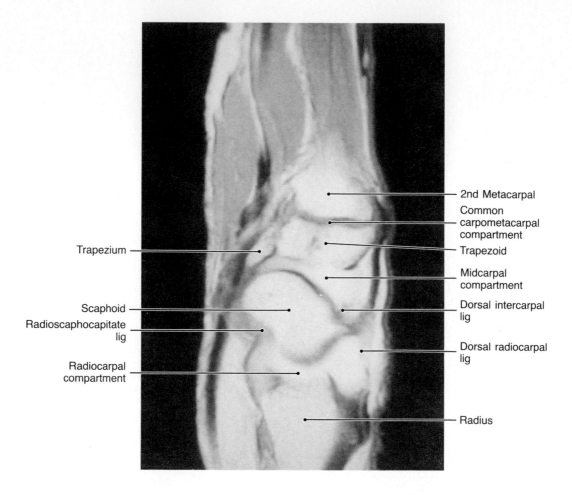

Trapezium

Scaphoid

Radioscaphocapitate lig

Radiocarpal compartment

2nd Metacarpal

Common carpometacarpal compartment

Trapezoid

Midcarpal compartment

Dorsal intercarpal lig

Dorsal radiocarpal lig

Radius

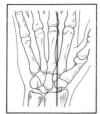

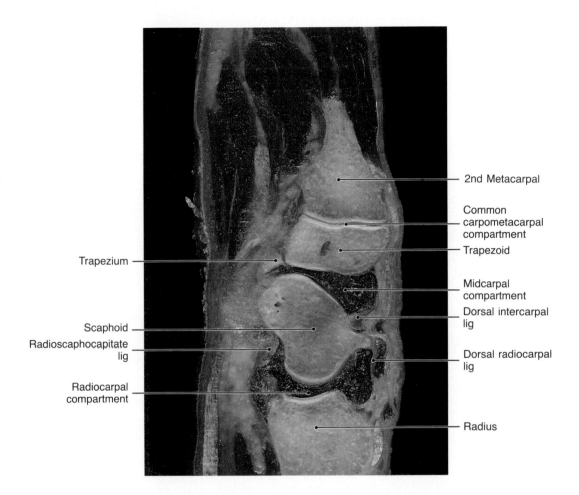

Trapezium

Scaphoid

Radioscaphocapitate
lig

Radiocarpal
compartment

2nd Metacarpal

Common
carpometacarpal
compartment

Trapezoid

Midcarpal
compartment

Dorsal intercarpal
lig

Dorsal radiocarpal
lig

Radius

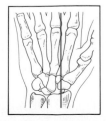

4 FINGER

FINGER, CORONAL

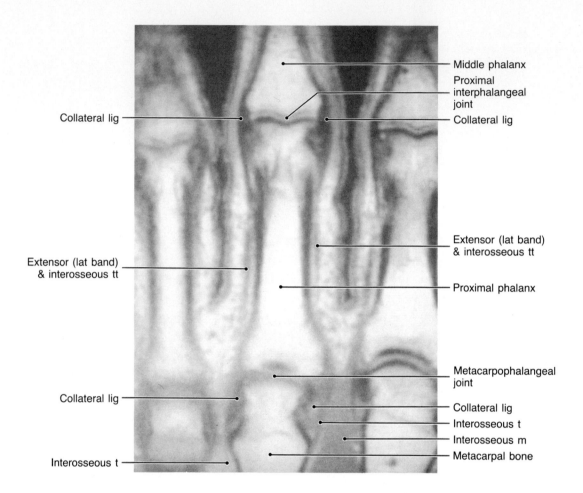

Collateral lig

Extensor (lat band)
& interosseous tt

Collateral lig

Interosseous t

Middle phalanx

Proximal
interphalangeal
joint

Collateral lig

Extensor (lat band)
& interosseous tt

Proximal phalanx

Metacarpophalangeal
joint

Collateral lig

Interosseous t

Interosseous m

Metacarpal bone

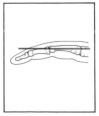

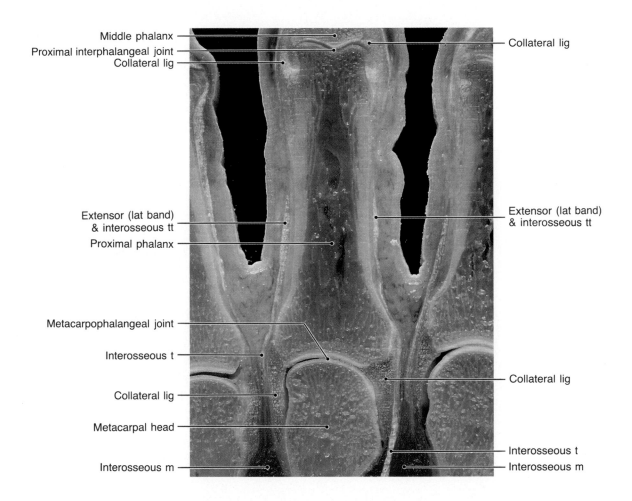

Middle phalanx

Proximal interphalangeal joint

Collateral lig

Collateral lig

Extensor (lat band) & interosseous tt

Extensor (lat band) & interosseous tt

Proximal phalanx

Metacarpophalangeal joint

Interosseous t

Collateral lig

Collateral lig

Metacarpal head

Interosseous t

Interosseous m

Interosseous m

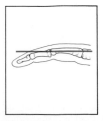

FINGER, CORONAL

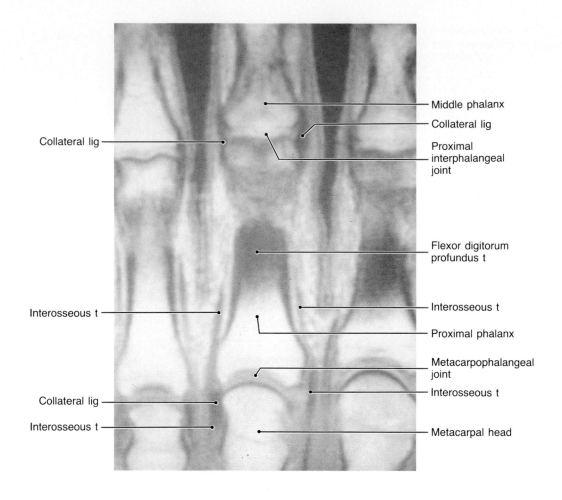

Collateral lig

Middle phalanx

Collateral lig

Proximal interphalangeal joint

Flexor digitorum profundus t

Interosseous t

Interosseous t

Proximal phalanx

Metacarpophalangeal joint

Collateral lig

Interosseous t

Interosseous t

Metacarpal head

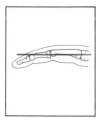

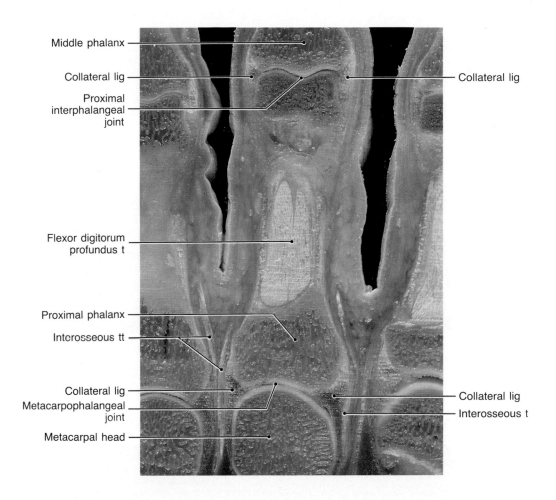

Middle phalanx

Collateral lig

Proximal interphalangeal joint

Collateral lig

Flexor digitorum profundus t

Proximal phalanx

Interosseous tt

Collateral lig

Metacarpophalangeal joint

Metacarpal head

Collateral lig

Interosseous t

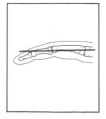

FINGER, TRANSVERSE

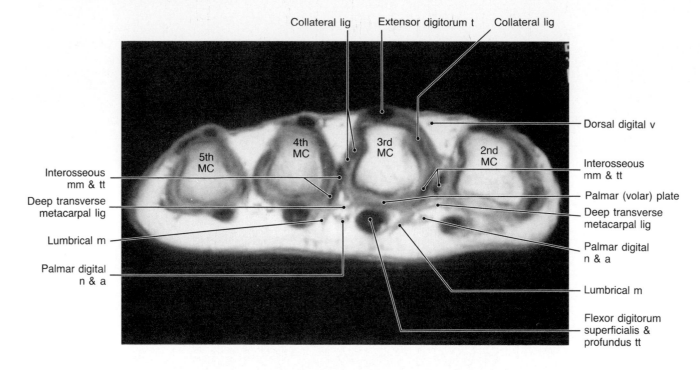

Collateral lig   Extensor digitorum t   Collateral lig

5th MC — 4th MC — 3rd MC — 2nd MC

Dorsal digital v

Interosseous mm & tt

Deep transverse metacarpal lig

Lumbrical m

Palmar digital n & a

Interosseous mm & tt

Palmar (volar) plate

Deep transverse metacarpal lig

Palmar digital n & a

Lumbrical m

Flexor digitorum superficialis & profundus tt

MC: Metacarpal

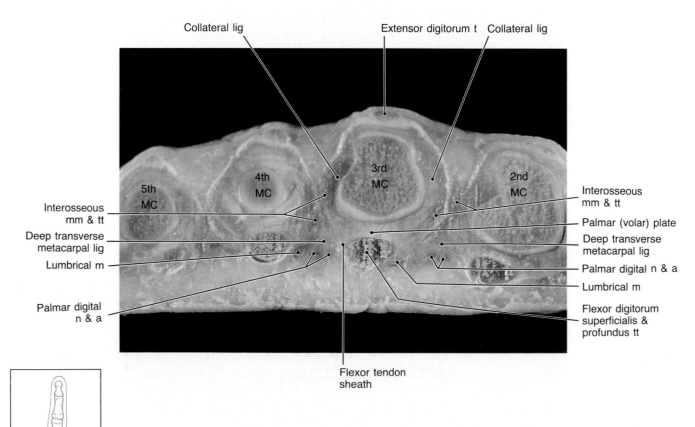

Collateral lig   Extensor digitorum t   Collateral lig

5th MC — 4th MC — 3rd MC — 2nd MC

Interosseous mm & tt

Deep transverse metacarpal lig

Lumbrical m

Palmar digital n & a

Interosseous mm & tt

Palmar (volar) plate

Deep transverse metacarpal lig

Palmar digital n & a

Lumbrical m

Flexor digitorum superficialis & profundus tt

Flexor tendon sheath

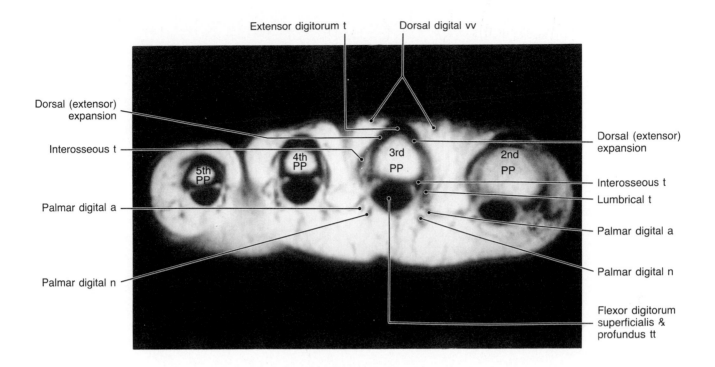

Extensor digitorum t

Dorsal digital vv

Dorsal (extensor) expansion

Dorsal (extensor) expansion

Interosseous t

Interosseous t

Lumbrical t

5th PP

4th PP

3rd PP

2nd PP

Palmar digital a

Palmar digital a

Palmar digital n

Palmar digital n

Flexor digitorum superficialis & profundus tt

PP: Proximal phalanx

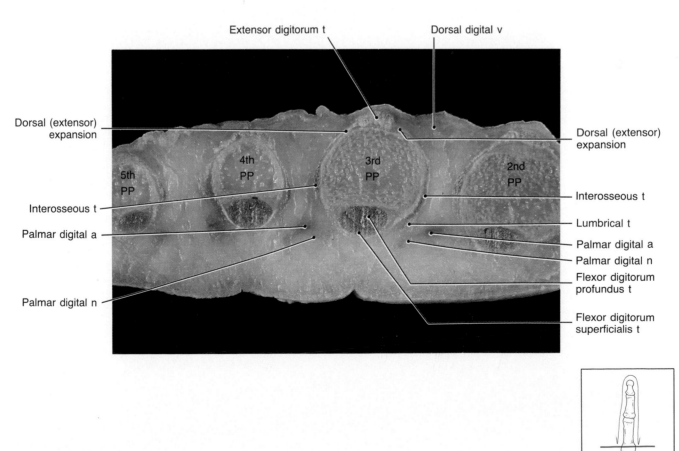

Extensor digitorum t

Dorsal digital v

Dorsal (extensor) expansion

Dorsal (extensor) expansion

5th PP

4th PP

3rd PP

2nd PP

Interosseous t

Interosseous t

Palmar digital a

Lumbrical t

Palmar digital a

Palmar digital n

Flexor digitorum profundus t

Palmar digital n

Flexor digitorum superficialis t

FINGER, TRANSVERSE

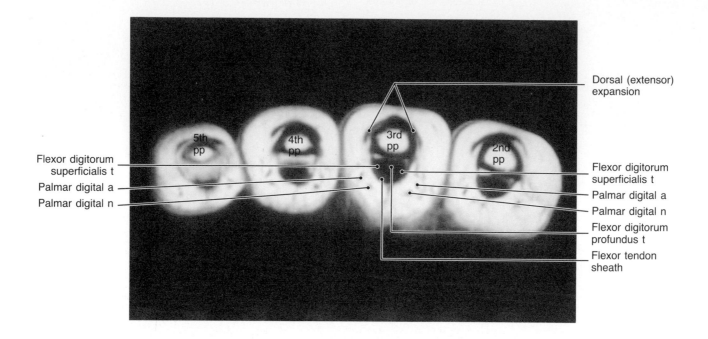

Dorsal (extensor) expansion

5th pp

4th pp

3rd pp

2nd pp

Flexor digitorum superficialis t

Palmar digital a

Palmar digital n

Flexor digitorum superficialis t

Palmar digital a

Palmar digital n

Flexor digitorum profundus t

Flexor tendon sheath

PP: Proximal phalanx

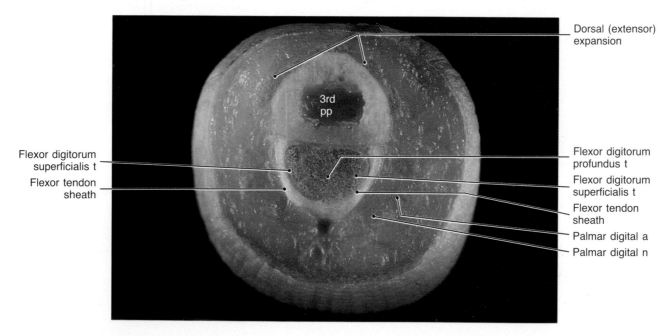

Dorsal (extensor) expansion

3rd pp

Flexor digitorum superficialis t

Flexor tendon sheath

Flexor digitorum profundus t

Flexor digitorum superficialis t

Flexor tendon sheath

Palmar digital a

Palmar digital n

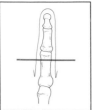

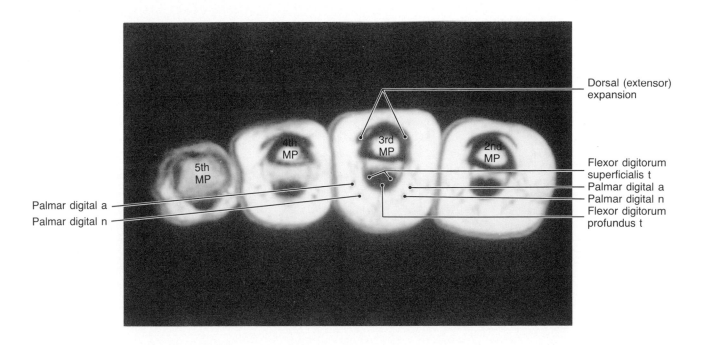

Dorsal (extensor) expansion

Flexor digitorum superficialis t
Palmar digital a
Palmar digital n
Flexor digitorum profundus t

Palmar digital a
Palmar digital n

MP: Middle phalanx

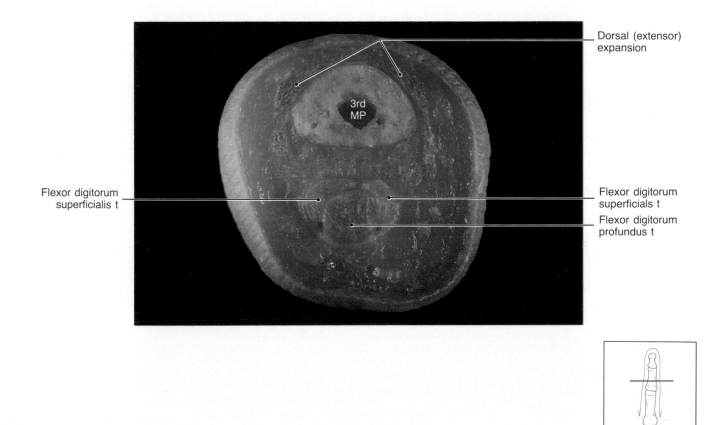

Dorsal (extensor) expansion

Flexor digitorum superficialis t

Flexor digitorum superficials t

Flexor digitorum profundus t

FINGER, SAGITTAL

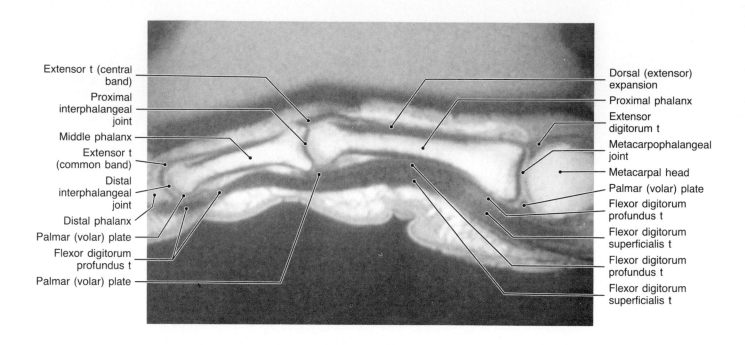

Extensor t (central band)

Proximal interphalangeal joint

Middle phalanx

Extensor t (common band)

Distal interphalangeal joint

Distal phalanx

Palmar (volar) plate

Flexor digitorum profundus t

Palmar (volar) plate

Dorsal (extensor) expansion

Proximal phalanx

Extensor digitorum t

Metacarpophalangeal joint

Metacarpal head

Palmar (volar) plate

Flexor digitorum profundus t

Flexor digitorum superficialis t

Flexor digitorum profundus t

Flexor digitorum superficialis t

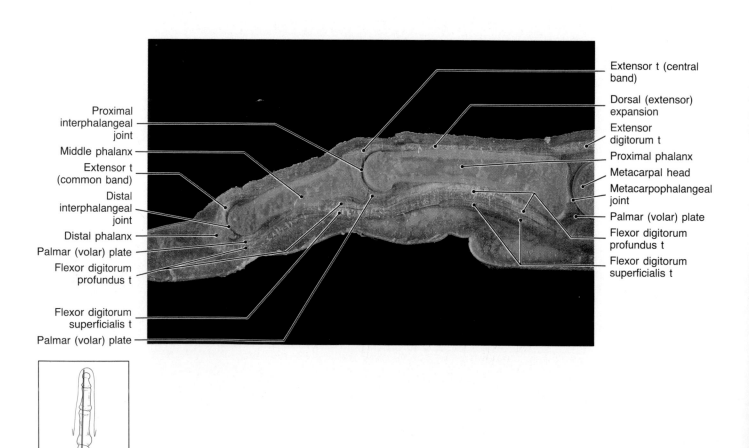

Proximal interphalangeal joint

Middle phalanx

Extensor t (common band)

Distal interphalangeal joint

Distal phalanx

Palmar (volar) plate

Flexor digitorum profundus t

Flexor digitorum superficialis t

Palmar (volar) plate

Extensor t (central band)

Dorsal (extensor) expansion

Extensor digitorum t

Proximal phalanx

Metacarpal head

Metacarpophalangeal joint

Palmar (volar) plate

Flexor digitorum profundus t

Flexor digitorum superficialis t

5 HIP

HIP, CORONAL

Gluteus minimus m

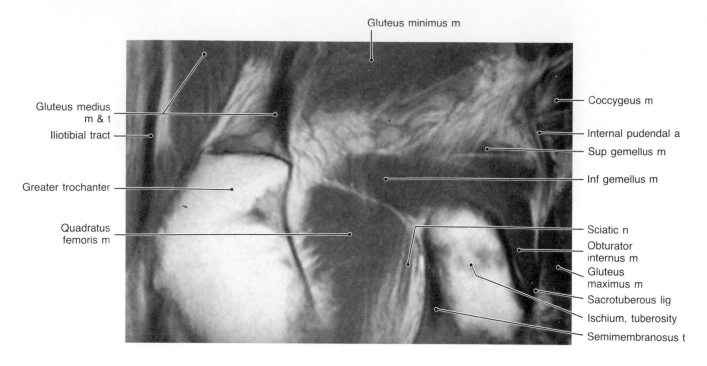

Gluteus medius m & t

Iliotibial tract

Greater trochanter

Quadratus femoris m

Coccygeus m

Internal pudendal a

Sup gemellus m

Inf gemellus m

Sciatic n

Obturator internus m

Gluteus maximus m

Sacrotuberous lig

Ischium, tuberosity

Semimembranosus t

Gluteus minimus m

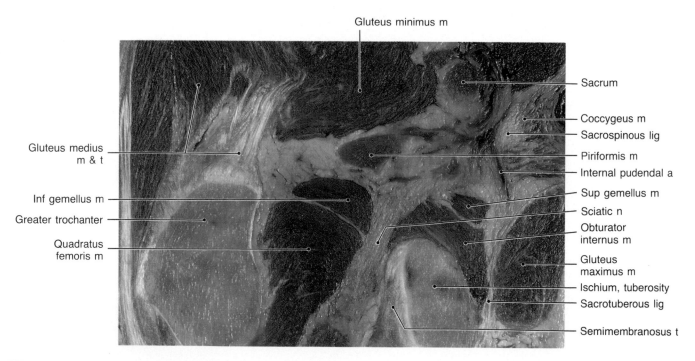

Gluteus medius m & t

Inf gemellus m

Greater trochanter

Quadratus femoris m

Sacrum

Coccygeus m

Sacrospinous lig

Piriformis m

Internal pudendal a

Sup gemellus m

Sciatic n

Obturator internus m

Gluteus maximus m

Ischium, tuberosity

Sacrotuberous lig

Semimembranosus t

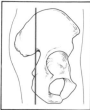

Gluteus minimus m

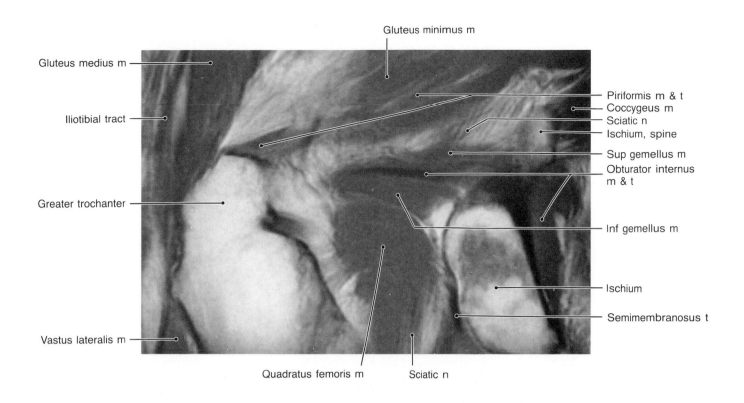

Gluteus medius m

Iliotibial tract

Greater trochanter

Vastus lateralis m

Quadratus femoris m

Sciatic n

Piriformis m & t
Coccygeus m
Sciatic n
Ischium, spine
Sup gemellus m
Obturator internus
m & t

Inf gemellus m

Ischium

Semimembranosus t

Gluteus minimus m

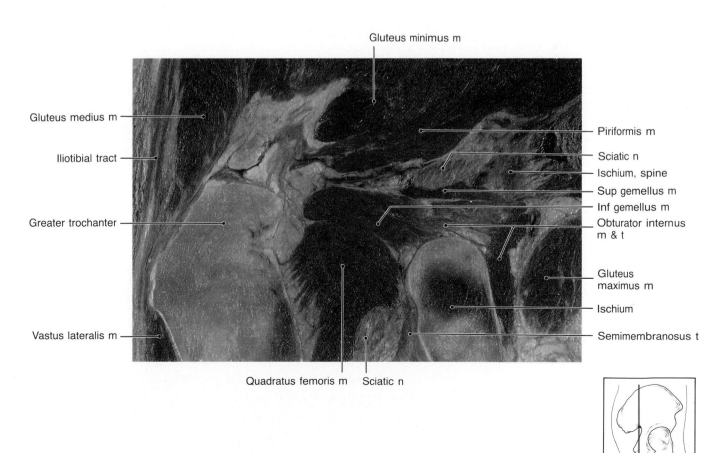

Gluteus medius m

Iliotibial tract

Greater trochanter

Vastus lateralis m

Quadratus femoris m

Sciatic n

Piriformis m

Sciatic n
Ischium, spine
Sup gemellus m
Inf gemellus m
Obturator internus
m & t

Gluteus
maximus m

Ischium

Semimembranosus t

HIP, CORONAL

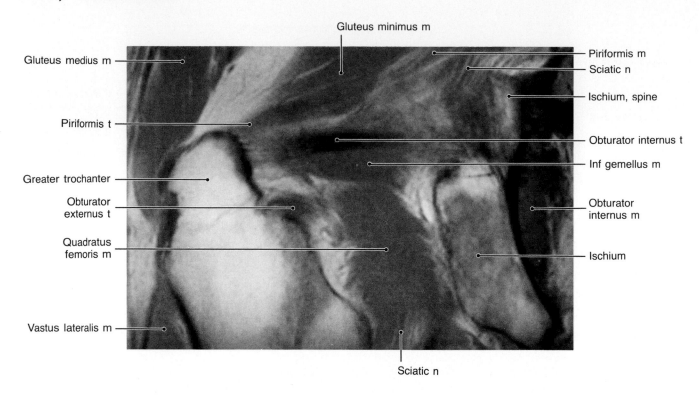

Gluteus minimus m

Gluteus medius m

Piriformis t

Greater trochanter

Obturator externus t

Quadratus femoris m

Vastus lateralis m

Piriformis m

Sciatic n

Ischium, spine

Obturator internus t

Inf gemellus m

Obturator internus m

Ischium

Sciatic n

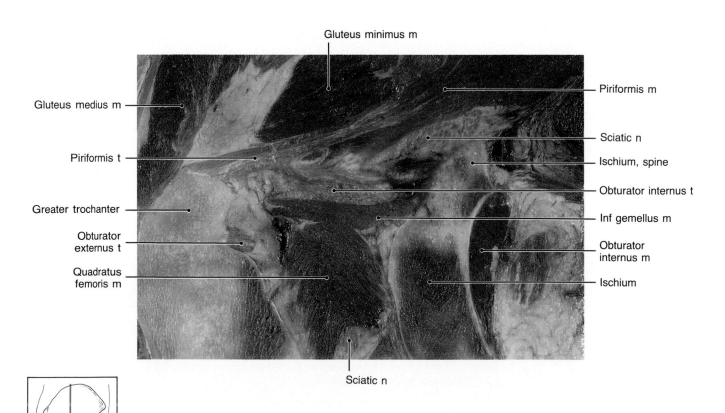

Gluteus minimus m

Gluteus medius m

Piriformis t

Greater trochanter

Obturator externus t

Quadratus femoris m

Piriformis m

Sciatic n

Ischium, spine

Obturator internus t

Inf gemellus m

Obturator internus m

Ischium

Sciatic n

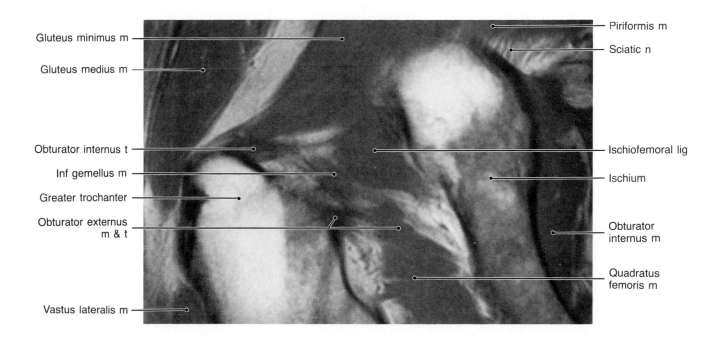

Gluteus minimus m

Gluteus medius m

Obturator internus t

Inf gemellus m

Greater trochanter

Obturator externus
m & t

Vastus lateralis m

Piriformis m

Sciatic n

Ischiofemoral lig

Ischium

Obturator
internus m

Quadratus
femoris m

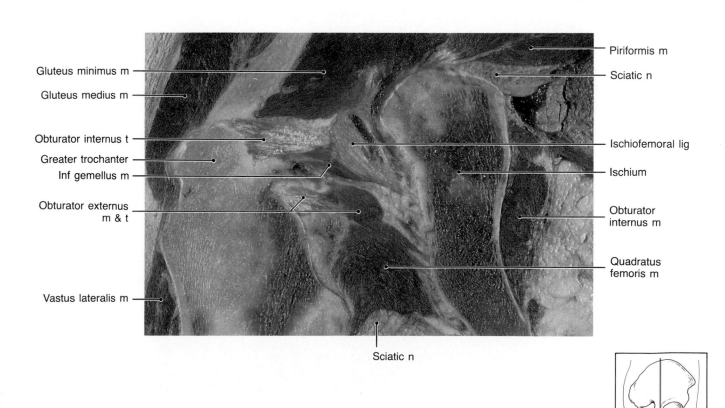

Gluteus minimus m

Gluteus medius m

Obturator internus t

Greater trochanter

Inf gemellus m

Obturator externus
m & t

Vastus lateralis m

Piriformis m

Sciatic n

Ischiofemoral lig

Ischium

Obturator
internus m

Quadratus
femoris m

Sciatic n

HIP, CORONAL

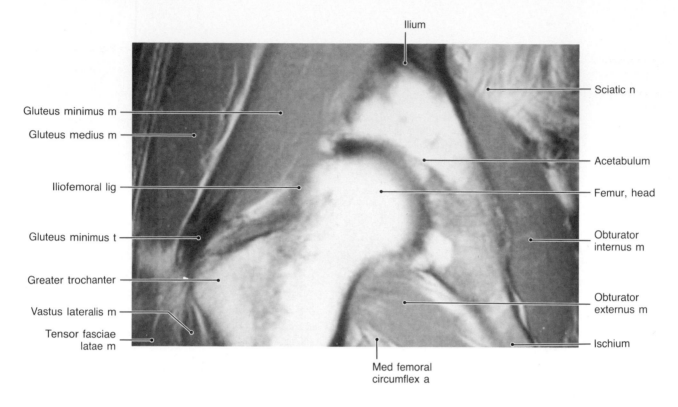

Ilium

Gluteus minimus m

Gluteus medius m

Iliofemoral lig

Gluteus minimus t

Greater trochanter

Vastus lateralis m

Tensor fasciae latae m

Med femoral circumflex a

Sciatic n

Acetabulum

Femur, head

Obturator internus m

Obturator externus m

Ischium

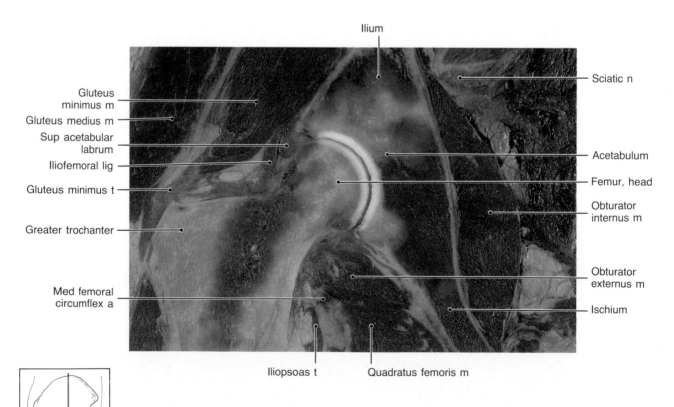

Ilium

Gluteus minimus m

Gluteus medius m

Sup acetabular labrum

Iliofemoral lig

Gluteus minimus t

Greater trochanter

Med femoral circumflex a

Iliopsoas t

Quadratus femoris m

Sciatic n

Acetabulum

Femur, head

Obturator internus m

Obturator externus m

Ischium

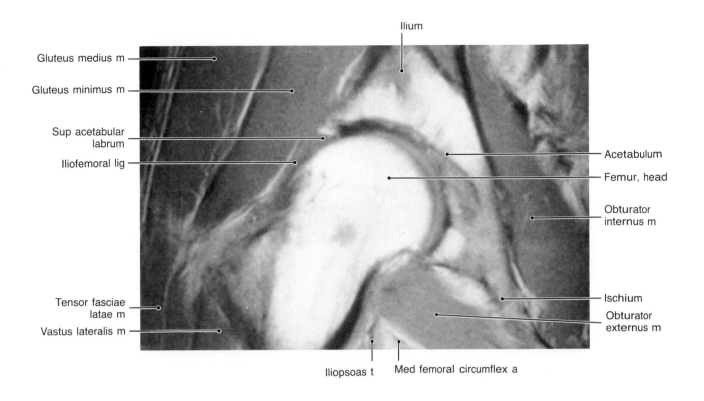

Ilium

Gluteus medius m

Gluteus minimus m

Sup acetabular labrum

Iliofemoral lig

Acetabulum

Femur, head

Obturator internus m

Tensor fasciae latae m

Vastus lateralis m

Ischium

Obturator externus m

Iliopsoas t

Med femoral circumflex a

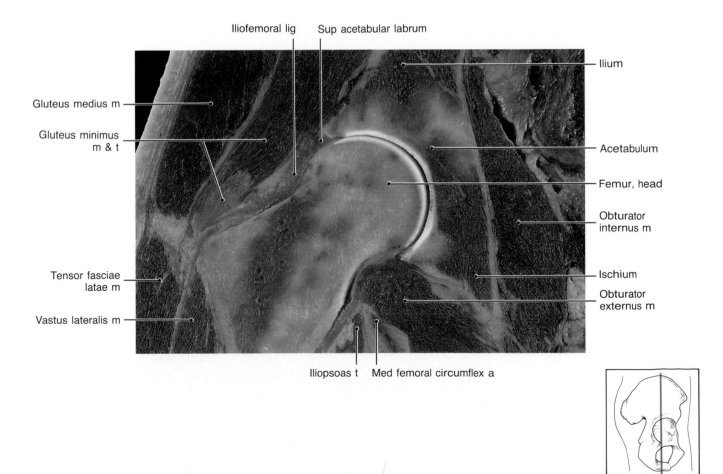

Iliofemoral lig

Sup acetabular labrum

Ilium

Gluteus medius m

Gluteus minimus m & t

Acetabulum

Femur, head

Obturator internus m

Tensor fasciae latae m

Ischium

Obturator externus m

Vastus lateralis m

Iliopsoas t

Med femoral circumflex a

HIP, CORONAL

Ilium

Gluteus medius m

Gluteus minimus m

Sup acetabular labrum

Iliofemoral lig

Acetabulum

Femur, head

Synovial membrane, acetabular fossa

Obturator internus m

Tensor fasciae latae m

Rectus femoris m

Obturator externus m

Med femoral circumflex a

Ischium

Iliopsoas m & t

Pectineus & adductor mm

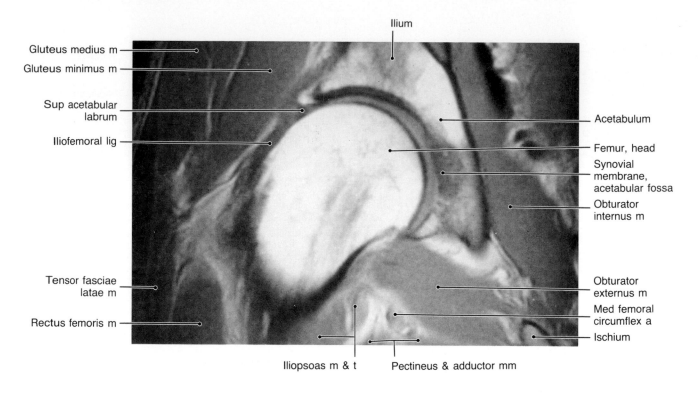

Sup acetabular labrum

Gluteus medius m

Gluteus minimus m

Iliofemoral lig

Tensor fasciae latae m

Rectus femoris m

Vastus lateralis m

Acetabulum

Femur, head

Synovial membrane, acetabular fossa

Obturator internus m

Inf acetabular labrum

Obturator externus m

Med femoral circumflex a

Iliopsoas m & t

Pectineus & adductor mm

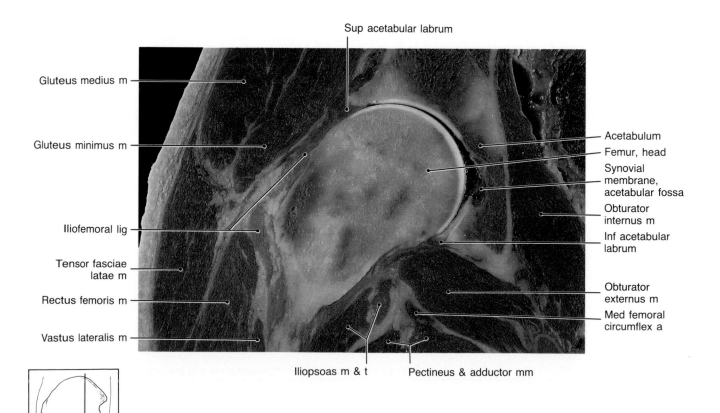

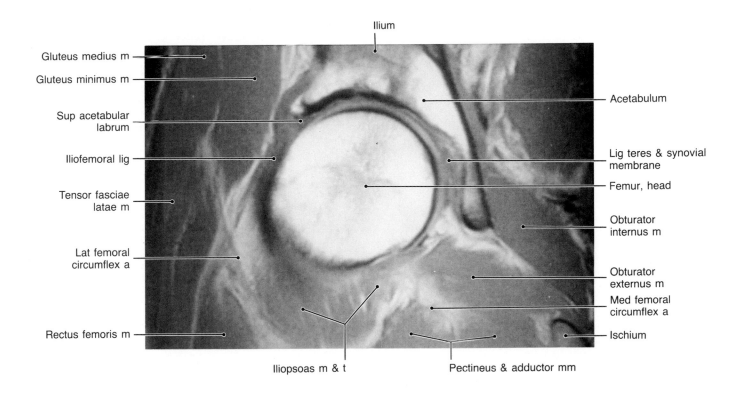

Ilium

Gluteus medius m

Gluteus minimus m

Sup acetabular labrum

Iliofemoral lig

Tensor fasciae latae m

Lat femoral circumflex a

Rectus femoris m

Iliopsoas m & t

Acetabulum

Lig teres & synovial membrane

Femur, head

Obturator internus m

Obturator externus m

Med femoral circumflex a

Ischium

Pectineus & adductor mm

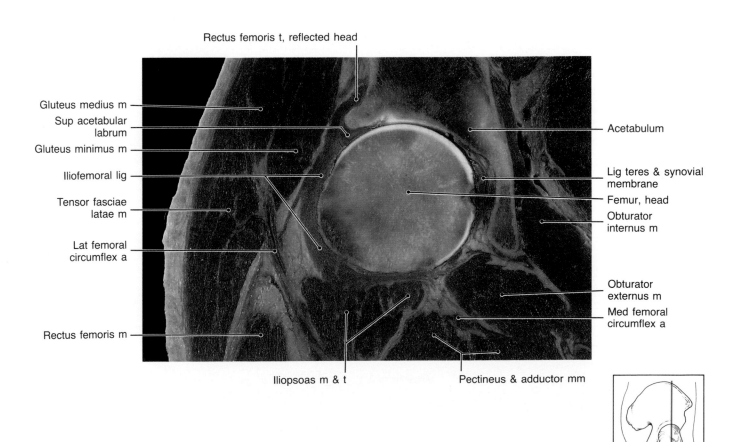

Rectus femoris t, reflected head

Gluteus medius m

Sup acetabular labrum

Gluteus minimus m

Iliofemoral lig

Tensor fasciae latae m

Lat femoral circumflex a

Rectus femoris m

Iliopsoas m & t

Acetabulum

Lig teres & synovial membrane

Femur, head

Obturator internus m

Obturator externus m

Med femoral circumflex a

Pectineus & adductor mm

HIP, CORONAL

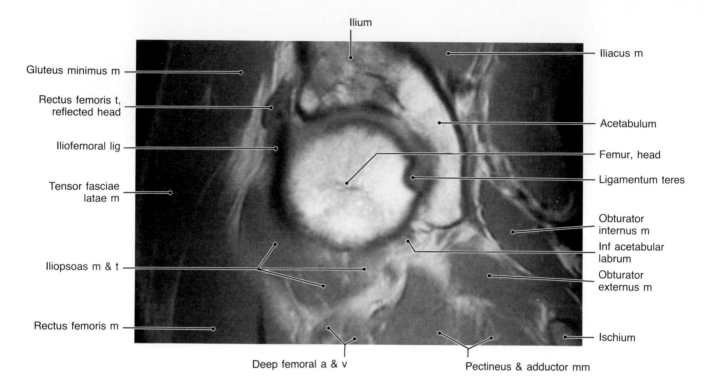

Ilium

Iliacus m

Gluteus minimus m

Rectus femoris t, reflected head

Acetabulum

Iliofemoral lig

Femur, head

Tensor fasciae latae m

Ligamentum teres

Obturator internus m

Inf acetabular labrum

Iliopsoas m & t

Obturator externus m

Rectus femoris m

Ischium

Deep femoral a & v

Pectineus & adductor mm

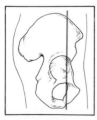

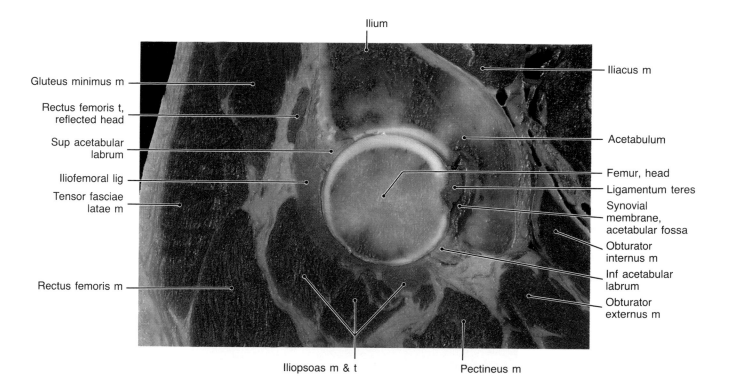

Ilium

Gluteus minimus m

Rectus femoris t, reflected head

Sup acetabular labrum

Iliofemoral lig

Tensor fasciae latae m

Rectus femoris m

Iliacus m

Acetabulum

Femur, head

Ligamentum teres

Synovial membrane, acetabular fossa

Obturator internus m

Inf acetabular labrum

Obturator externus m

Iliopsoas m & t

Pectineus m

Gluteus minimus m

Ilium

Rectus femoris m & t

Femoral n, branches

Sartorius m

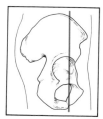

HIP, CORONAL

Gluteus minimus m

Ilium

Rectus femoris
m &

Sartorius m

Femoral r
branche

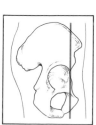

HIP, TRANSVERSE

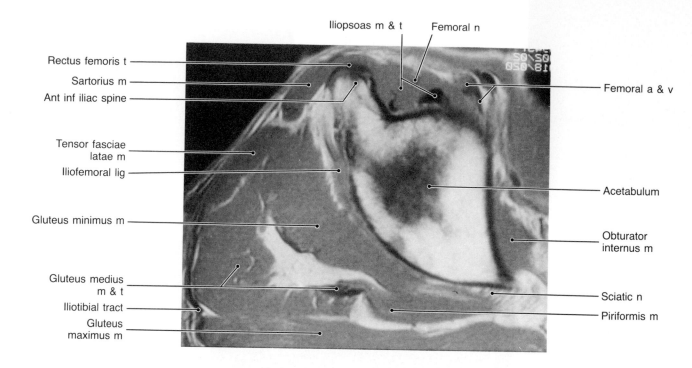

Iliopsoas m & t

Femoral n

Rectus femoris t

Sartorius m

Ant inf iliac spine

Tensor fasciae latae m

Iliofemoral lig

Gluteus minimus m

Gluteus medius m & t

Iliotibial tract

Gluteus maximus m

Femoral a & v

Acetabulum

Obturator internus m

Sciatic n

Piriformis m

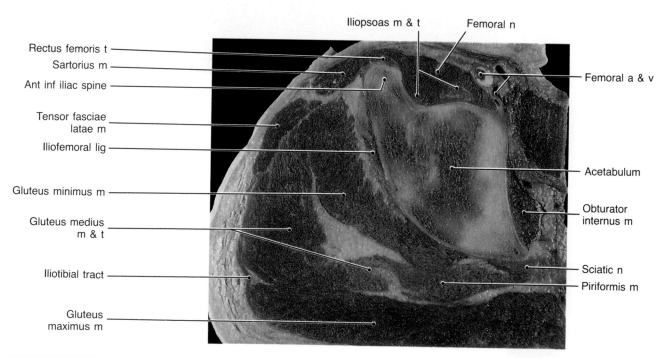

Iliopsoas m & t

Femoral n

Rectus femoris t

Sartorius m

Ant inf iliac spine

Tensor fasciae latae m

Iliofemoral lig

Gluteus minimus m

Gluteus medius m & t

Iliotibial tract

Gluteus maximus m

Femoral a & v

Acetabulum

Obturator internus m

Sciatic n

Piriformis m

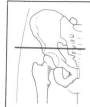

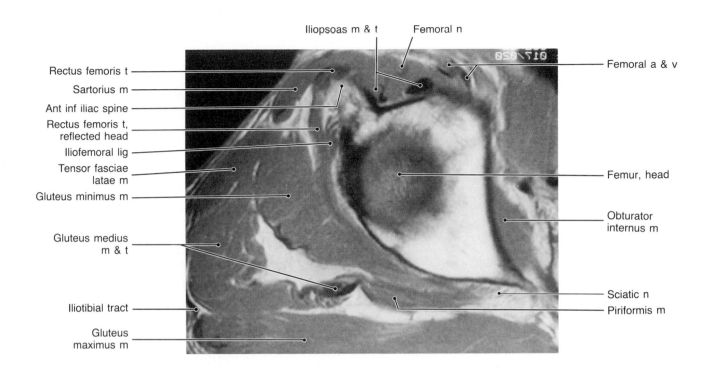

Iliopsoas m & t
Femoral n
Femoral a & v
Rectus femoris t
Sartorius m
Ant inf iliac spine
Rectus femoris t, reflected head
Iliofemoral lig
Tensor fasciae latae m
Femur, head
Gluteus minimus m
Obturator internus m
Gluteus medius m & t
Iliotibial tract
Sciatic n
Piriformis m
Gluteus maximus m

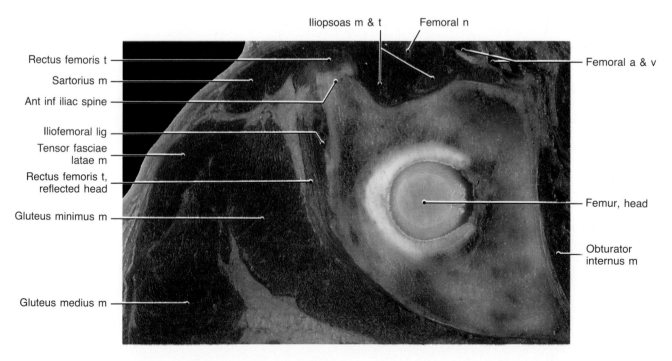

Iliopsoas m & t
Femoral n
Femoral a & v
Rectus femoris t
Sartorius m
Ant inf iliac spine
Iliofemoral lig
Tensor fasciae latae m
Rectus femoris t, reflected head
Femur, head
Gluteus minimus m
Obturator internus m
Gluteus medius m

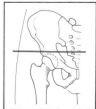

HIP, TRANSVERSE

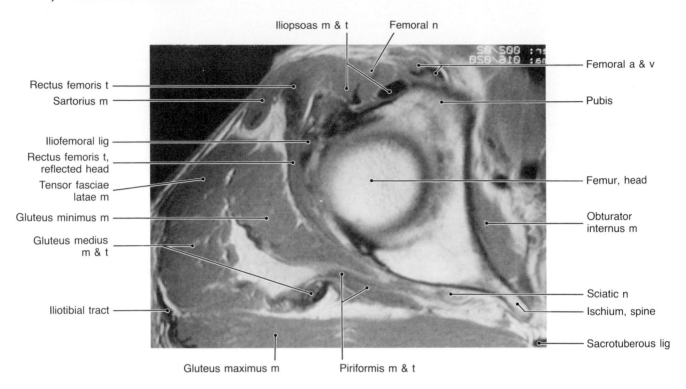

Iliopsoas m & t
Femoral n
Rectus femoris t
Sartorius m
Femoral a & v
Pubis
Iliofemoral lig
Rectus femoris t, reflected head
Tensor fasciae latae m
Femur, head
Gluteus minimus m
Obturator internus m
Gluteus medius m & t
Iliotibial tract
Sciatic n
Ischium, spine
Sacrotuberous lig
Gluteus maximus m
Piriformis m & t

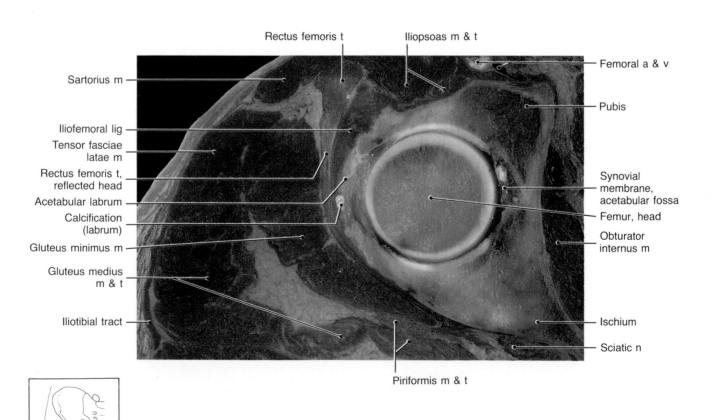

Rectus femoris t
Iliopsoas m & t
Sartorius m
Femoral a & v
Pubis
Iliofemoral lig
Tensor fasciae latae m
Rectus femoris t, reflected head
Acetabular labrum
Synovial membrane, acetabular fossa
Femur, head
Calcification (labrum)
Gluteus minimus m
Obturator internus m
Gluteus medius m & t
Iliotibial tract
Ischium
Sciatic n
Piriformis m & t

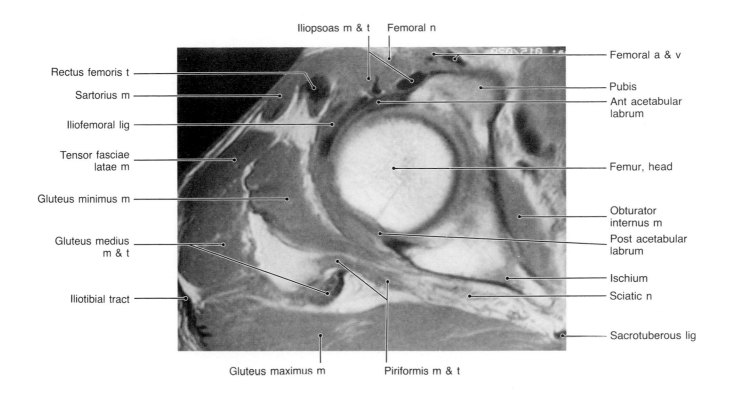

Iliopsoas m & t
Femoral n
Rectus femoris t
Sartorius m
Iliofemoral lig
Tensor fasciae latae m
Gluteus minimus m
Gluteus medius m & t
Iliotibial tract
Femoral a & v
Pubis
Ant acetabular labrum
Femur, head
Obturator internus m
Post acetabular labrum
Ischium
Sciatic n
Sacrotuberous lig
Gluteus maximus m
Piriformis m & t

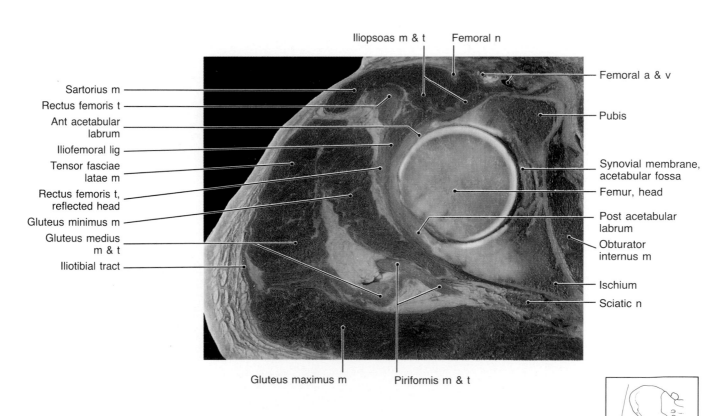

Iliopsoas m & t
Femoral n
Sartorius m
Rectus femoris t
Ant acetabular labrum
Iliofemoral lig
Tensor fasciae latae m
Rectus femoris t, reflected head
Gluteus minimus m
Gluteus medius m & t
Iliotibial tract
Femoral a & v
Pubis
Synovial membrane, acetabular fossa
Femur, head
Post acetabular labrum
Obturator internus m
Ischium
Sciatic n
Gluteus maximus m
Piriformis m & t

HIP, TRANSVERSE

Iliopsoas m & t   Femoral n

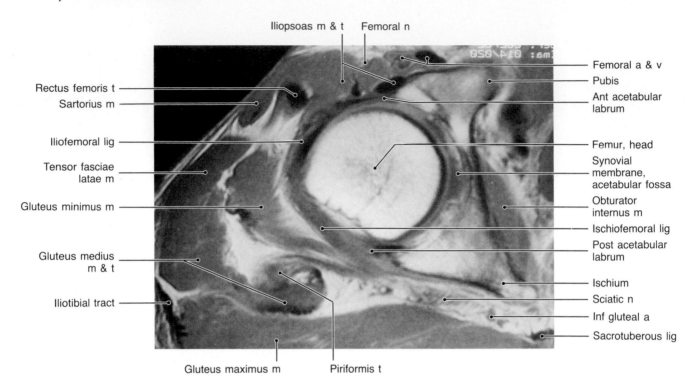

Rectus femoris t

Sartorius m

Iliofemoral lig

Tensor fasciae latae m

Gluteus minimus m

Gluteus medius m & t

Iliotibial tract

Femoral a & v

Pubis

Ant acetabular labrum

Femur, head

Synovial membrane, acetabular fossa

Obturator internus m

Ischiofemoral lig

Post acetabular labrum

Ischium

Sciatic n

Inf gluteal a

Sacrotuberous lig

Gluteus maximus m   Piriformis t

Iliopsoas m & t   Femoral n

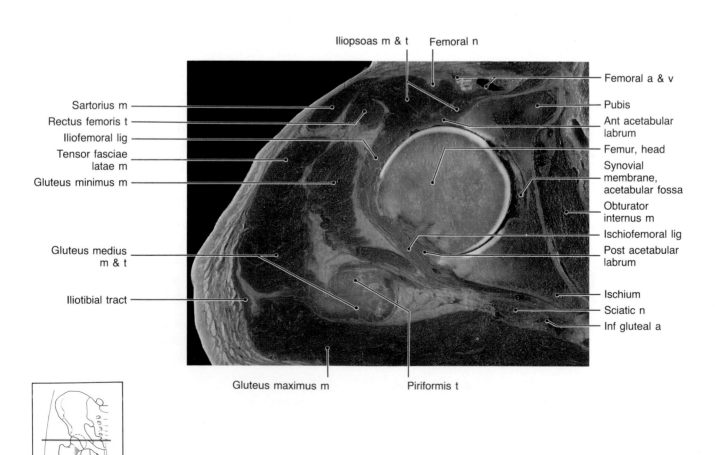

Sartorius m

Rectus femoris t

Iliofemoral lig

Tensor fasciae latae m

Gluteus minimus m

Gluteus medius m & t

Iliotibial tract

Femoral a & v

Pubis

Ant acetabular labrum

Femur, head

Synovial membrane, acetabular fossa

Obturator internus m

Ischiofemoral lig

Post acetabular labrum

Ischium

Sciatic n

Inf gluteal a

Gluteus maximus m   Piriformis t

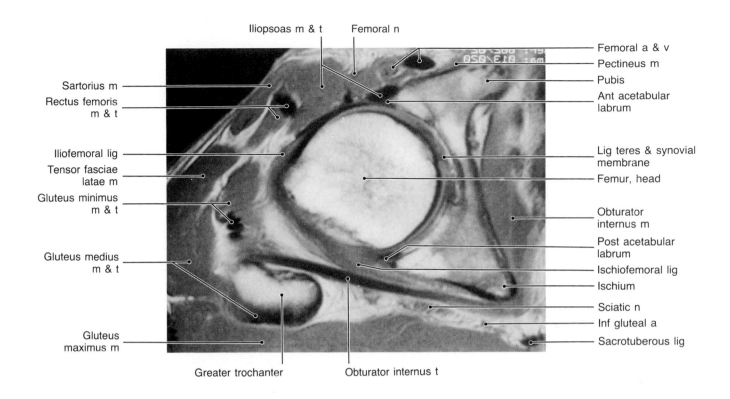

Iliopsoas m & t   Femoral n

Femoral a & v
Pectineus m
Pubis
Ant acetabular labrum

Sartorius m
Rectus femoris m & t

Iliofemoral lig
Tensor fasciae latae m

Gluteus minimus m & t

Lig teres & synovial membrane
Femur, head

Obturator internus m

Gluteus medius m & t

Post acetabular labrum
Ischiofemoral lig
Ischium
Sciatic n
Inf gluteal a
Sacrotuberous lig

Gluteus maximus m

Greater trochanter   Obturator internus t

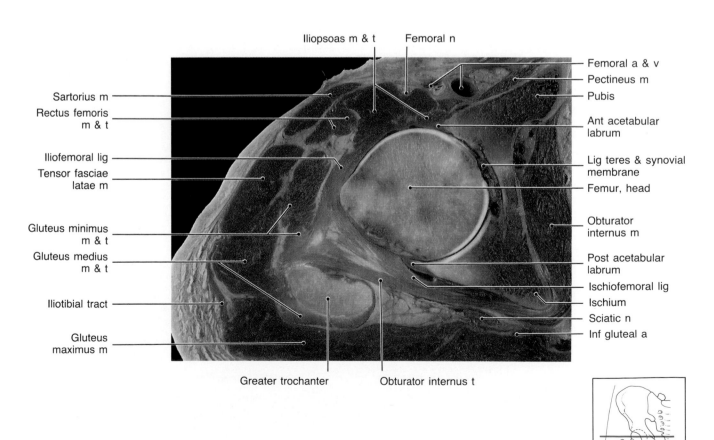

Iliopsoas m & t   Femoral n

Femoral a & v
Pectineus m
Pubis

Sartorius m
Rectus femoris m & t

Ant acetabular labrum

Iliofemoral lig
Tensor fasciae latae m

Lig teres & synovial membrane
Femur, head

Obturator internus m

Gluteus minimus m & t
Gluteus medius m & t

Iliotibial tract

Post acetabular labrum
Ischiofemoral lig
Ischium
Sciatic n
Inf gluteal a

Gluteus maximus m

Greater trochanter   Obturator internus t

HIP, TRANSVERSE

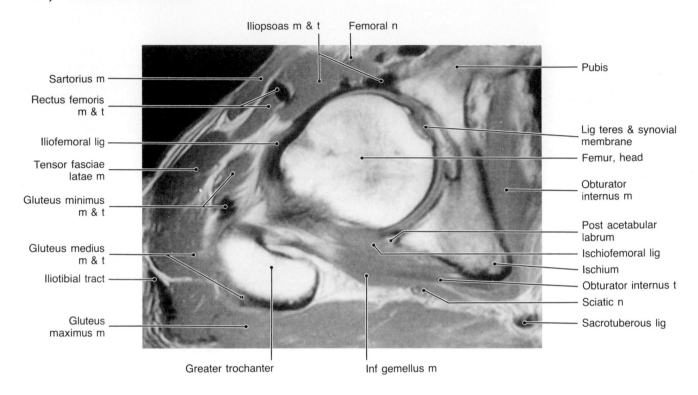

Iliopsoas m & t

Femoral n

Pubis

Sartorius m

Rectus femoris m & t

Lig teres & synovial membrane

Iliofemoral lig

Femur, head

Tensor fasciae latae m

Obturator internus m

Gluteus minimus m & t

Post acetabular labrum

Gluteus medius m & t

Ischiofemoral lig

Iliotibial tract

Ischium

Obturator internus t

Sciatic n

Gluteus maximus m

Sacrotuberous lig

Greater trochanter

Inf gemellus m

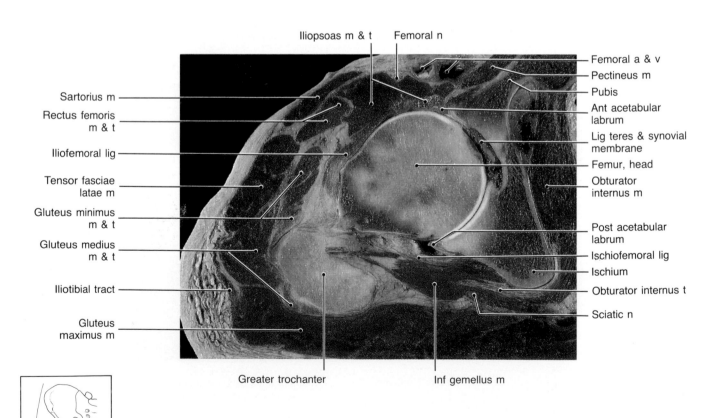

Iliopsoas m & t

Femoral n

Femoral a & v

Pectineus m

Sartorius m

Pubis

Rectus femoris m & t

Ant acetabular labrum

Iliofemoral lig

Lig teres & synovial membrane

Tensor fasciae latae m

Femur, head

Gluteus minimus m & t

Obturator internus m

Gluteus medius m & t

Post acetabular labrum

Iliotibial tract

Ischiofemoral lig

Ischium

Obturator internus t

Gluteus maximus m

Sciatic n

Greater trochanter

Inf gemellus m

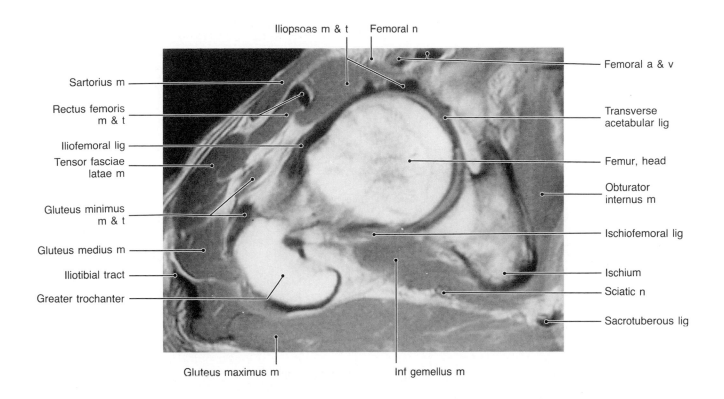

Iliopsoas m & t   Femoral n

Sartorius m

Rectus femoris m & t

Iliofemoral lig

Tensor fasciae latae m

Gluteus minimus m & t

Gluteus medius m

Iliotibial tract

Greater trochanter

Femoral a & v

Transverse acetabular lig

Femur, head

Obturator internus m

Ischiofemoral lig

Ischium

Sciatic n

Sacrotuberous lig

Gluteus maximus m

Inf gemellus m

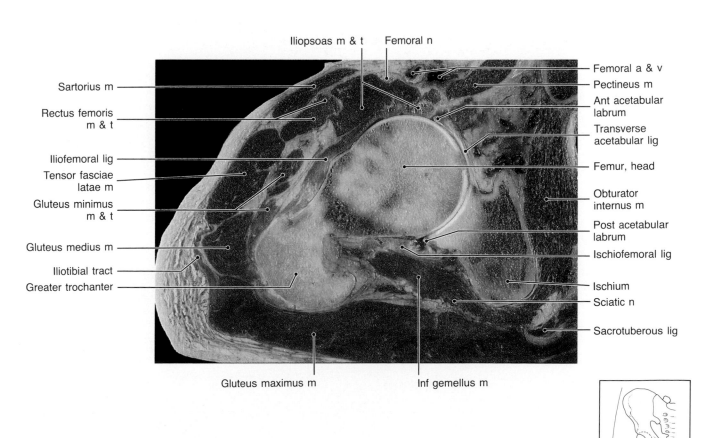

Iliopsoas m & t   Femoral n

Sartorius m

Rectus femoris m & t

Iliofemoral lig

Tensor fasciae latae m

Gluteus minimus m & t

Gluteus medius m

Iliotibial tract

Greater trochanter

Femoral a & v

Pectineus m

Ant acetabular labrum

Transverse acetabular lig

Femur, head

Obturator internus m

Post acetabular labrum

Ischiofemoral lig

Ischium

Sciatic n

Sacrotuberous lig

Gluteus maximus m

Inf gemellus m

HIP, TRANSVERSE

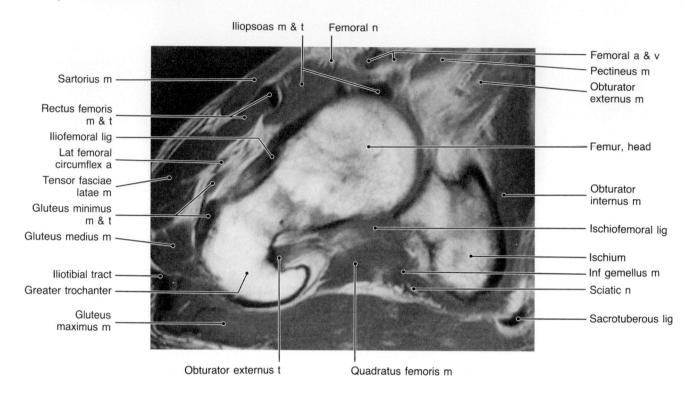

Iliopsoas m & t   Femoral n

Sartorius m

Rectus femoris m & t

Iliofemoral lig

Lat femoral circumflex a

Tensor fasciae latae m

Gluteus minimus m & t

Gluteus medius m

Iliotibial tract

Greater trochanter

Gluteus maximus m

Femoral a & v

Pectineus m

Obturator externus m

Femur, head

Obturator internus m

Ischiofemoral lig

Ischium

Inf gemellus m

Sciatic n

Sacrotuberous lig

Obturator externus t   Quadratus femoris m

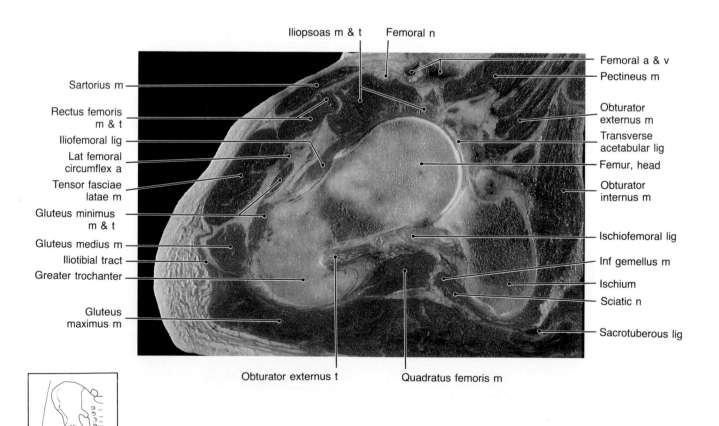

Iliopsoas m & t   Femoral n

Sartorius m

Rectus femoris m & t

Iliofemoral lig

Lat femoral circumflex a

Tensor fasciae latae m

Gluteus minimus m & t

Gluteus medius m

Iliotibial tract

Greater trochanter

Gluteus maximus m

Femoral a & v

Pectineus m

Obturator externus m

Transverse acetabular lig

Femur, head

Obturator internus m

Ischiofemoral lig

Inf gemellus m

Ischium

Sciatic n

Sacrotuberous lig

Obturator externus t   Quadratus femoris m

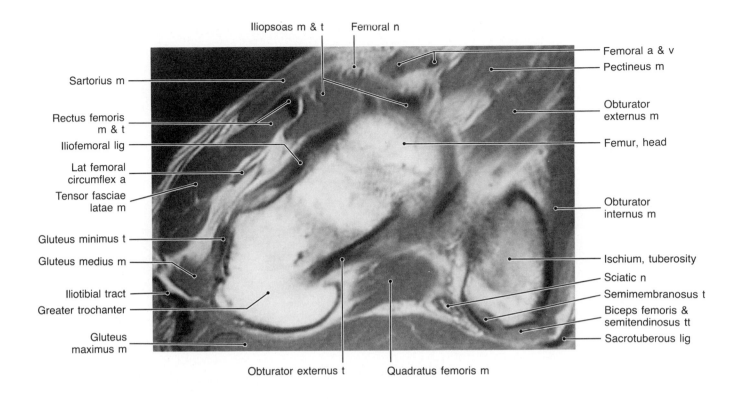

Iliopsoas m & t   Femoral n

Sartorius m

Rectus femoris m & t

Iliofemoral lig

Lat femoral circumflex a

Tensor fasciae latae m

Gluteus minimus t

Gluteus medius m

Iliotibial tract

Greater trochanter

Gluteus maximus m

Femoral a & v

Pectineus m

Obturator externus m

Femur, head

Obturator internus m

Ischium, tuberosity

Sciatic n

Semimembranosus t

Biceps femoris & semitendinosus tt

Sacrotuberous lig

Obturator externus t   Quadratus femoris m

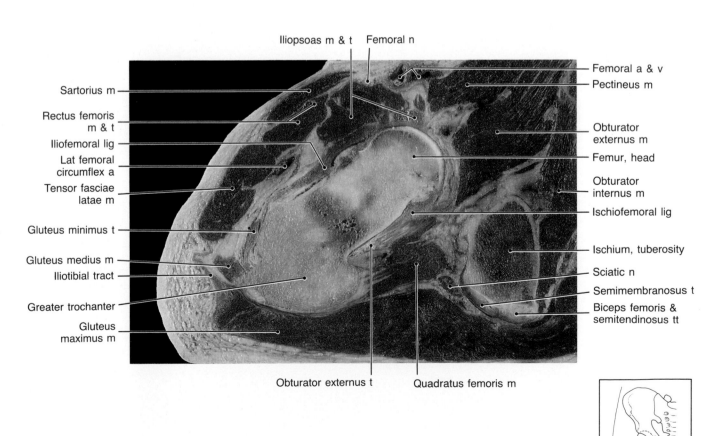

Iliopsoas m & t   Femoral n

Sartorius m

Rectus femoris m & t

Iliofemoral lig

Lat femoral circumflex a

Tensor fasciae latae m

Gluteus minimus t

Gluteus medius m

Iliotibial tract

Greater trochanter

Gluteus maximus m

Femoral a & v

Pectineus m

Obturator externus m

Femur, head

Obturator internus m

Ischiofemoral lig

Ischium, tuberosity

Sciatic n

Semimembranosus t

Biceps femoris & semitendinosus tt

Obturator externus t   Quadratus femoris m

HIP, TRANSVERSE

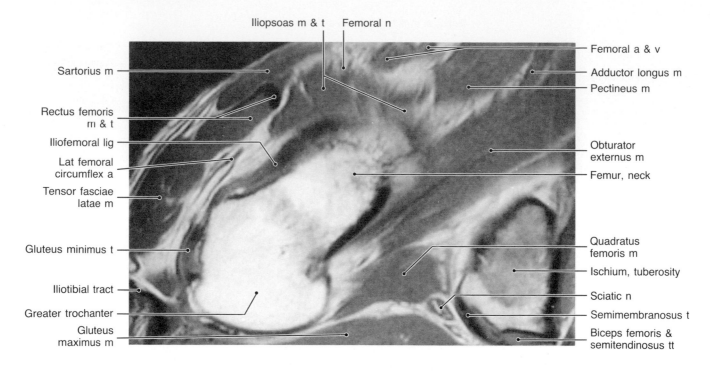

Iliopsoas m & t   Femoral n

Sartorius m

Rectus femoris m & t

Iliofemoral lig

Lat femoral circumflex a

Tensor fasciae latae m

Gluteus minimus t

Iliotibial tract

Greater trochanter

Gluteus maximus m

Femoral a & v

Adductor longus m

Pectineus m

Obturator externus m

Femur, neck

Quadratus femoris m

Ischium, tuberosity

Sciatic n

Semimembranosus t

Biceps femoris & semitendinosus tt

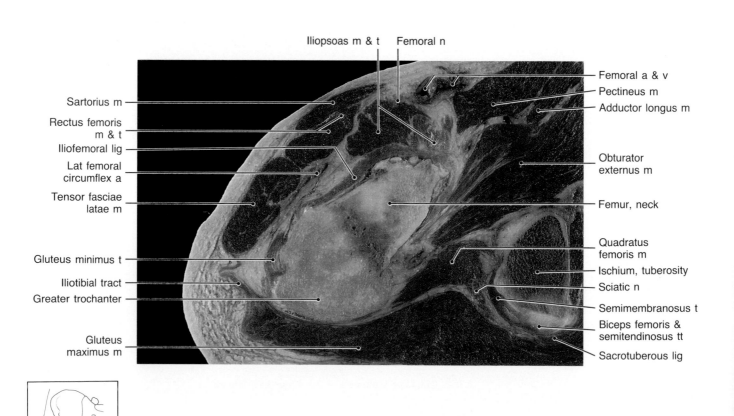

Iliopsoas m & t   Femoral n

Sartorius m

Rectus femoris m & t

Iliofemoral lig

Lat femoral circumflex a

Tensor fasciae latae m

Gluteus minimus t

Iliotibial tract

Greater trochanter

Gluteus maximus m

Femoral a & v

Pectineus m

Adductor longus m

Obturator externus m

Femur, neck

Quadratus femoris m

Ischium, tuberosity

Sciatic n

Semimembranosus t

Biceps femoris & semitendinosus tt

Sacrotuberous lig

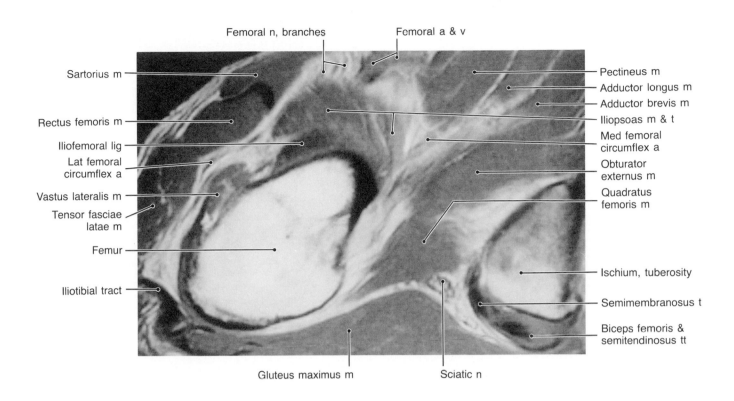

Femoral n, branches
Femoral a & v

Sartorius m
Rectus femoris m
Iliofemoral lig
Lat femoral circumflex a
Vastus lateralis m
Tensor fasciae latae m
Femur
Iliotibial tract

Pectineus m
Adductor longus m
Adductor brevis m
Iliopsoas m & t
Med femoral circumflex a
Obturator externus m
Quadratus femoris m
Ischium, tuberosity
Semimembranosus t
Biceps femoris & semitendinosus tt

Gluteus maximus m
Sciatic n

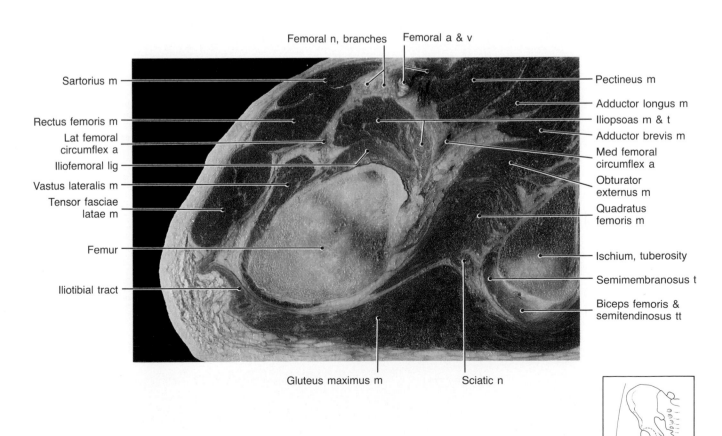

Femoral n, branches
Femoral a & v

Sartorius m
Rectus femoris m
Lat femoral circumflex a
Iliofemoral lig
Vastus lateralis m
Tensor fasciae latae m
Femur
Iliotibial tract

Pectineus m
Adductor longus m
Iliopsoas m & t
Adductor brevis m
Med femoral circumflex a
Obturator externus m
Quadratus femoris m
Ischium, tuberosity
Semimembranosus t
Biceps femoris & semitendinosus tt

Gluteus maximus m
Sciatic n

Hɪᴘ, Tʀᴀɴsᴠᴇʀsᴇ

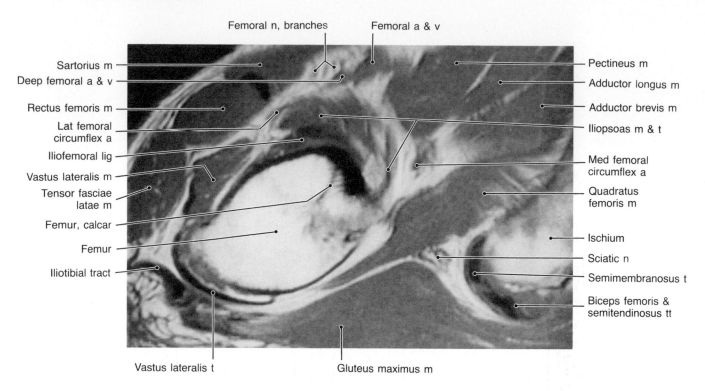

Femoral n, branches

Femoral a & v

Sartorius m

Deep femoral a & v

Rectus femoris m

Lat femoral circumflex a

Iliofemoral lig

Vastus lateralis m

Tensor fasciae latae m

Femur, calcar

Femur

Iliotibial tract

Pectineus m

Adductor longus m

Adductor brevis m

Iliopsoas m & t

Med femoral circumflex a

Quadratus femoris m

Ischium

Sciatic n

Semimembranosus t

Biceps femoris & semitendinosus tt

Vastus lateralis t

Gluteus maximus m

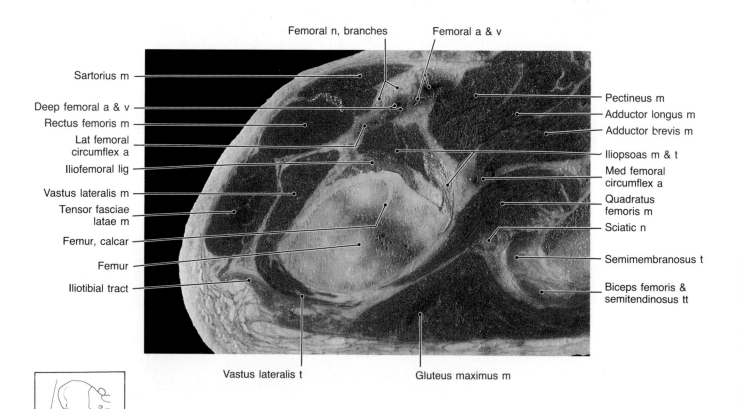

Femoral n, branches

Femoral a & v

Sartorius m

Deep femoral a & v

Rectus femoris m

Lat femoral circumflex a

Iliofemoral lig

Vastus lateralis m

Tensor fasciae latae m

Femur, calcar

Femur

Iliotibial tract

Pectineus m

Adductor longus m

Adductor brevis m

Iliopsoas m & t

Med femoral circumflex a

Quadratus femoris m

Sciatic n

Semimembranosus t

Biceps femoris & semitendinosus tt

Vastus lateralis t

Gluteus maximus m

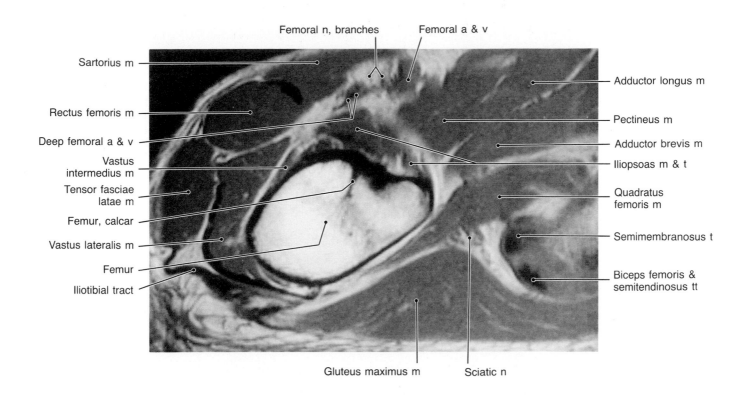

Femoral n, branches

Femoral a & v

Sartorius m

Rectus femoris m

Deep femoral a & v

Vastus intermedius m

Tensor fasciae latae m

Femur, calcar

Vastus lateralis m

Femur

Iliotibial tract

Adductor longus m

Pectineus m

Adductor brevis m

Iliopsoas m & t

Quadratus femoris m

Semimembranosus t

Biceps femoris & semitendinosus tt

Gluteus maximus m

Sciatic n

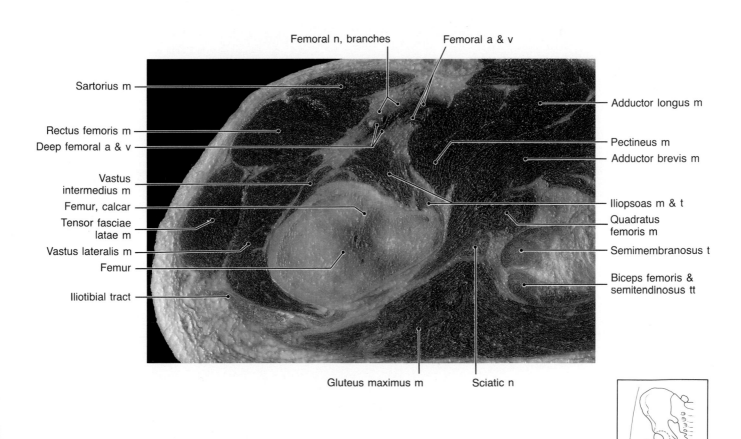

Femoral n, branches

Femoral a & v

Sartorius m

Rectus femoris m

Deep femoral a & v

Vastus intermedius m

Femur, calcar

Tensor fasciae latae m

Vastus lateralis m

Femur

Iliotibial tract

Adductor longus m

Pectineus m

Adductor brevis m

Iliopsoas m & t

Quadratus femoris m

Semimembranosus t

Biceps femoris & semitendlnosus tt

Gluteus maximus m

Sciatic n

HIP, SAGITTAL

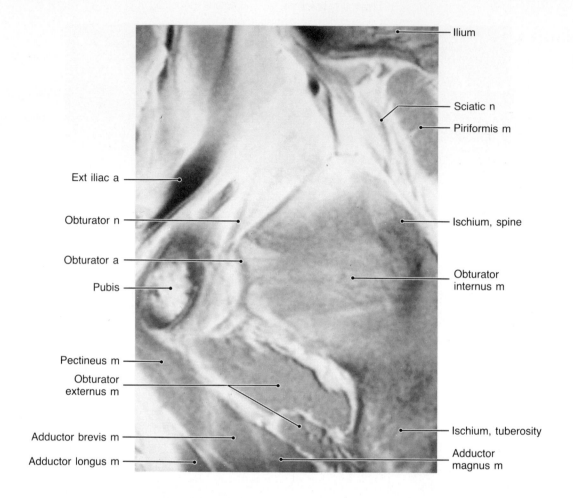

Ilium

Sciatic n

Piriformis m

Ext iliac a

Obturator n

Ischium, spine

Obturator a

Pubis

Obturator
internus m

Pectineus m

Obturator
externus m

Adductor brevis m

Ischium, tuberosity

Adductor longus m

Adductor
magnus m

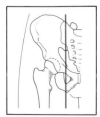

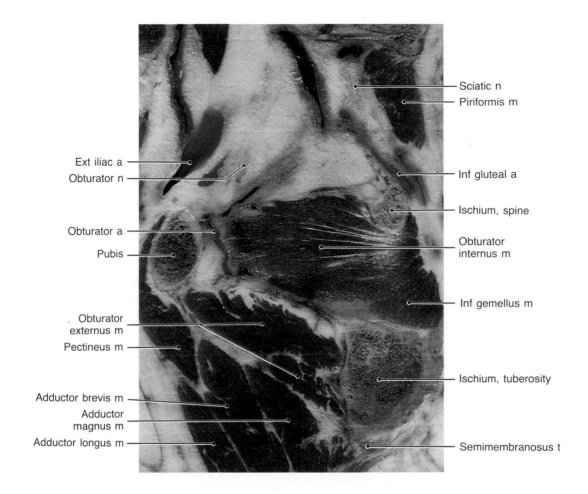

Sciatic n

Piriformis m

Ext iliac a

Obturator n

Inf gluteal a

Ischium, spine

Obturator a

Pubis

Obturator
internus m

Obturator
externus m

Inf gemellus m

Pectineus m

Ischium, tuberosity

Adductor brevis m

Adductor
magnus m

Adductor longus m

Semimembranosus t

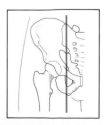

HIP, SAGITTAL

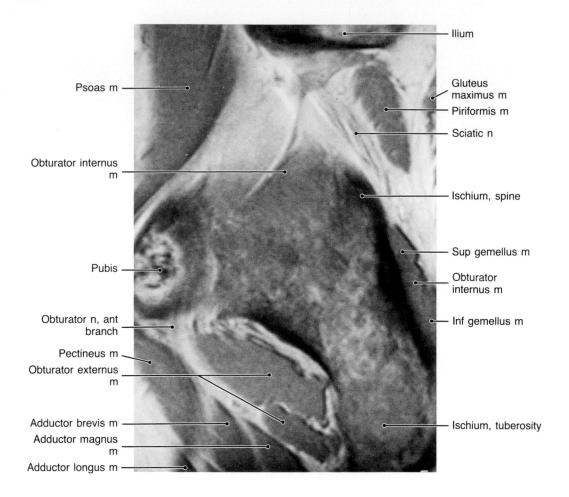

Psoas m

Ilium

Gluteus maximus m

Piriformis m

Sciatic n

Obturator internus m

Ischium, spine

Sup gemellus m

Pubis

Obturator internus m

Obturator n, ant branch

Inf gemellus m

Pectineus m

Obturator externus m

Adductor brevis m

Ischium, tuberosity

Adductor magnus m

Adductor longus m

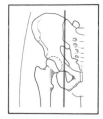

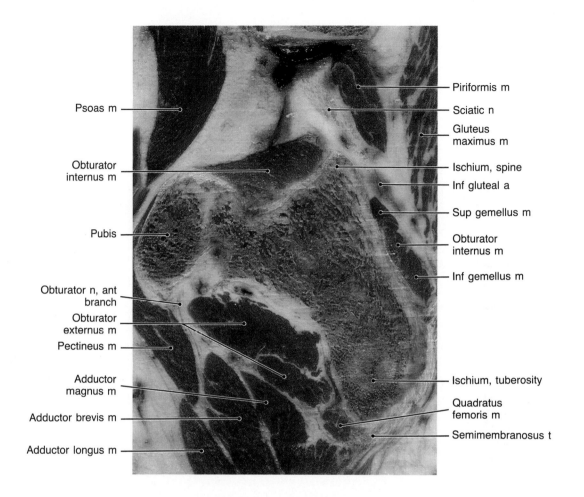

Psoas m

Obturator
internus m

Pubis

Obturator n, ant
branch

Obturator
externus m

Pectineus m

Adductor
magnus m

Adductor brevis m

Adductor longus m

Piriformis m

Sciatic n

Gluteus
maximus m

Ischium, spine

Inf gluteal a

Sup gemellus m

Obturator
internus m

Inf gemellus m

Ischium, tuberosity

Quadratus
femoris m

Semimembranosus t

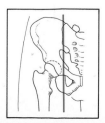

HIP, SAGITTAL

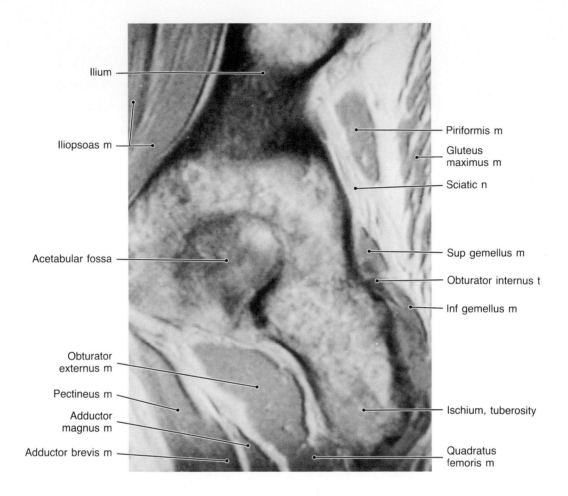

Ilium

Iliopsoas m

Piriformis m

Gluteus maximus m

Sciatic n

Acetabular fossa

Sup gemellus m

Obturator internus t

Inf gemellus m

Obturator externus m

Pectineus m

Adductor magnus m

Adductor brevis m

Ischium, tuberosity

Quadratus femoris m

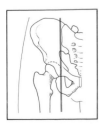

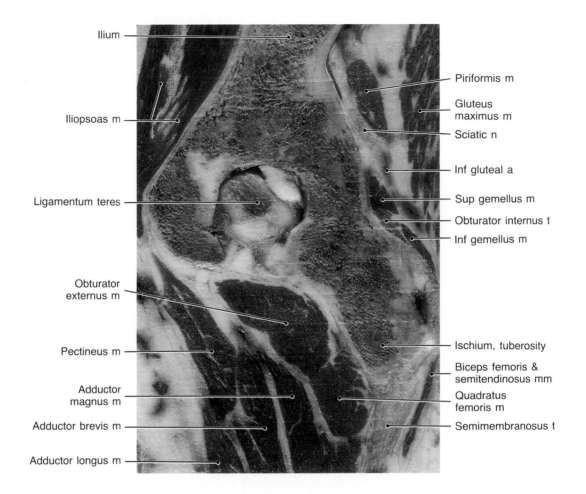

Ilium

Iliopsoas m

Ligamentum teres

Obturator
externus m

Pectineus m

Adductor
magnus m

Adductor brevis m

Adductor longus m

Piriformis m

Gluteus
maximus m

Sciatic n

Inf gluteal a

Sup gemellus m

Obturator internus t

Inf gemellus m

Ischium, tuberosity

Biceps femoris &
semitendinosus mm

Quadratus
femoris m

Semimembranosus t

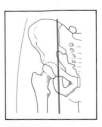

HIP, SAGITTAL

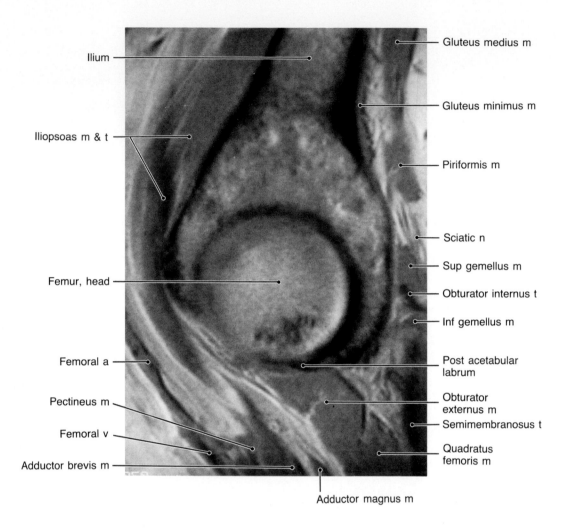

Ilium

Iliopsoas m & t

Femur, head

Femoral a

Pectineus m

Femoral v

Adductor brevis m

Adductor magnus m

Gluteus medius m

Gluteus minimus m

Piriformis m

Sciatic n

Sup gemellus m

Obturator internus t

Inf gemellus m

Post acetabular labrum

Obturator externus m

Semimembranosus t

Quadratus femoris m

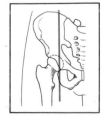

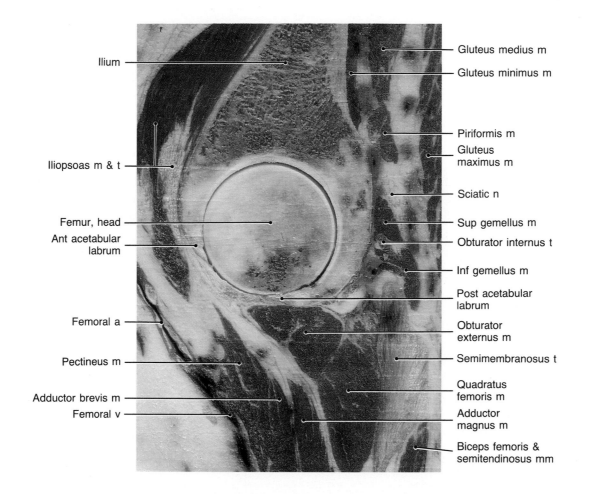

Ilium

Iliopsoas m & t

Femur, head

Ant acetabular labrum

Femoral a

Pectineus m

Adductor brevis m

Femoral v

Gluteus medius m

Gluteus minimus m

Piriformis m

Gluteus maximus m

Sciatic n

Sup gemellus m

Obturator internus t

Inf gemellus m

Post acetabular labrum

Obturator externus m

Semimembranosus t

Quadratus femoris m

Adductor magnus m

Biceps femoris & semitendinosus mm

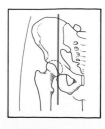

HIP, SAGITTAL

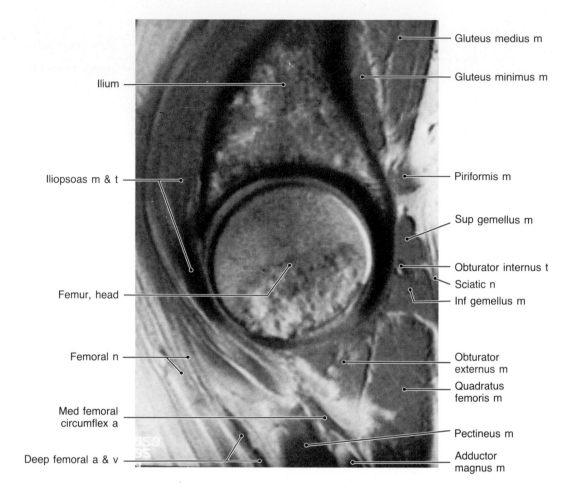

Gluteus medius m

Gluteus minimus m

Ilium

Piriformis m

Iliopsoas m & t

Sup gemellus m

Obturator internus t

Sciatic n

Femur, head

Inf gemellus m

Femoral n

Obturator externus m

Quadratus femoris m

Med femoral circumflex a

Pectineus m

Deep femoral a & v

Adductor magnus m

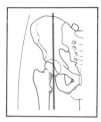

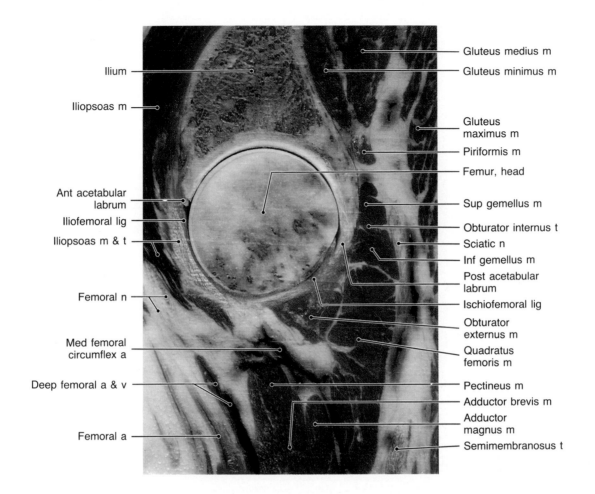

Ilium

Iliopsoas m

Ant acetabular labrum

Iliofemoral lig

Iliopsoas m & t

Femoral n

Med femoral circumflex a

Deep femoral a & v

Femoral a

Gluteus medius m

Gluteus minimus m

Gluteus maximus m

Piriformis m

Femur, head

Sup gemellus m

Obturator internus t

Sciatic n

Inf gemellus m

Post acetabular labrum

Ischiofemoral lig

Obturator externus m

Quadratus femoris m

Pectineus m

Adductor brevis m

Adductor magnus m

Semimembranosus t

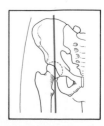

HIP, SAGITTAL

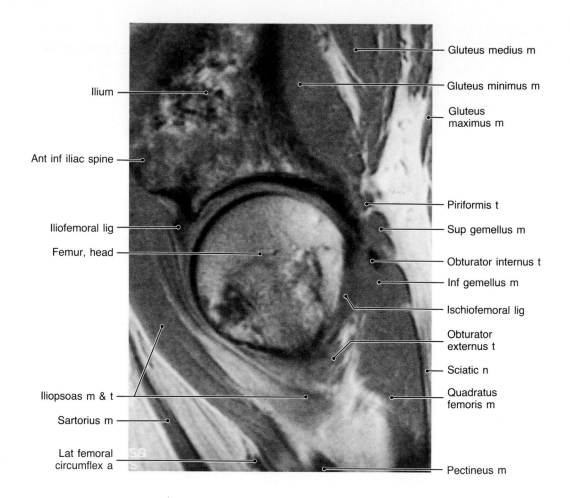

Ilium

Ant inf iliac spine

Iliofemoral lig

Femur, head

Iliopsoas m & t

Sartorius m

Lat femoral circumflex a

Gluteus medius m

Gluteus minimus m

Gluteus maximus m

Piriformis t

Sup gemellus m

Obturator internus t

Inf gemellus m

Ischiofemoral lig

Obturator externus t

Sciatic n

Quadratus femoris m

Pectineus m

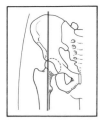

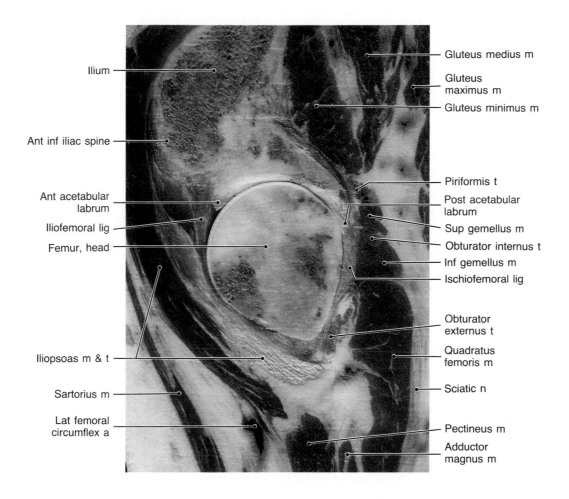

Ilium

Ant inf iliac spine

Ant acetabular labrum

Iliofemoral lig

Femur, head

Iliopsoas m & t

Sartorius m

Lat femoral circumflex a

Gluteus medius m

Gluteus maximus m

Gluteus minimus m

Piriformis t

Post acetabular labrum

Sup gemellus m

Obturator internus t

Inf gemellus m

Ischiofemoral lig

Obturator externus t

Quadratus femoris m

Sciatic n

Pectineus m

Adductor magnus m

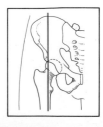

HIP, SAGITTAL

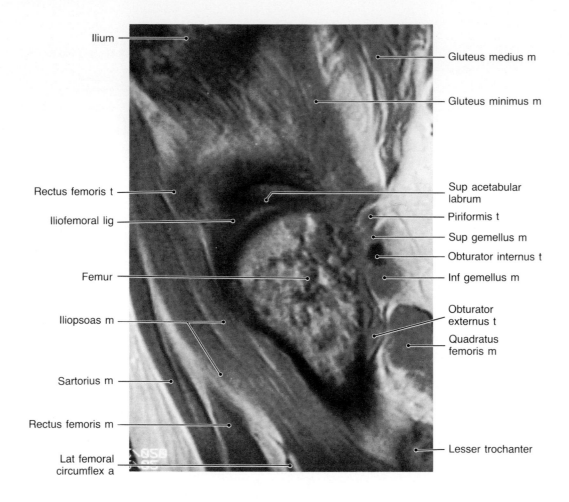

Ilium

Gluteus medius m

Gluteus minimus m

Rectus femoris t

Sup acetabular labrum

Iliofemoral lig

Piriformis t

Sup gemellus m

Obturator internus t

Femur

Inf gemellus m

Iliopsoas m

Obturator externus t

Quadratus femoris m

Sartorius m

Rectus femoris m

Lesser trochanter

Lat femoral circumflex a

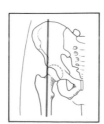

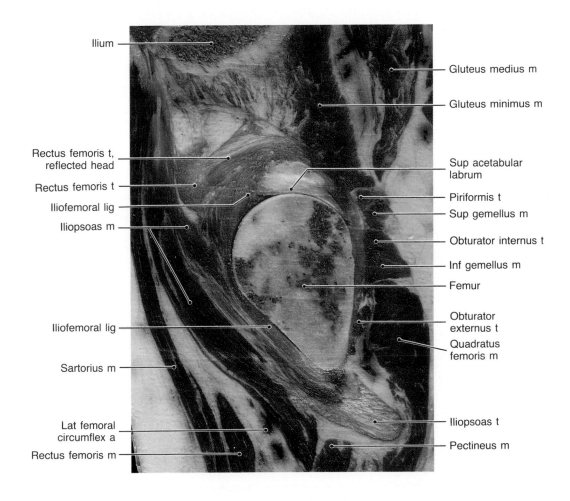

Ilium

Gluteus medius m

Gluteus minimus m

Rectus femoris t, reflected head

Sup acetabular labrum

Rectus femoris t

Piriformis t

Iliofemoral lig

Sup gemellus m

Iliopsoas m

Obturator internus t

Inf gemellus m

Femur

Obturator externus t

Iliofemoral lig

Quadratus femoris m

Sartorius m

Lat femoral circumflex a

Iliopsoas t

Rectus femoris m

Pectineus m

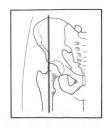

HIP, SAGITTAL

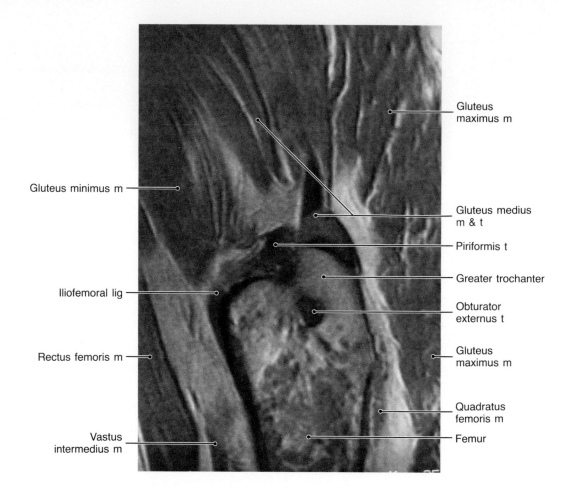

Gluteus minimus m

Iliofemoral lig

Rectus femoris m

Vastus intermedius m

Gluteus maximus m

Gluteus medius m & t

Piriformis t

Greater trochanter

Obturator externus t

Gluteus maximus m

Quadratus femoris m

Femur

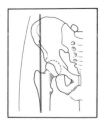

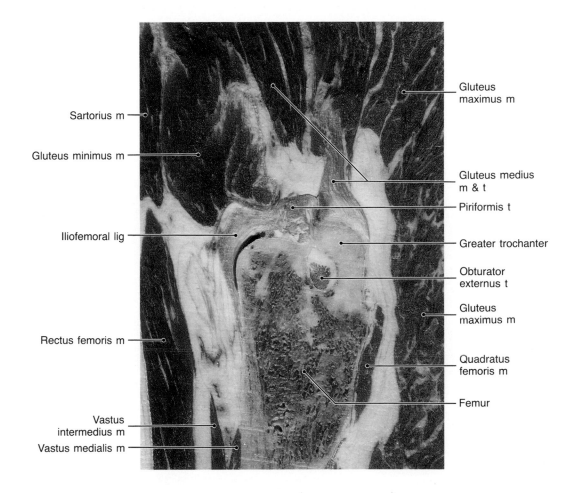

Sartorius m

Gluteus minimus m

Iliofemoral lig

Rectus femoris m

Vastus
intermedius m

Vastus medialis m

Gluteus
maximus m

Gluteus medius
m & t

Piriformis t

Greater trochanter

Obturator
externus t

Gluteus
maximus m

Quadratus
femoris m

Femur

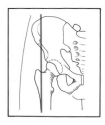

6 KNEE

KNEE, CORONAL

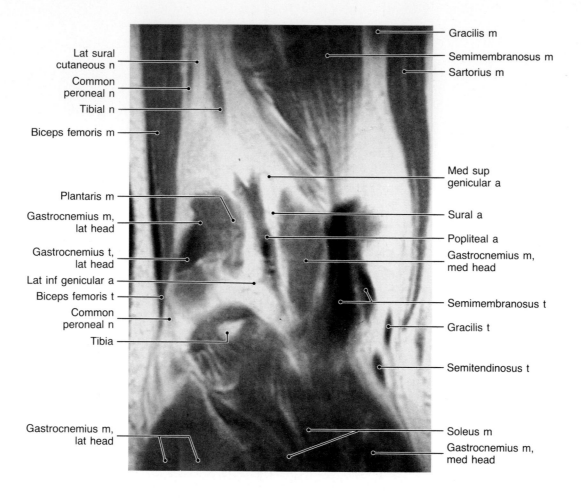

Lat sural cutaneous n

Common peroneal n

Tibial n

Biceps femoris m

Plantaris m

Gastrocnemius m, lat head

Gastrocnemius t, lat head

Lat inf genicular a

Biceps femoris t

Common peroneal n

Tibia

Gastrocnemius m, lat head

Gracilis m

Semimembranosus m

Sartorius m

Med sup genicular a

Sural a

Popliteal a

Gastrocnemius m, med head

Semimembranosus t

Gracilis t

Semitendinosus t

Soleus m

Gastrocnemius m, med head

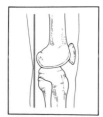

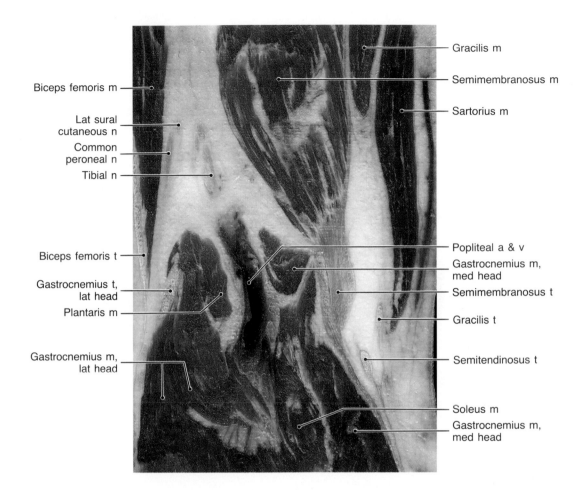

Gracilis m

Semimembranosus m

Sartorius m

Biceps femoris m

Lat sural
cutaneous n

Common
peroneal n

Tibial n

Biceps femoris t

Gastrocnemius t,
lat head

Plantaris m

Gastrocnemius m,
lat head

Popliteal a & v

Gastrocnemius m,
med head

Semimembranosus t

Gracilis t

Semitendinosus t

Soleus m

Gastrocnemius m,
med head

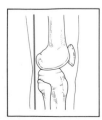

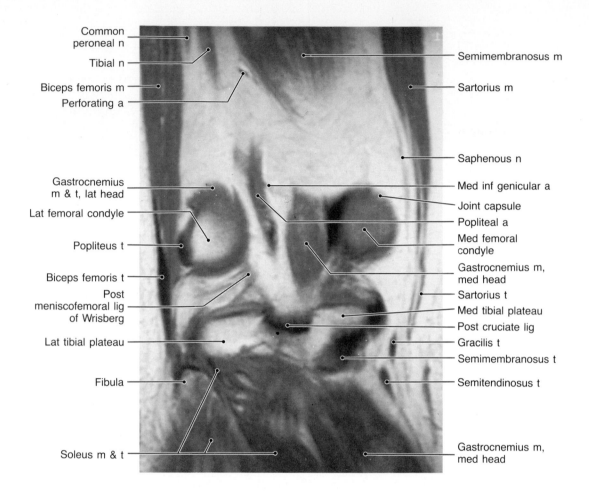

Common peroneal n

Tibial n

Biceps femoris m

Perforating a

Gastrocnemius m & t, lat head

Lat femoral condyle

Popliteus t

Biceps femoris t

Post meniscofemoral lig of Wrisberg

Lat tibial plateau

Fibula

Soleus m & t

Semimembranosus m

Sartorius m

Saphenous n

Med inf genicular a

Joint capsule

Popliteal a

Med femoral condyle

Gastrocnemius m, med head

Sartorius t

Med tibial plateau

Post cruciate lig

Gracilis t

Semimembranosus t

Semitendinosus t

Gastrocnemius m, med head

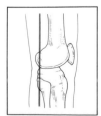

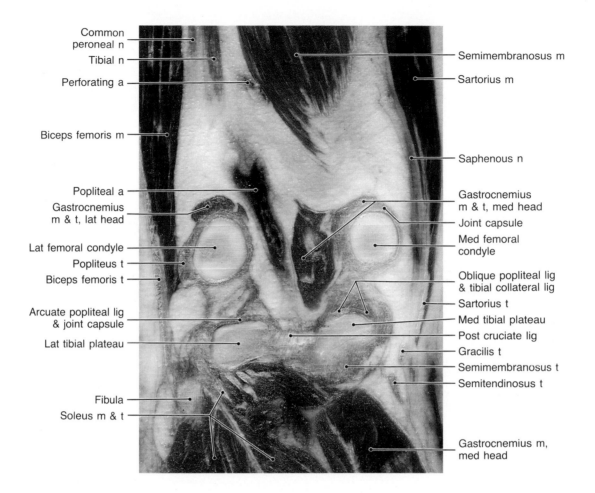

Common peroneal n

Tibial n

Perforating a

Biceps femoris m

Popliteal a

Gastrocnemius m & t, lat head

Lat femoral condyle

Popliteus t

Biceps femoris t

Arcuate popliteal lig & joint capsule

Lat tibial plateau

Fibula

Soleus m & t

Semimembranosus m

Sartorius m

Saphenous n

Gastrocnemius m & t, med head

Joint capsule

Med femoral condyle

Oblique popliteal lig & tibial collateral lig

Sartorius t

Med tibial plateau

Post cruciate lig

Gracilis t

Semimembranosus t

Semitendinosus t

Gastrocnemius m, med head

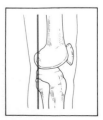

KNEE, CORONAL

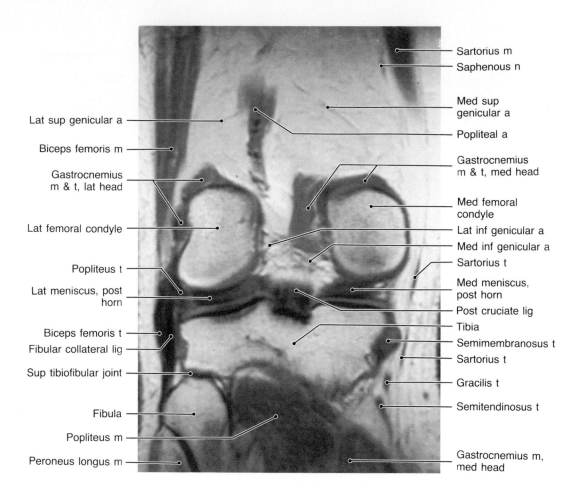

Lat sup genicular a

Biceps femoris m

Gastrocnemius m & t, lat head

Lat femoral condyle

Popliteus t

Lat meniscus, post horn

Biceps femoris t

Fibular collateral lig

Sup tibiofibular joint

Fibula

Popliteus m

Peroneus longus m

Sartorius m

Saphenous n

Med sup genicular a

Popliteal a

Gastrocnemius m & t, med head

Med femoral condyle

Lat inf genicular a

Med inf genicular a

Sartorius t

Med meniscus, post horn

Post cruciate lig

Tibia

Semimembranosus t

Sartorius t

Gracilis t

Semitendinosus t

Gastrocnemius m, med head

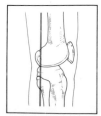

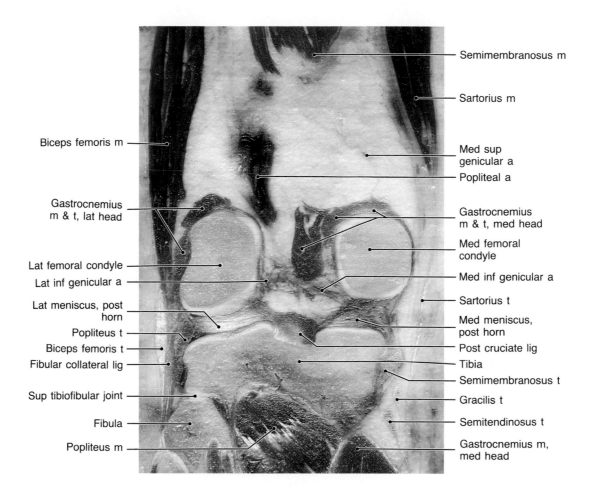

Semimembranosus m

Sartorius m

Biceps femoris m

Med sup genicular a

Popliteal a

Gastrocnemius m & t, lat head

Gastrocnemius m & t, med head

Med femoral condyle

Lat femoral condyle

Lat inf genicular a

Med inf genicular a

Sartorius t

Lat meniscus, post horn

Med meniscus, post horn

Popliteus t

Biceps femoris t

Post cruciate lig

Fibular collateral lig

Tibia

Semimembranosus t

Sup tibiofibular joint

Gracilis t

Fibula

Semitendinosus t

Popliteus m

Gastrocnemius m, med head

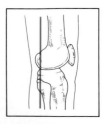

KNEE, CORONAL

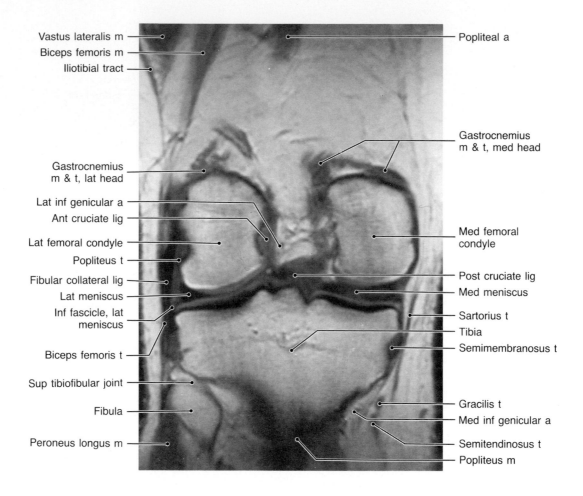

Vastus lateralis m

Biceps femoris m

Iliotibial tract

Popliteal a

Gastrocnemius
m & t, med head

Gastrocnemius
m & t, lat head

Lat inf genicular a

Ant cruciate lig

Lat femoral condyle

Popliteus t

Fibular collateral lig

Lat meniscus

Inf fascicle, lat
meniscus

Biceps femoris t

Sup tibiofibular joint

Fibula

Peroneus longus m

Med femoral
condyle

Post cruciate lig

Med meniscus

Sartorius t

Tibia

Semimembranosus t

Gracilis t

Med inf genicular a

Semitendinosus t

Popliteus m

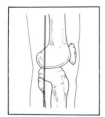

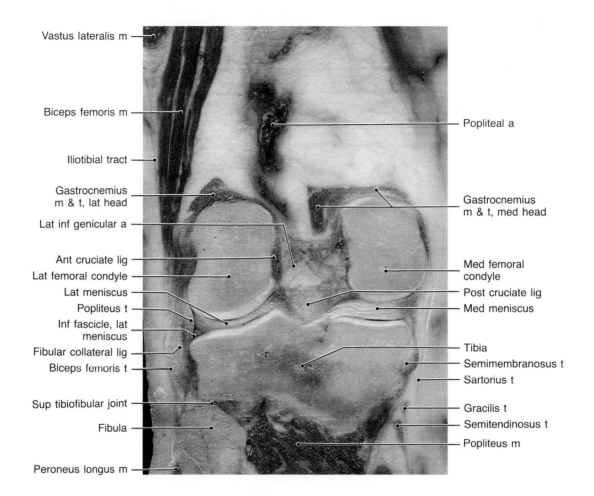

Vastus lateralis m

Biceps femoris m

Iliotibial tract

Gastrocnemius m & t, lat head

Lat inf genicular a

Ant cruciate lig

Lat femoral condyle

Lat meniscus

Popliteus t

Inf fascicle, lat meniscus

Fibular collateral lig

Biceps femoris t

Sup tibiofibular joint

Fibula

Peroneus longus m

Popliteal a

Gastrocnemius m & t, med head

Med femoral condyle

Post cruciate lig

Med meniscus

Tibia

Semimembranosus t

Sartorius t

Gracilis t

Semitendinosus t

Popliteus m

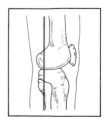

KNEE, CORONAL

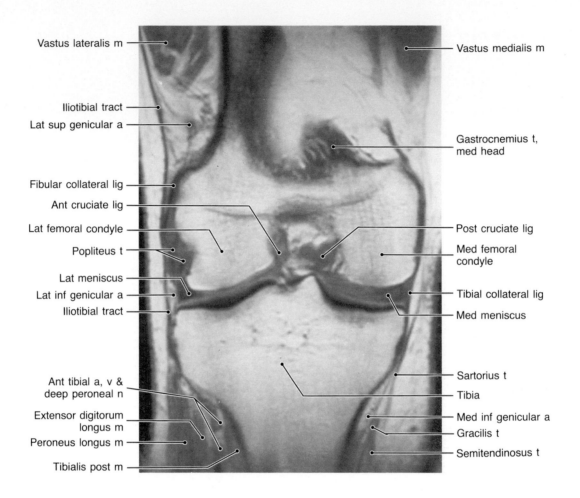

Vastus lateralis m

Iliotibial tract

Lat sup genicular a

Fibular collateral lig

Ant cruciate lig

Lat femoral condyle

Popliteus t

Lat meniscus

Lat inf genicular a

Iliotibial tract

Ant tibial a, v &
deep peroneal n

Extensor digitorum
longus m

Peroneus longus m

Tibialis post m

Vastus medialis m

Gastrocnemius t,
med head

Post cruciate lig

Med femoral
condyle

Tibial collateral lig

Med meniscus

Sartorius t

Tibia

Med inf genicular a

Gracilis t

Semitendinosus t

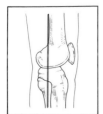

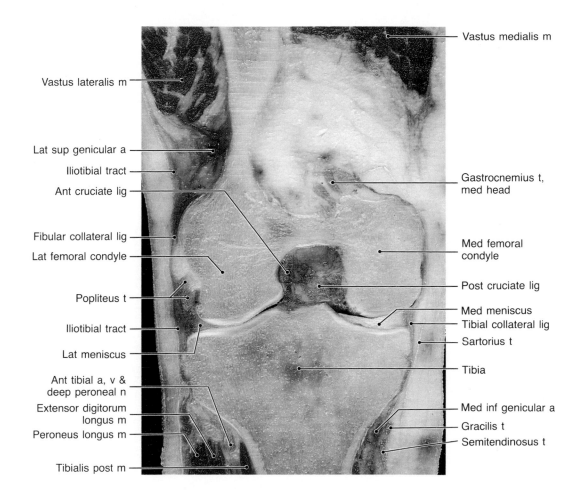

Vastus medialis m

Vastus lateralis m

Lat sup genicular a

Iliotibial tract

Ant cruciate lig

Gastrocnemius t, med head

Fibular collateral lig

Lat femoral condyle

Med femoral condyle

Popliteus t

Post cruciate lig

Iliotibial tract

Med meniscus

Tibial collateral lig

Lat meniscus

Sartorius t

Ant tibial a, v & deep peroneal n

Tibia

Extensor digitorum longus m

Med inf genicular a

Gracilis t

Peroneus longus m

Semitendinosus t

Tibialis post m

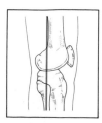

KNEE, CORONAL

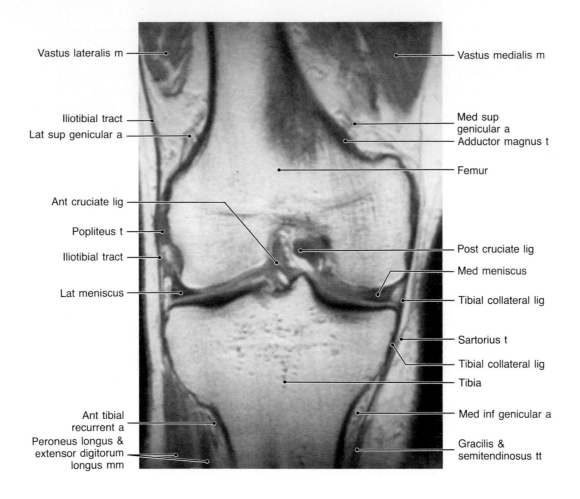

Vastus lateralis m

Iliotibial tract

Lat sup genicular a

Ant cruciate lig

Popliteus t

Iliotibial tract

Lat meniscus

Ant tibial recurrent a

Peroneus longus & extensor digitorum longus mm

Vastus medialis m

Med sup genicular a

Adductor magnus t

Femur

Post cruciate lig

Med meniscus

Tibial collateral lig

Sartorius t

Tibial collateral lig

Tibia

Med inf genicular a

Gracilis & semitendinosus tt

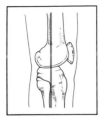

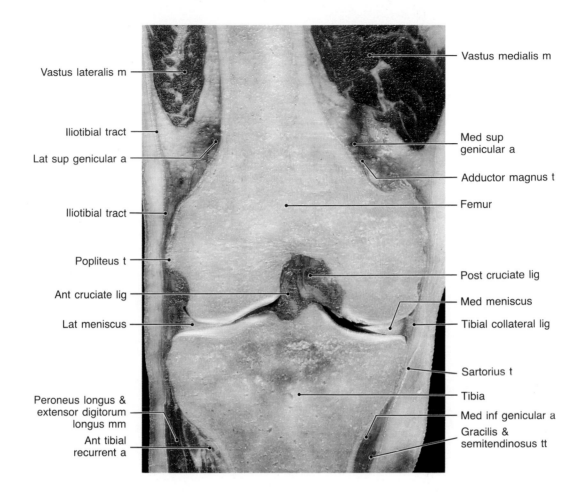

Vastus lateralis m

Iliotibial tract

Lat sup genicular a

Iliotibial tract

Popliteus t

Ant cruciate lig

Lat meniscus

Peroneus longus &
extensor digitorum
longus mm

Ant tibial
recurrent a

Vastus medialis m

Med sup
genicular a

Adductor magnus t

Femur

Post cruciate lig

Med meniscus

Tibial collateral lig

Sartorius t

Tibia

Med inf genicular a

Gracilis &
semitendinosus tt

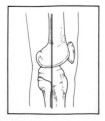

KNEE, CORONAL

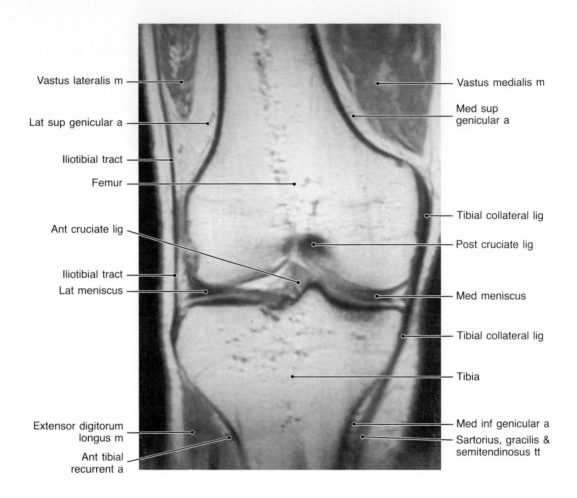

Vastus lateralis m

Lat sup genicular a

Iliotibial tract

Femur

Ant cruciate lig

Iliotibial tract

Lat meniscus

Extensor digitorum longus m

Ant tibial recurrent a

Vastus medialis m

Med sup genicular a

Tibial collateral lig

Post cruciate lig

Med meniscus

Tibial collateral lig

Tibia

Med inf genicular a

Sartorius, gracilis & semitendinosus tt

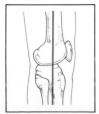

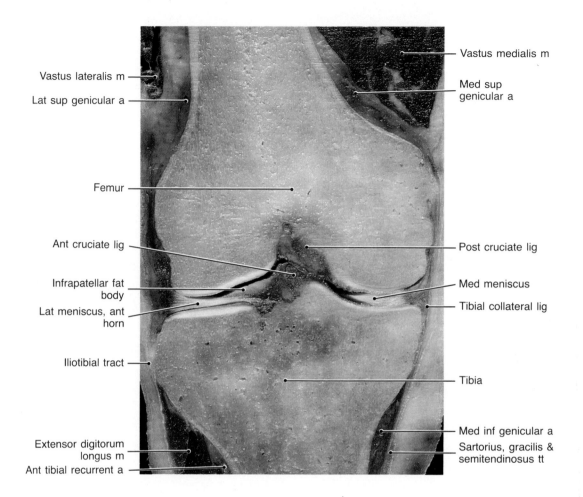

Vastus lateralis m

Lat sup genicular a

Femur

Ant cruciate lig

Infrapatellar fat body

Lat meniscus, ant horn

Iliotibial tract

Extensor digitorum longus m

Ant tibial recurrent a

Vastus medialis m

Med sup genicular a

Post cruciate lig

Med meniscus

Tibial collateral lig

Tibia

Med inf genicular a

Sartorius, gracilis & semitendinosus tt

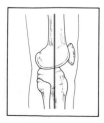

KNEE, CORONAL

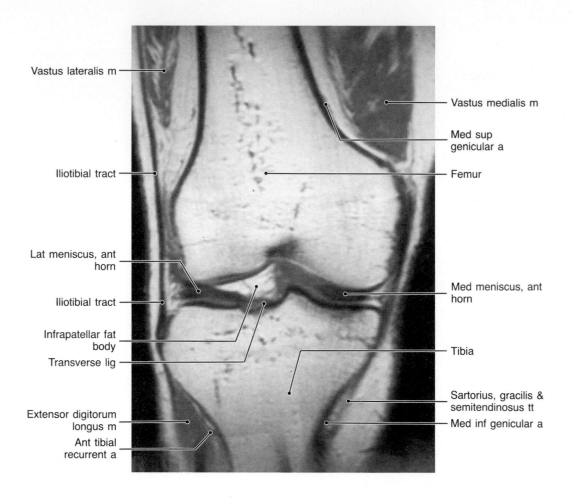

Vastus lateralis m

Iliotibial tract

Lat meniscus, ant horn

Iliotibial tract

Infrapatellar fat body

Transverse lig

Extensor digitorum longus m

Ant tibial recurrent a

Vastus medialis m

Med sup genicular a

Femur

Med meniscus, ant horn

Tibia

Sartorius, gracilis & semitendinosus tt

Med inf genicular a

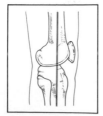

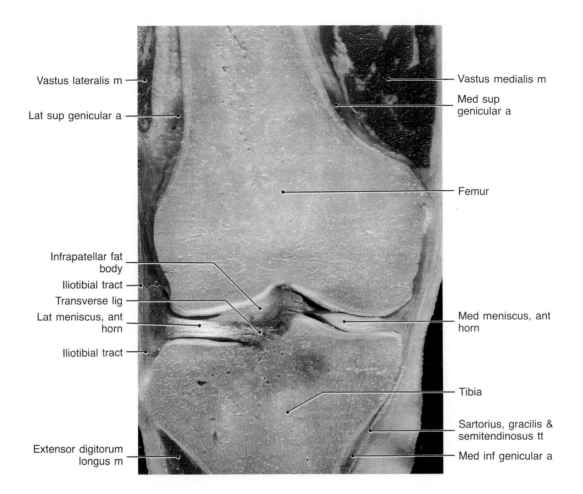

Vastus lateralis m

Lat sup genicular a

Vastus medialis m

Med sup genicular a

Femur

Infrapatellar fat body

Iliotibial tract

Transverse lig

Lat meniscus, ant horn

Iliotibial tract

Med meniscus, ant horn

Tibia

Sartorius, gracilis & semitendinosus tt

Extensor digitorum longus m

Med inf genicular a

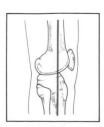

KNEE, CORONAL

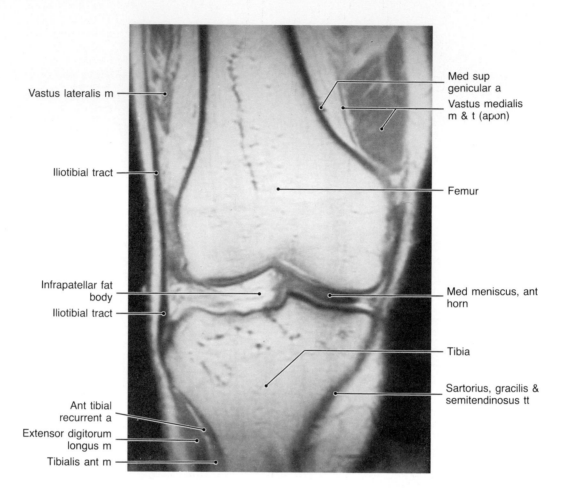

Vastus lateralis m

Iliotibial tract

Infrapatellar fat body

Iliotibial tract

Ant tibial recurrent a

Extensor digitorum longus m

Tibialis ant m

Med sup genicular a

Vastus medialis m & t (apon)

Femur

Med meniscus, ant horn

Tibia

Sartorius, gracilis & semitendinosus tt

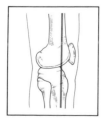

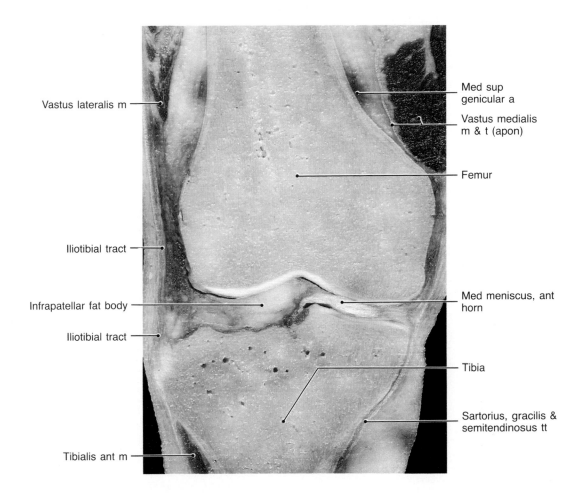

Vastus lateralis m

Iliotibial tract

Infrapatellar fat body

Iliotibial tract

Tibialis ant m

Med sup genicular a

Vastus medialis m & t (apon)

Femur

Med meniscus, ant horn

Tibia

Sartorius, gracilis & semitendinosus tt

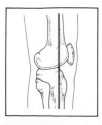

KNEE, CORONAL

Vastus lateralis m

Vastus medialis
m & t (apon)

Femur

Iliotibial tract,
vastus lateralis t
(apon) & lat patellar
retinaculum

Med meniscus, ant
horn

Lat inf genicular a

Med inf genicular a

Infrapatellar fat
body

Sartorius, gracilis &
semitendinosus tt &
med patellar
retinaculum

Tibia

Lat patellar
retinaculum

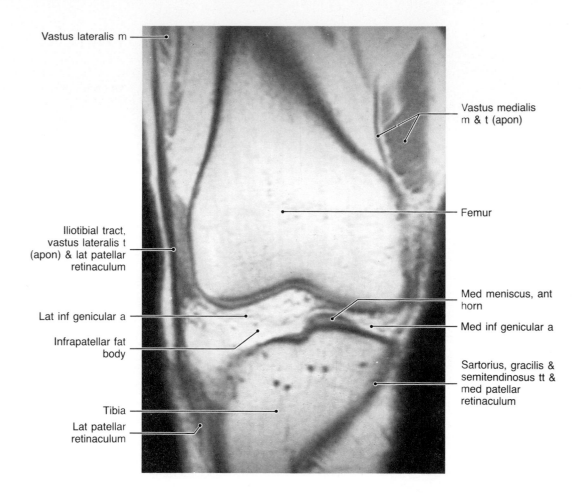

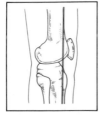

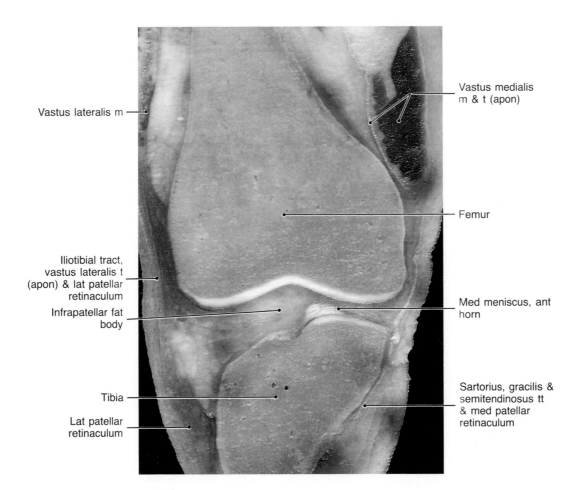

Vastus medialis
m & t (apon)

Vastus lateralis m

Femur

Iliotibial tract,
vastus lateralis t
(apon) & lat patellar
retinaculum

Infrapatellar fat
body

Med meniscus, ant
horn

Tibia

Sartorius, gracilis &
semitendinosus tt
& med patellar
retinaculum

Lat patellar
retinaculum

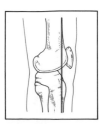

KNEE, CORONAL

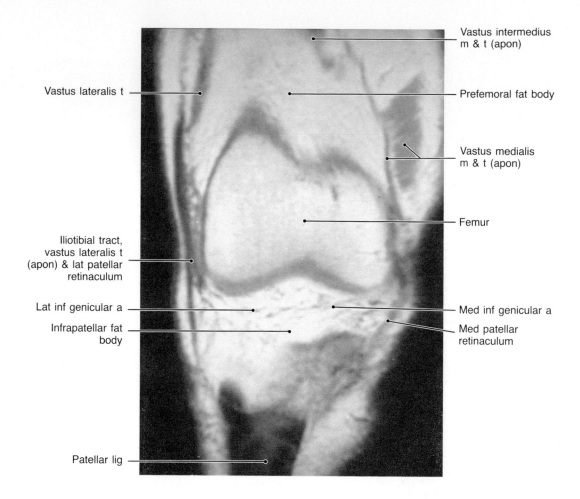

Vastus intermedius m & t (apon)

Vastus lateralis t

Prefemoral fat body

Vastus medialis m & t (apon)

Iliotibial tract, vastus lateralis t (apon) & lat patellar retinaculum

Femur

Lat inf genicular a

Infrapatellar fat body

Med inf genicular a

Med patellar retinaculum

Patellar lig

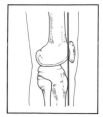

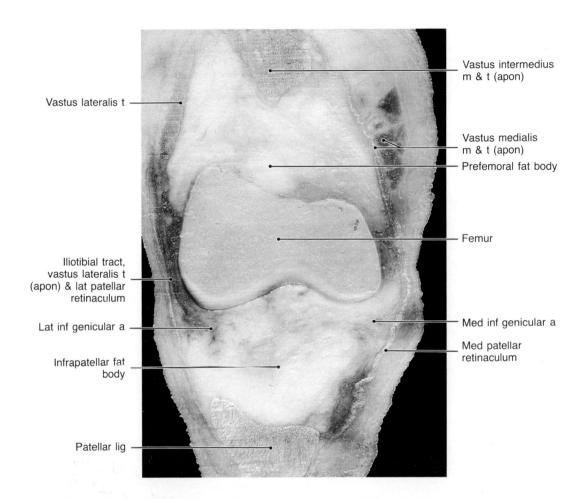

Vastus lateralis t

Iliotibial tract, vastus lateralis t (apon) & lat patellar retinaculum

Lat inf genicular a

Infrapatellar fat body

Patellar lig

Vastus intermedius m & t (apon)

Vastus medialis m & t (apon)

Prefemoral fat body

Femur

Med inf genicular a

Med patellar retinaculum

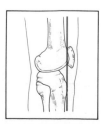

KNEE, TRANSVERSE

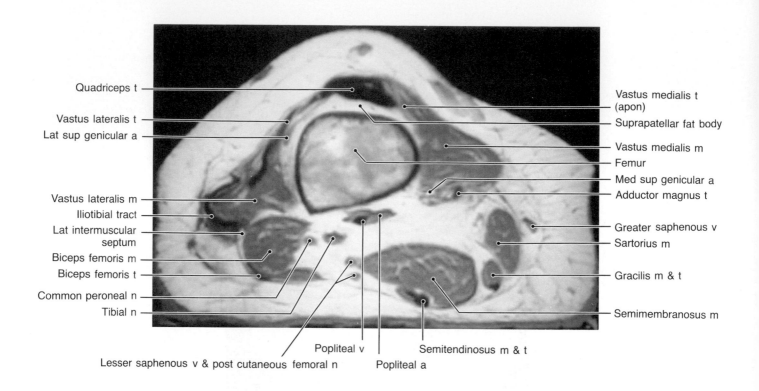

Quadriceps t
Vastus lateralis t
Lat sup genicular a

Vastus lateralis m
Iliotibial tract
Lat intermuscular septum
Biceps femoris m
Biceps femoris t
Common peroneal n
Tibial n

Lesser saphenous v & post cutaneous femoral n

Popliteal v
Popliteal a

Semitendinosus m & t

Vastus medialis t (apon)
Suprapatellar fat body
Vastus medialis m
Femur
Med sup genicular a
Adductor magnus t
Greater saphenous v
Sartorius m
Gracilis m & t
Semimembranosus m

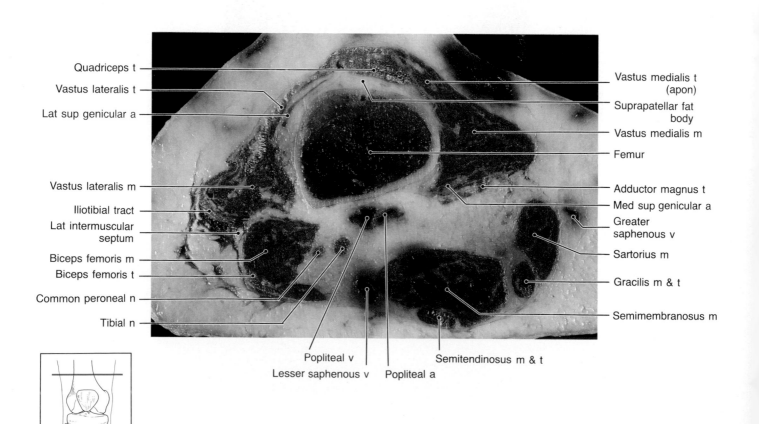

Quadriceps t
Vastus lateralis t
Lat sup genicular a

Vastus lateralis m
Iliotibial tract
Lat intermuscular septum
Biceps femoris m
Biceps femoris t
Common peroneal n
Tibial n

Popliteal v
Lesser saphenous v
Popliteal a

Semitendinosus m & t

Vastus medialis t (apon)
Suprapatellar fat body
Vastus medialis m
Femur
Adductor magnus t
Med sup genicular a
Greater saphenous v
Sartorius m
Gracilis m & t
Semimembranosus m

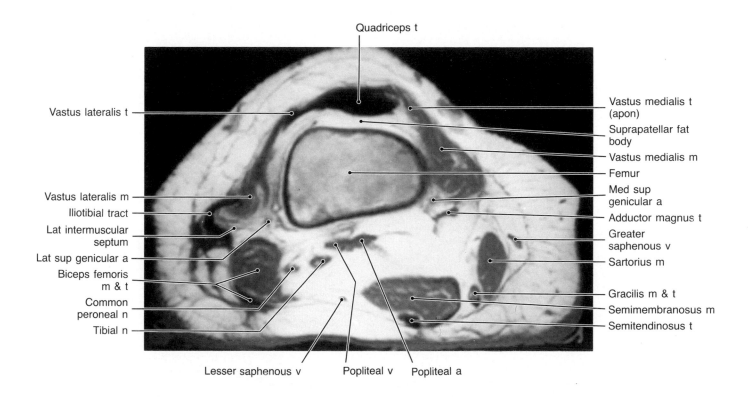

Quadriceps t

Vastus lateralis t

Vastus lateralis m

Iliotibial tract

Lat intermuscular septum

Lat sup genicular a

Biceps femoris m & t

Common peroneal n

Tibial n

Vastus medialis t (apon)

Suprapatellar fat body

Vastus medialis m

Femur

Med sup genicular a

Adductor magnus t

Greater saphenous v

Sartorius m

Gracilis m & t

Semimembranosus m

Semitendinosus t

Lesser saphenous v   Popliteal v   Popliteal a

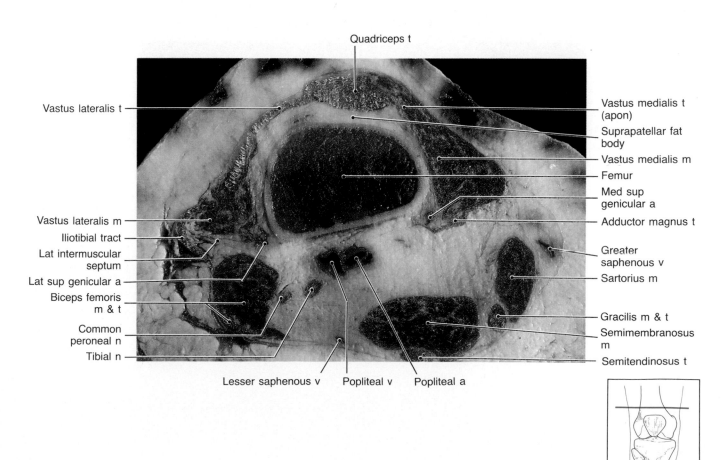

Quadriceps t

Vastus lateralis t

Vastus lateralis m

Iliotibial tract

Lat intermuscular septum

Lat sup genicular a

Biceps femoris m & t

Common peroneal n

Tibial n

Vastus medialis t (apon)

Suprapatellar fat body

Vastus medialis m

Femur

Med sup genicular a

Adductor magnus t

Greater saphenous v

Sartorius m

Gracilis m & t

Semimembranosus m

Semitendinosus t

Lesser saphenous v   Popliteal v   Popliteal a

KNEE, TRANSVERSE

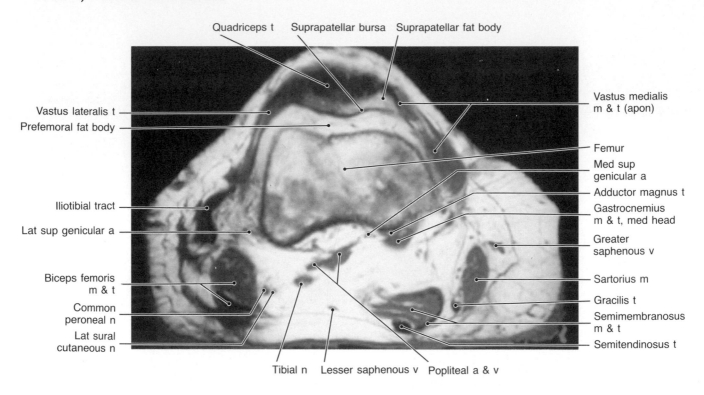

Quadriceps t   Suprapatellar bursa   Suprapatellar fat body

Vastus lateralis t
Prefemoral fat body

Vastus medialis
m & t (apon)

Femur

Med sup
genicular a

Adductor magnus t

Iliotibial tract

Lat sup genicular a

Gastrocnemius
m & t, med head

Greater
saphenous v

Biceps femoris
m & t

Sartorius m

Common
peroneal n

Gracilis t

Semimembranosus
m & t

Lat sural
cutaneous n

Semitendinosus t

Tibial n   Lesser saphenous v   Popliteal a & v

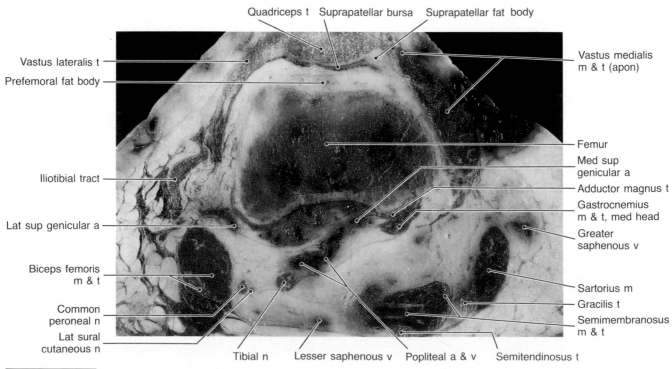

Quadriceps t   Suprapatellar bursa   Suprapatellar fat body

Vastus lateralis t
Prefemoral fat body

Vastus medialis
m & t (apon)

Femur

Med sup
genicular a

Adductor magnus t

Iliotibial tract

Gastrocnemius
m & t, med head

Greater
saphenous v

Lat sup genicular a

Biceps femoris
m & t

Sartorius m

Common
peroneal n

Gracilis t

Semimembranosus
m & t

Lat sural
cutaneous n

Tibial n   Lesser saphenous v   Popliteal a & v   Semitendinosus t

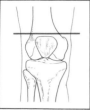

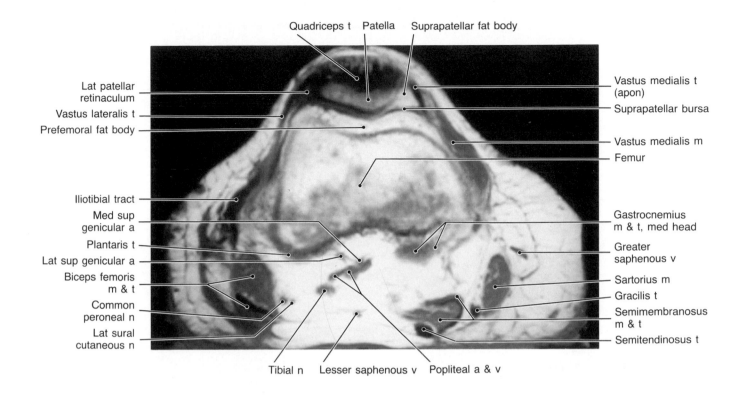

Quadriceps t   Patella   Suprapatellar fat body

Lat patellar retinaculum

Vastus lateralis t

Prefemoral fat body

Iliotibial tract

Med sup genicular a

Plantaris t

Lat sup genicular a

Biceps femoris m & t

Common peroneal n

Lat sural cutaneous n

Vastus medialis t (apon)

Suprapatellar bursa

Vastus medialis m

Femur

Gastrocnemius m & t, med head

Greater saphenous v

Sartorius m

Gracilis t

Semimembranosus m & t

Semitendinosus t

Tibial n   Lesser saphenous v   Popliteal a & v

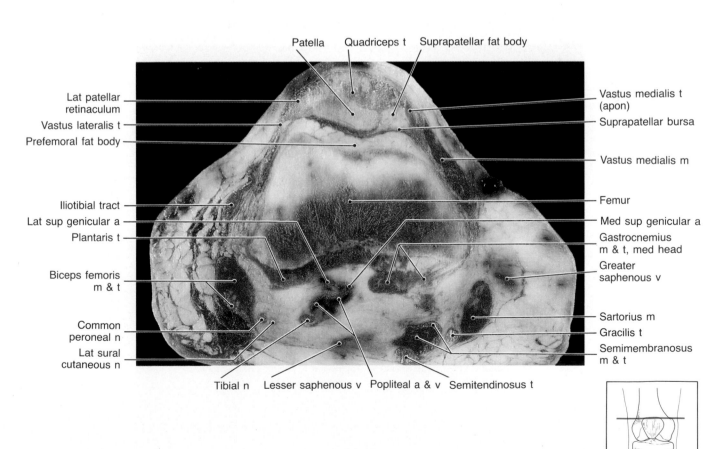

Patella   Quadriceps t   Suprapatellar fat body

Lat patellar retinaculum

Vastus lateralis t

Prefemoral fat body

Iliotibial tract

Lat sup genicular a

Plantaris t

Biceps femoris m & t

Common peroneal n

Lat sural cutaneous n

Vastus medialis t (apon)

Suprapatellar bursa

Vastus medialis m

Femur

Med sup genicular a

Gastrocnemius m & t, med head

Greater saphenous v

Sartorius m

Gracilis t

Semimembranosus m & t

Tibial n   Lesser saphenous v   Popliteal a & v   Semitendinosus t

KNEE, TRANSVERSE

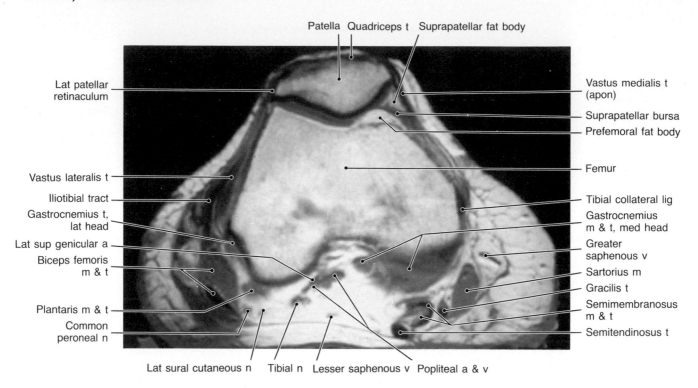

Patella Quadriceps t Suprapatellar fat body

Lat patellar retinaculum

Vastus medialis t (apon)

Suprapatellar bursa

Prefemoral fat body

Vastus lateralis t

Iliotibial tract

Gastrocnemius t, lat head

Lat sup genicular a

Biceps femoris m & t

Plantaris m & t

Common peroneal n

Femur

Tibial collateral lig

Gastrocnemius m & t, med head

Greater saphenous v

Sartorius m

Gracilis t

Semimembranosus m & t

Semitendinosus t

Lat sural cutaneous n   Tibial n   Lesser saphenous v Popliteal a & v

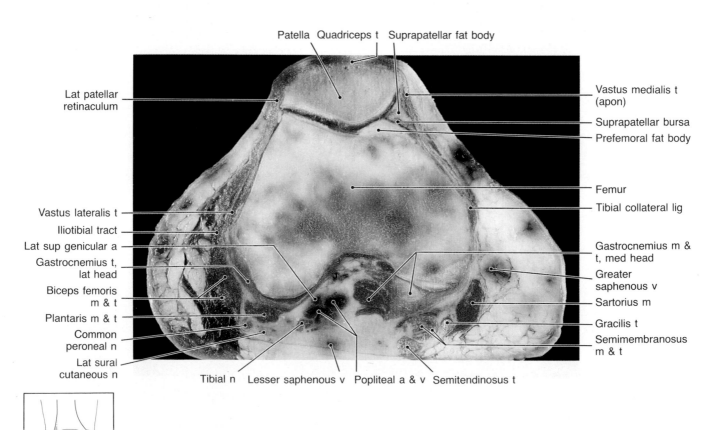

Patella Quadriceps t Suprapatellar fat body

Lat patellar retinaculum

Vastus medialis t (apon)

Suprapatellar bursa

Prefemoral fat body

Vastus lateralis t

Iliotibial tract

Lat sup genicular a

Gastrocnemius t, lat head

Biceps femoris m & t

Plantaris m & t

Common peroneal n

Lat sural cutaneous n

Femur

Tibial collateral lig

Gastrocnemius m & t, med head

Greater saphenous v

Sartorius m

Gracilis t

Semimembranosus m & t

Tibial n   Lesser saphenous v Popliteal a & v   Semitendinosus t

Quadriceps t   Patella   Alar synovial fold & fat

Lat patellar retinaculum

Vastus lateralis t

Iliotibial tract

Lat sup genicular a

Fibular collateral lig

Gastrocnemius t, lat head

Biceps femoris m & t

Plantaris m

Common peroneal n

Lat sural cutaneous n

Vastus medialis t (apon)

Infrapatellar fat body

Femur

Tibial collateral lig

Ant cruciate lig

Greater saphenous v

Gastrocnemius m & t, med head

Sartorius m & t

Gracilis t

Semimembranosus t

Semitendinosus t

Tibial n   Lesser saphenous v   Popliteal a & v

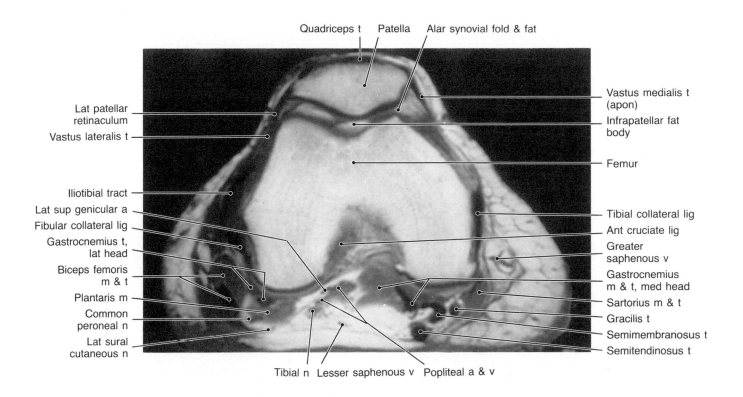

Patella   Quadriceps t   Alar synovial fold & fat

Lat patellar retinaculum

Vastus lateralis t

Iliotibial tract

Lat sup genicular a

Fibular collateral lig

Gastrocnemius t, lat head

Biceps femoris m & t

Common peroneal n

Plantaris m

Vastus medialis t (apon)

Infrapatellar fat body

Femur

Tibial collateral lig

Ant cruciate lig

Greater saphenous v

Gastrocnemius m & t, med head

Sartorius m & t

Gracilis t

Semimembranosus t

Tibial n   Popliteal a & v   Semitendinosus t

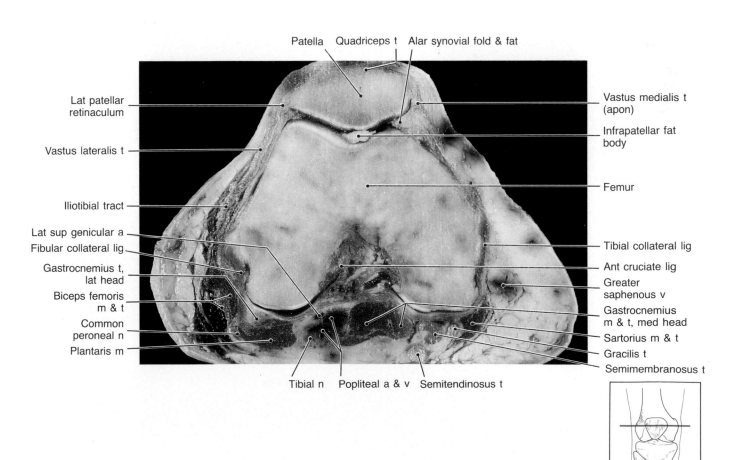

KNEE, TRANSVERSE

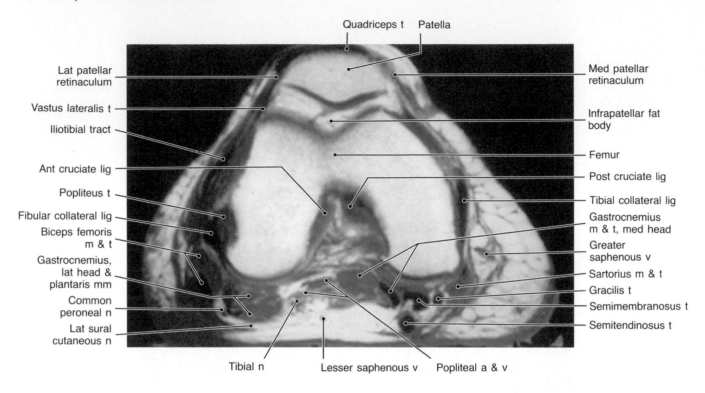

Quadriceps t   Patella

Lat patellar retinaculum

Vastus lateralis t

Iliotibial tract

Ant cruciate lig

Popliteus t

Fibular collateral lig

Biceps femoris m & t

Gastrocnemius, lat head & plantaris mm

Common peroneal n

Lat sural cutaneous n

Med patellar retinaculum

Infrapatellar fat body

Femur

Post cruciate lig

Tibial collateral lig

Gastrocnemius m & t, med head

Greater saphenous v

Sartorius m & t

Gracilis t

Semimembranosus t

Semitendinosus t

Tibial n   Lesser saphenous v   Popliteal a & v

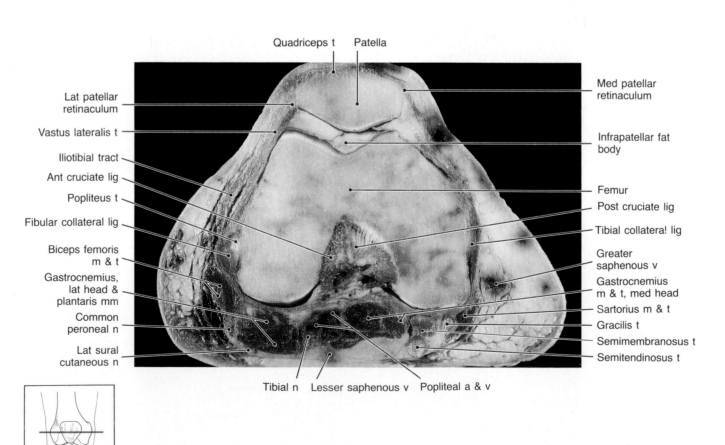

Quadriceps t   Patella

Lat patellar retinaculum

Vastus lateralis t

Iliotibial tract

Ant cruciate lig

Popliteus t

Fibular collateral lig

Biceps femoris m & t

Gastrocnemius, lat head & plantaris mm

Common peroneal n

Lat sural cutaneous n

Med patellar retinaculum

Infrapatellar fat body

Femur

Post cruciate lig

Tibial collateral lig

Greater saphenous v

Gastrocnemius m & t, med head

Sartorius m & t

Gracilis t

Semimembranosus t

Semitendinosus t

Tibial n   Lesser saphenous v   Popliteal a & v

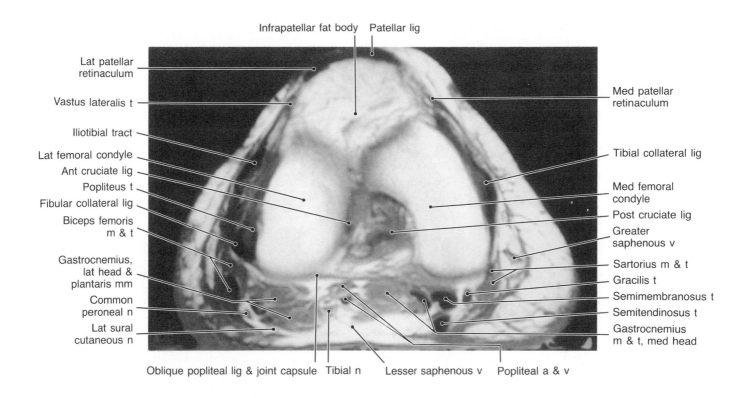

Infrapatellar fat body   Patellar lig

Lat patellar retinaculum

Vastus lateralis t

Iliotibial tract

Lat femoral condyle

Ant cruciate lig

Popliteus t

Fibular collateral lig

Biceps femoris m & t

Gastrocnemius, lat head & plantaris mm

Common peroneal n

Lat sural cutaneous n

Med patellar retinaculum

Tibial collateral lig

Med femoral condyle

Post cruciate lig

Greater saphenous v

Sartorius m & t

Gracilis t

Semimembranosus t

Semitendinosus t

Gastrocnemius m & t, med head

Oblique popliteal lig & joint capsule   Tibial n   Lesser saphenous v   Popliteal a & v

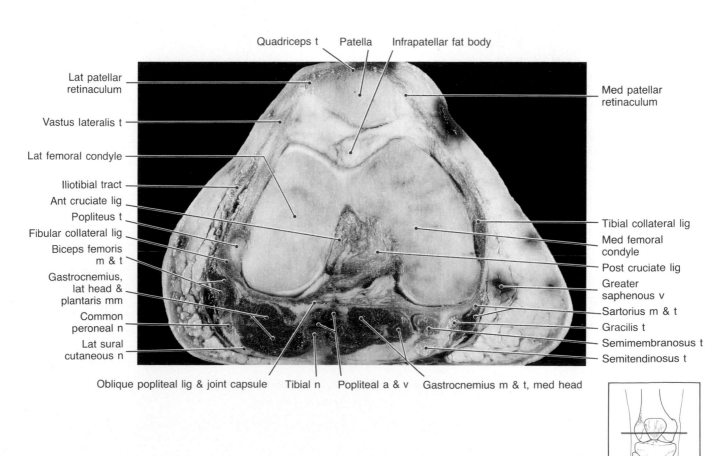

Quadriceps t   Patella   Infrapatellar fat body

Lat patellar retinaculum

Vastus lateralis t

Lat femoral condyle

Iliotibial tract

Ant cruciate lig

Popliteus t

Fibular collateral lig

Biceps femoris m & t

Gastrocnemius, lat head & plantaris mm

Common peroneal n

Lat sural cutaneous n

Med patellar retinaculum

Tibial collateral lig

Med femoral condyle

Post cruciate lig

Greater saphenous v

Sartorius m & t

Gracilis t

Semimembranosus t

Semitendinosus t

Oblique popliteal lig & joint capsule   Tibial n   Popliteal a & v   Gastrocnemius m & t, med head

KNEE, TRANSVERSE

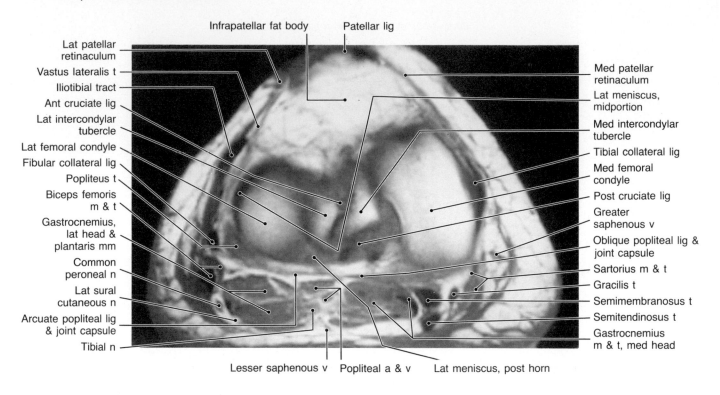

Infrapatellar fat body   Patellar lig

Lat patellar retinaculum
Vastus lateralis t
Iliotibial tract
Ant cruciate lig
Lat intercondylar tubercle
Lat femoral condyle
Fibular collateral lig
Popliteus t
Biceps femoris m & t
Gastrocnemius, lat head & plantaris mm
Common peroneal n
Lat sural cutaneous n
Arcuate popliteal lig & joint capsule
Tibial n

Med patellar retinaculum
Lat meniscus, midportion
Med intercondylar tubercle
Tibial collateral lig
Med femoral condyle
Post cruciate lig
Greater saphenous v
Oblique popliteal lig & joint capsule
Sartorius m & t
Gracilis t
Semimembranosus t
Semitendinosus t
Gastrocnemius m & t, med head

Lesser saphenous v   Popliteal a & v   Lat meniscus, post horn

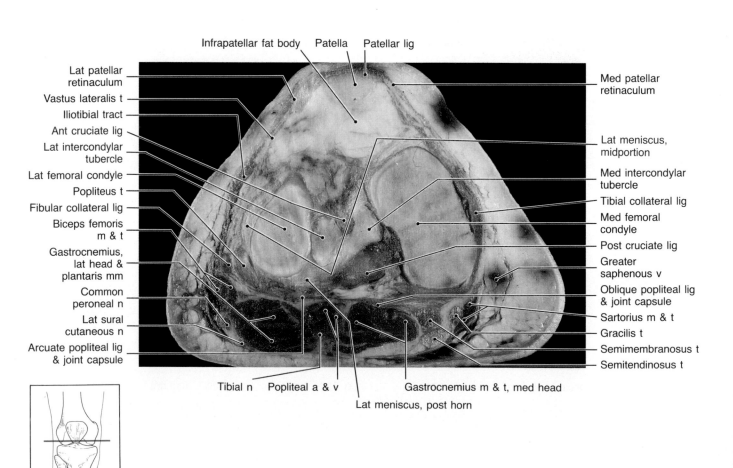

Infrapatellar fat body   Patella   Patellar lig

Lat patellar retinaculum
Vastus lateralis t
Iliotibial tract
Ant cruciate lig
Lat intercondylar tubercle
Lat femoral condyle
Popliteus t
Fibular collateral lig
Biceps femoris m & t
Gastrocnemius, lat head & plantaris mm
Common peroneal n
Lat sural cutaneous n
Arcuate popliteal lig & joint capsule

Med patellar retinaculum
Lat meniscus, midportion
Med intercondylar tubercle
Tibial collateral lig
Med femoral condyle
Post cruciate lig
Greater saphenous v
Oblique popliteal lig & joint capsule
Sartorius m & t
Gracilis t
Semimembranosus t
Semitendinosus t

Tibial n   Popliteal a & v   Gastrocnemius m & t, med head

Lat meniscus, post horn

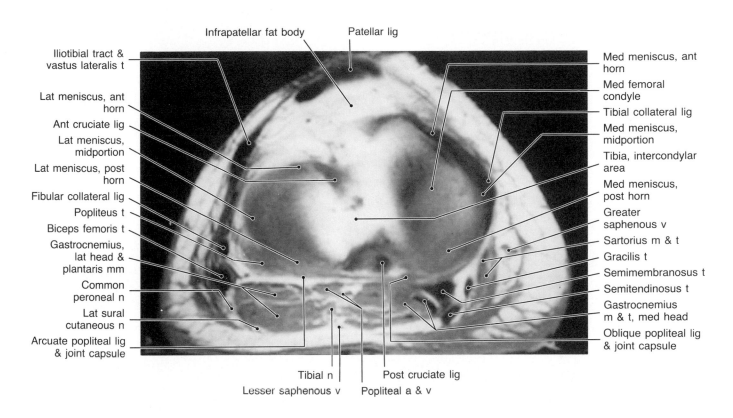

Infrapatellar fat body

Patellar lig

Iliotibial tract & vastus lateralis t

Lat meniscus, ant horn

Ant cruciate lig

Lat meniscus, midportion

Lat meniscus, post horn

Fibular collateral lig

Popliteus t

Biceps femoris t

Gastrocnemius, lat head & plantaris mm

Common peroneal n

Lat sural cutaneous n

Arcuate popliteal lig & joint capsule

Med meniscus, ant horn

Med femoral condyle

Tibial collateral lig

Med meniscus, midportion

Tibia, intercondylar area

Med meniscus, post horn

Greater saphenous v

Sartorius m & t

Gracilis t

Semimembranosus t

Semitendinosus t

Gastrocnemius m & t, med head

Oblique popliteal lig & joint capsule

Tibial n

Lesser saphenous v

Post cruciate lig

Popliteal a & v

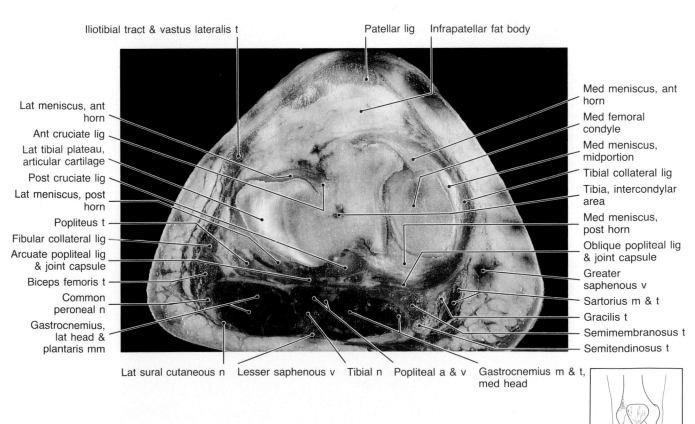

Iliotibial tract & vastus lateralis t

Patellar lig

Infrapatellar fat body

Lat meniscus, ant horn

Ant cruciate lig

Lat tibial plateau, articular cartilage

Post cruciate lig

Lat meniscus, post horn

Popliteus t

Fibular collateral lig

Arcuate popliteal lig & joint capsule

Biceps femoris t

Common peroneal n

Gastrocnemius, lat head & plantaris mm

Med meniscus, ant horn

Med femoral condyle

Med meniscus, midportion

Tibial collateral lig

Tibia, intercondylar area

Med meniscus, post horn

Oblique popliteal lig & joint capsule

Greater saphenous v

Sartorius m & t

Gracilis t

Semimembranosus t

Semitendinosus t

Lat sural cutaneous n

Lesser saphenous v

Tibial n

Popliteal a & v

Gastrocnemius m & t, med head

KNEE, TRANSVERSE

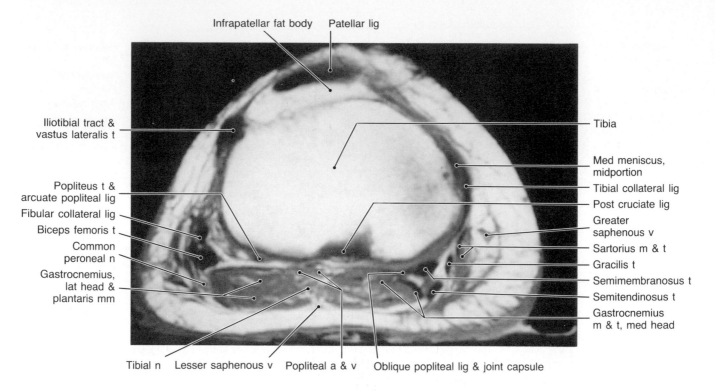

Infrapatellar fat body Patellar lig

Iliotibial tract &
vastus lateralis t

Popliteus t &
arcuate popliteal lig

Fibular collateral lig

Biceps femoris t

Common
peroneal n

Gastrocnemius,
lat head &
plantaris mm

Tibia

Med meniscus,
midportion

Tibial collateral lig

Post cruciate lig

Greater
saphenous v

Sartorius m & t

Gracilis t

Semimembranosus t

Semitendinosus t

Gastrocnemius
m & t, med head

Tibial n Lesser saphenous v Popliteal a & v Oblique popliteal lig & joint capsule

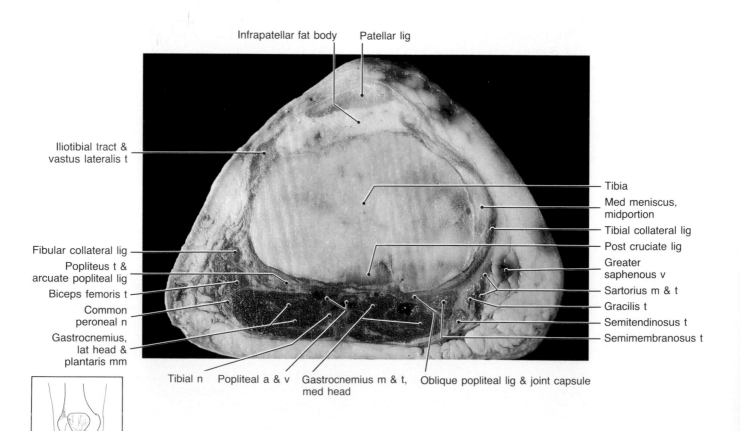

Infrapatellar fat body Patellar lig

Iliotibial tract &
vastus lateralis t

Fibular collateral lig

Popliteus t &
arcuate popliteal lig

Biceps femoris t

Common
peroneal n

Gastrocnemius,
lat head &
plantaris mm

Tibia

Med meniscus,
midportion

Tibial collateral lig

Post cruciate lig

Greater
saphenous v

Sartorius m & t

Gracilis t

Semitendinosus t

Semimembranosus t

Tibial n Popliteal a & v Gastrocnemius m & t,
med head Oblique popliteal lig & joint capsule

Patellar lig

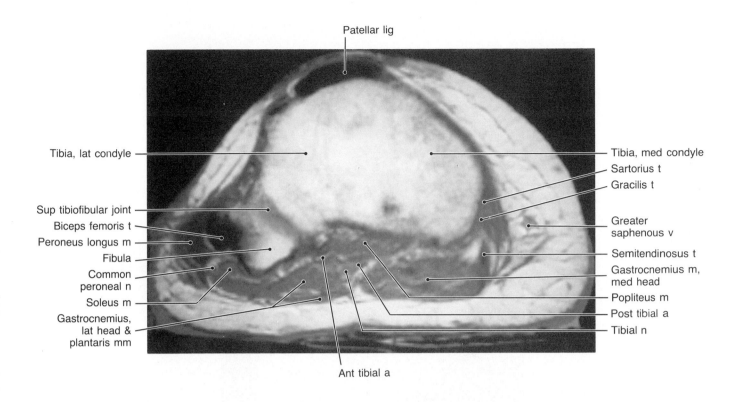

Tibia, lat condyle

Sup tibiofibular joint

Biceps femoris t

Peroneus longus m

Fibula

Common peroneal n

Soleus m

Gastrocnemius, lat head & plantaris mm

Tibia, med condyle

Sartorius t

Gracilis t

Greater saphenous v

Semitendinosus t

Gastrocnemius m, med head

Popliteus m

Post tibial a

Tibial n

Ant tibial a

Patellar lig

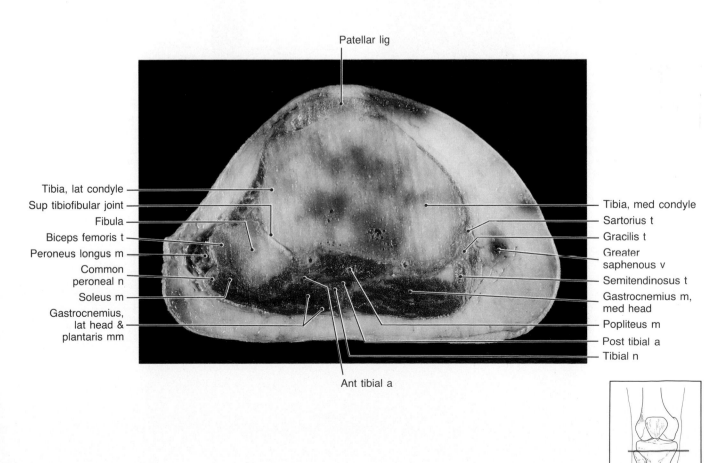

Tibia, lat condyle

Sup tibiofibular joint

Fibula

Biceps femoris t

Peroneus longus m

Common peroneal n

Soleus m

Gastrocnemius, lat head & plantaris mm

Tibia, med condyle

Sartorius t

Gracilis t

Greater saphenous v

Semitendinosus t

Gastrocnemius m, med head

Popliteus m

Post tibial a

Tibial n

Ant tibial a

KNEE, SAGITTAL

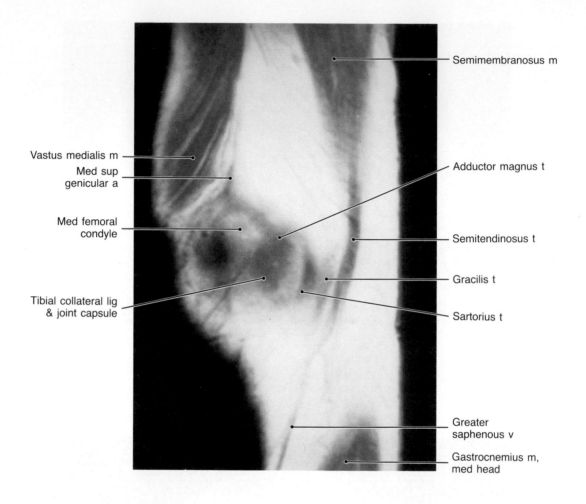

Semimembranosus m

Vastus medialis m

Med sup
genicular a

Adductor magnus t

Med femoral
condyle

Semitendinosus t

Gracilis t

Tibial collateral lig
& joint capsule

Sartorius t

Greater
saphenous v

Gastrocnemius m,
med head

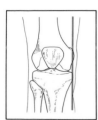

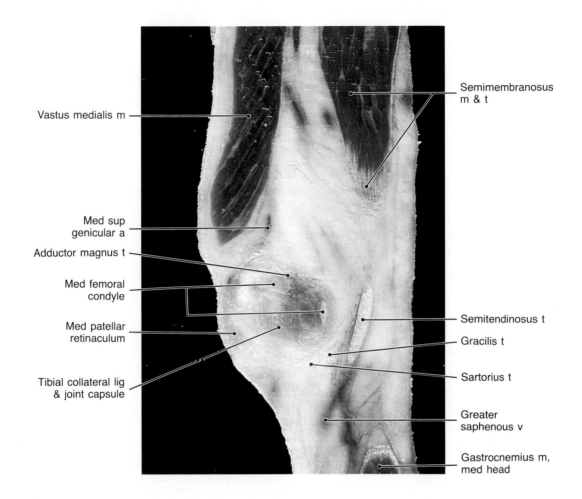

Vastus medialis m

Semimembranosus
m & t

Med sup
genicular a

Adductor magnus t

Med femoral
condyle

Med patellar
retinaculum

Tibial collateral lig
& joint capsule

Semitendinosus t

Gracilis t

Sartorius t

Greater
saphenous v

Gastrocnemius m,
med head

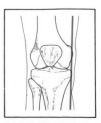

KNEE, SAGITTAL

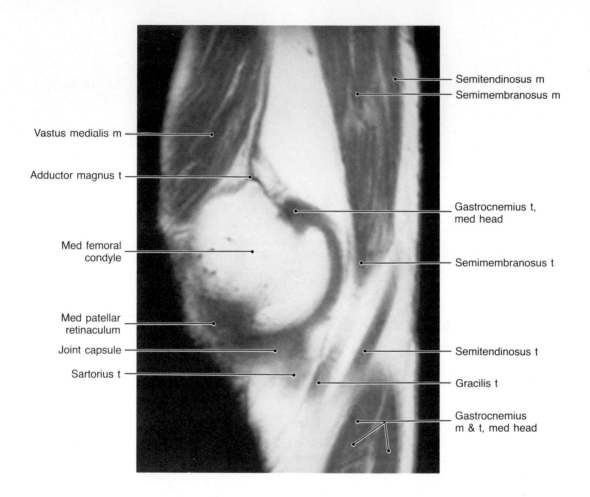

Vastus medialis m

Adductor magnus t

Med femoral
condyle

Med patellar
retinaculum

Joint capsule

Sartorius t

Semitendinosus m

Semimembranosus m

Gastrocnemius t,
med head

Semimembranosus t

Semitendinosus t

Gracilis t

Gastrocnemius
m & t, med head

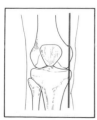

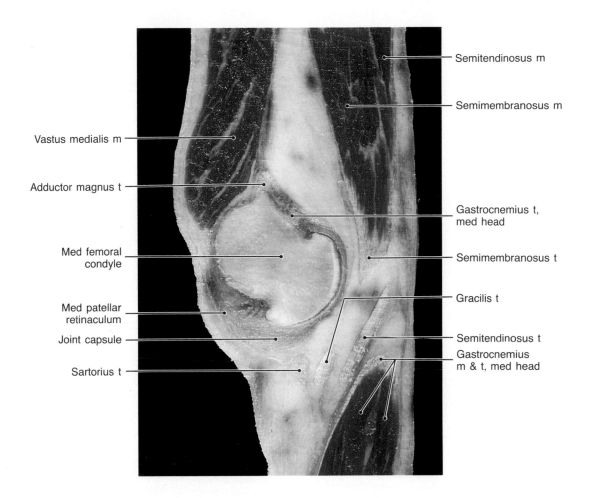

Vastus medialis m

Adductor magnus t

Med femoral condyle

Med patellar retinaculum

Joint capsule

Sartorius t

Semitendinosus m

Semimembranosus m

Gastrocnemius t, med head

Semimembranosus t

Gracilis t

Semitendinosus t

Gastrocnemius m & t, med head

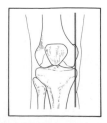

KNEE, SAGITTAL

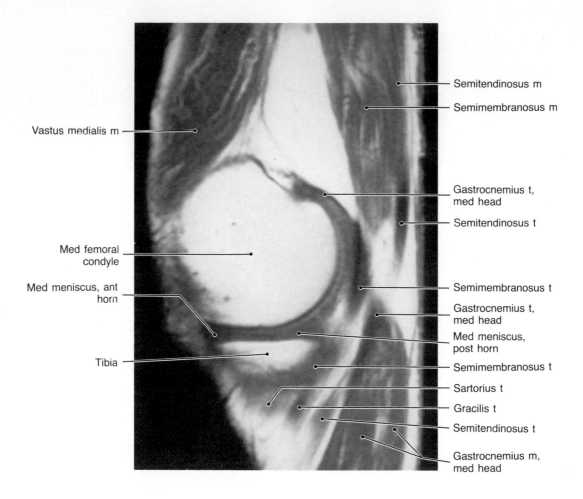

Vastus medialis m

Med femoral condyle

Med meniscus, ant horn

Tibia

Semitendinosus m

Semimembranosus m

Gastrocnemius t, med head

Semitendinosus t

Semimembranosus t

Gastrocnemius t, med head

Med meniscus, post horn

Semimembranosus t

Sartorius t

Gracilis t

Semitendinosus t

Gastrocnemius m, med head

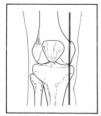

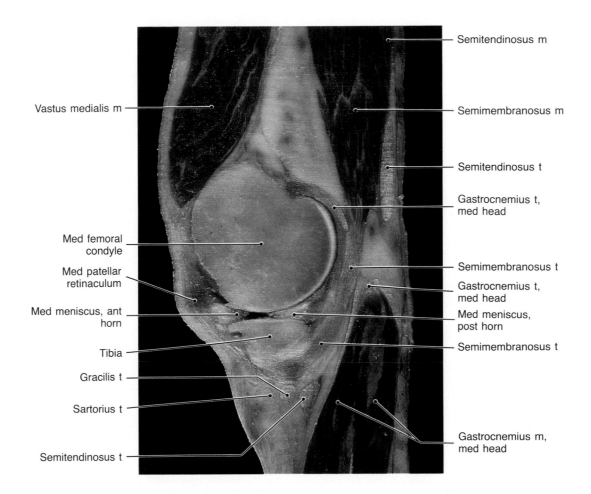

Semitendinosus m

Vastus medialis m

Semimembranosus m

Semitendinosus t

Gastrocnemius t,
med head

Med femoral
condyle

Med patellar
retinaculum

Semimembranosus t

Gastrocnemius t,
med head

Med meniscus, ant
horn

Med meniscus,
post horn

Tibia

Semimembranosus t

Gracilis t

Sartorius t

Gastrocnemius m,
med head

Semitendinosus t

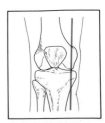

KNEE, SAGITTAL

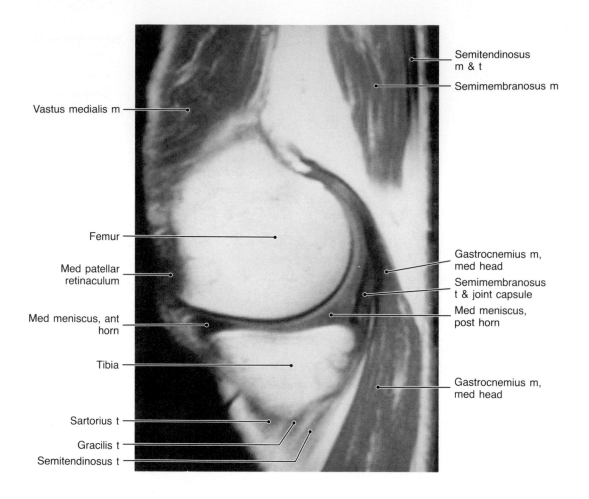

Vastus medialis m

Femur

Med patellar retinaculum

Med meniscus, ant horn

Tibia

Sartorius t

Gracilis t

Semitendinosus t

Semitendinosus m & t

Semimembranosus m

Gastrocnemius m, med head

Semimembranosus t & joint capsule

Med meniscus, post horn

Gastrocnemius m, med head

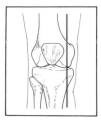

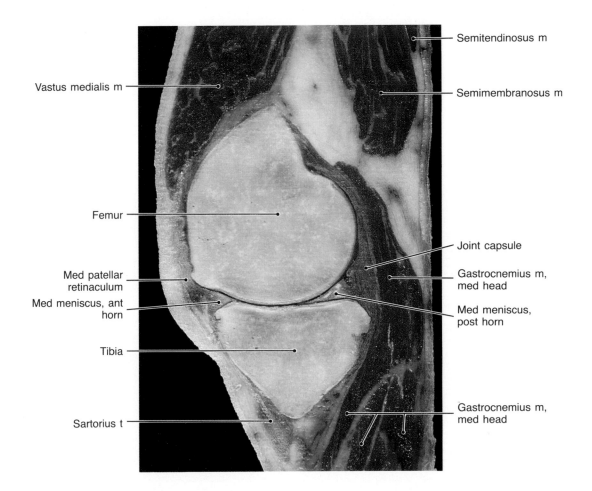

Semitendinosus m

Vastus medialis m

Semimembranosus m

Femur

Joint capsule

Med patellar
retinaculum

Gastrocnemius m,
med head

Med meniscus, ant
horn

Med meniscus,
post horn

Tibia

Sartorius t

Gastrocnemius m,
med head

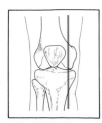

KNEE, SAGITTAL

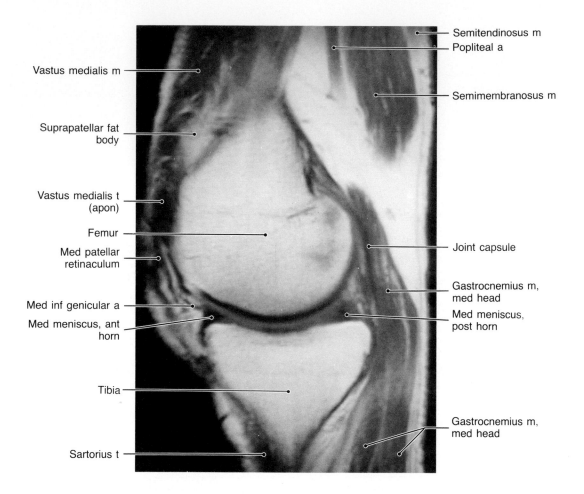

Vastus medialis m

Suprapatellar fat body

Vastus medialis t (apon)

Femur

Med patellar retinaculum

Med inf genicular a

Med meniscus, ant horn

Tibia

Sartorius t

Semitendinosus m

Popliteal a

Semimembranosus m

Joint capsule

Gastrocnemius m, med head

Med meniscus, post horn

Gastrocnemius m, med head

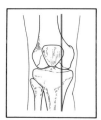

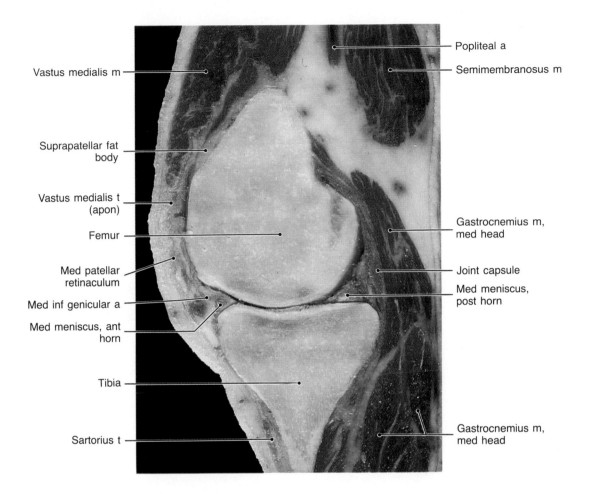

Vastus medialis m

Suprapatellar fat body

Vastus medialis t (apon)

Femur

Med patellar retinaculum

Med inf genicular a

Med meniscus, ant horn

Tibia

Sartorius t

Popliteal a

Semimembranosus m

Gastrocnemius m, med head

Joint capsule

Med meniscus, post horn

Gastrocnemius m, med head

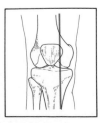

KNEE, SAGITTAL

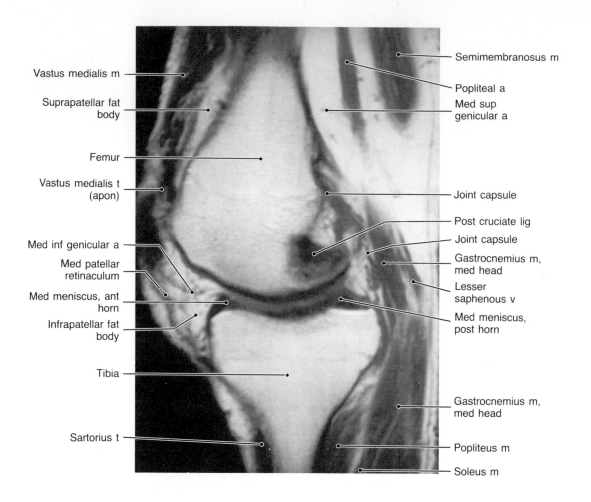

Vastus medialis m

Suprapatellar fat body

Femur

Vastus medialis t (apon)

Med inf genicular a

Med patellar retinaculum

Med meniscus, ant horn

Infrapatellar fat body

Tibia

Sartorius t

Semimembranosus m

Popliteal a

Med sup genicular a

Joint capsule

Post cruciate lig

Joint capsule

Gastrocnemius m, med head

Lesser saphenous v

Med meniscus, post horn

Gastrocnemius m, med head

Popliteus m

Soleus m

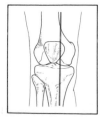

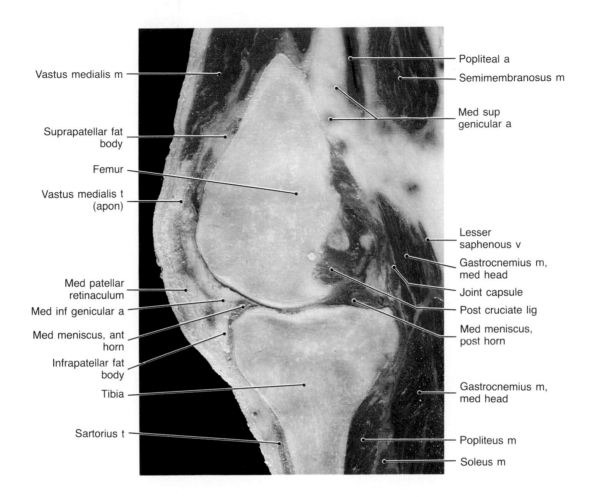

Vastus medialis m

Suprapatellar fat body

Femur

Vastus medialis t (apon)

Med patellar retinaculum

Med inf genicular a

Med meniscus, ant horn

Infrapatellar fat body

Tibia

Sartorius t

Popliteal a

Semimembranosus m

Med sup genicular a

Lesser saphenous v

Gastrocnemius m, med head

Joint capsule

Post cruciate lig

Med meniscus, post horn

Gastrocnemius m, med head

Popliteus m

Soleus m

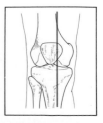

KNEE, SAGITTAL

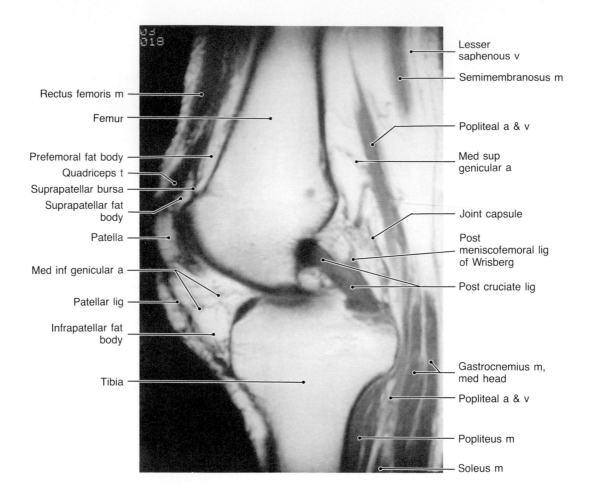

Rectus femoris m

Femur

Prefemoral fat body

Quadriceps t

Suprapatellar bursa

Suprapatellar fat body

Patella

Med inf genicular a

Patellar lig

Infrapatellar fat body

Tibia

Lesser saphenous v

Semimembranosus m

Popliteal a & v

Med sup genicular a

Joint capsule

Post meniscofemoral lig of Wrisberg

Post cruciate lig

Gastrocnemius m, med head

Popliteal a & v

Popliteus m

Soleus m

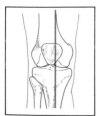

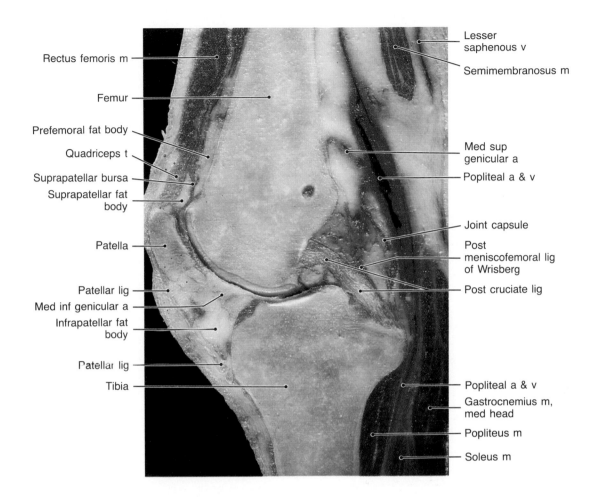

Rectus femoris m

Femur

Prefemoral fat body

Quadriceps t

Suprapatellar bursa

Suprapatellar fat body

Patella

Patellar lig

Med inf genicular a

Infrapatellar fat body

Patellar lig

Tibia

Lesser saphenous v

Semimembranosus m

Med sup genicular a

Popliteal a & v

Joint capsule

Post meniscofemoral lig of Wrisberg

Post cruciate lig

Popliteal a & v

Gastrocnemius m, med head

Popliteus m

Soleus m

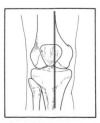

KNEE, SAGITTAL

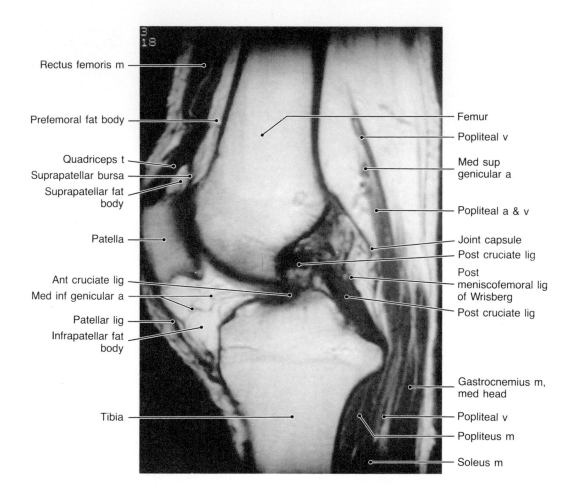

Rectus femoris m

Prefemoral fat body

Quadriceps t
Suprapatellar bursa
Suprapatellar fat body

Patella

Ant cruciate lig
Med inf genicular a

Patellar lig
Infrapatellar fat body

Tibia

Femur
Popliteal v

Med sup genicular a

Popliteal a & v

Joint capsule
Post cruciate lig

Post meniscofemoral lig of Wrisberg

Post cruciate lig

Gastrocnemius m, med head

Popliteal v
Popliteus m
Soleus m

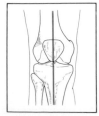

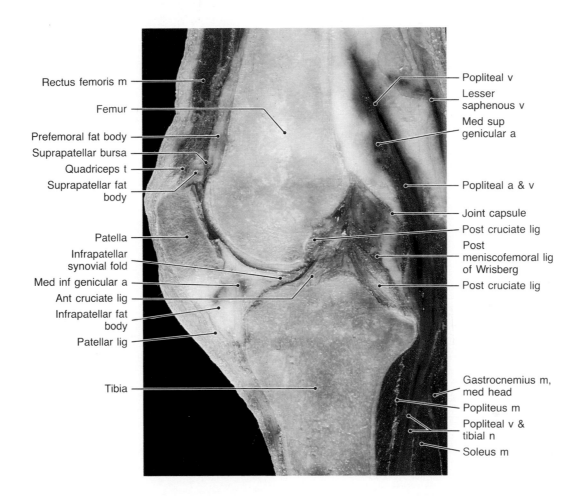

Rectus femoris m

Femur

Prefemoral fat body

Suprapatellar bursa

Quadriceps t

Suprapatellar fat body

Patella

Infrapatellar synovial fold

Med inf genicular a

Ant cruciate lig

Infrapatellar fat body

Patellar lig

Tibia

Popliteal v

Lesser saphenous v

Med sup genicular a

Popliteal a & v

Joint capsule

Post cruciate lig

Post meniscofemoral lig of Wrisberg

Post cruciate lig

Gastrocnemius m, med head

Popliteus m

Popliteal v & tibial n

Soleus m

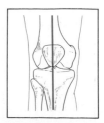

KNEE, SAGITTAL

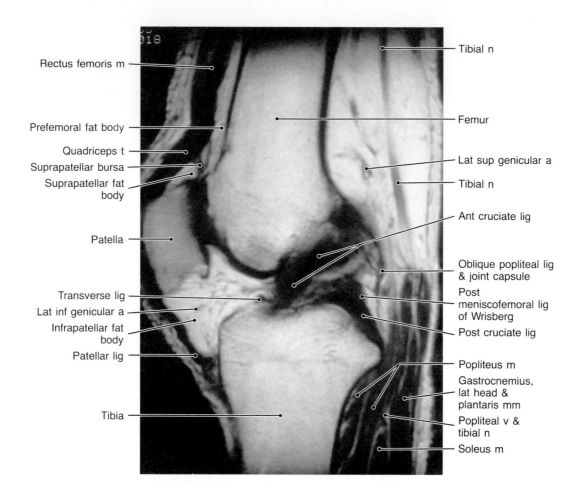

Rectus femoris m

Prefemoral fat body

Quadriceps t

Suprapatellar bursa

Suprapatellar fat body

Patella

Transverse lig

Lat inf genicular a

Infrapatellar fat body

Patellar lig

Tibia

Tibial n

Femur

Lat sup genicular a

Tibial n

Ant cruciate lig

Oblique popliteal lig & joint capsule

Post meniscofemoral lig of Wrisberg

Post cruciate lig

Popliteus m

Gastrocnemius, lat head & plantaris mm

Popliteal v & tibial n

Soleus m

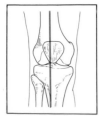

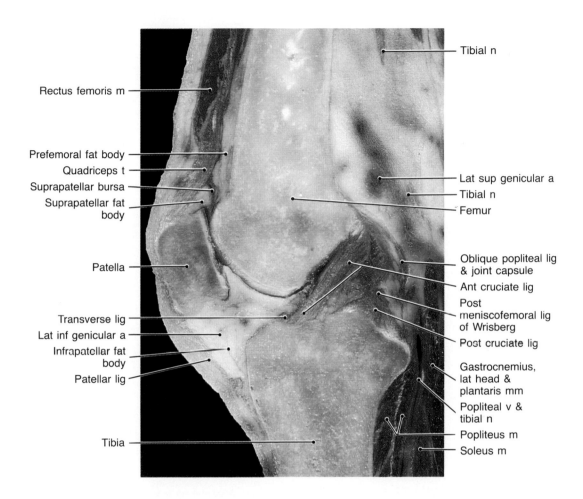

Rectus femoris m

Prefemoral fat body

Quadriceps t

Suprapatellar bursa

Suprapatellar fat body

Patella

Transverse lig

Lat inf genicular a

Infrapatellar fat body

Patellar lig

Tibia

Tibial n

Lat sup genicular a

Tibial n

Femur

Oblique popliteal lig & joint capsule

Ant cruciate lig

Post meniscofemoral lig of Wrisberg

Post cruciate lig

Gastrocnemius, lat head & plantaris mm

Popliteal v & tibial n

Popliteus m

Soleus m

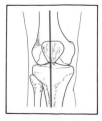

KNEE, SAGITTAL

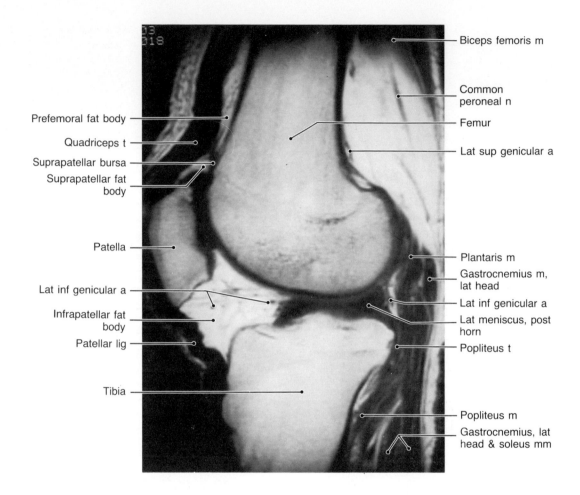

Biceps femoris m

Common peroneal n

Prefemoral fat body

Femur

Quadriceps t

Lat sup genicular a

Suprapatellar bursa

Suprapatellar fat body

Patella

Plantaris m

Gastrocnemius m, lat head

Lat inf genicular a

Lat inf genicular a

Infrapatellar fat body

Lat meniscus, post horn

Patellar lig

Popliteus t

Tibia

Popliteus m

Gastrocnemius, lat head & soleus mm

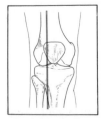

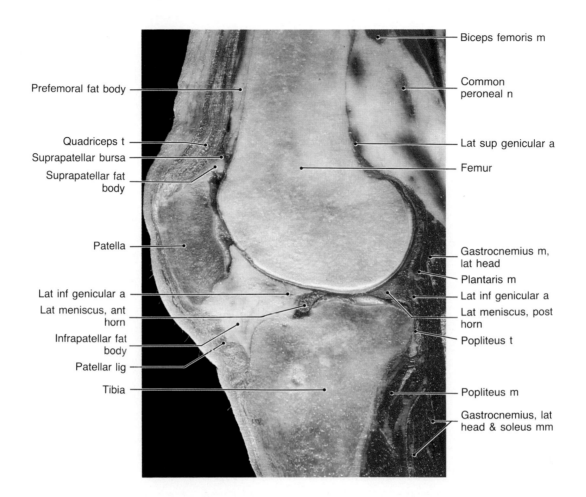

Prefemoral fat body

Quadriceps t
Suprapatellar bursa
Suprapatellar fat body

Patella

Lat inf genicular a
Lat meniscus, ant horn
Infrapatellar fat body
Patellar lig
Tibia

Biceps femoris m

Common peroneal n

Lat sup genicular a
Femur

Gastrocnemius m, lat head
Plantaris m
Lat inf genicular a
Lat meniscus, post horn
Popliteus t

Popliteus m

Gastrocnemius, lat head & soleus mm

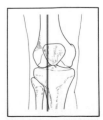

KNEE, SAGITTAL

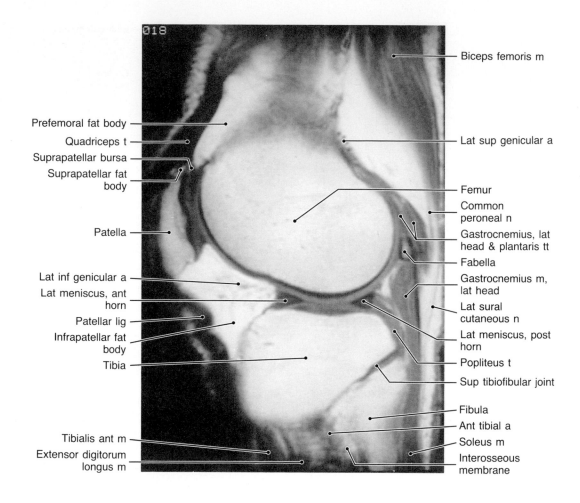

Biceps femoris m

Prefemoral fat body

Quadriceps t

Suprapatellar bursa

Suprapatellar fat body

Lat sup genicular a

Femur

Common peroneal n

Gastrocnemius, lat head & plantaris tt

Fabella

Gastrocnemius m, lat head

Lat sural cutaneous n

Lat meniscus, post horn

Popliteus t

Sup tibiofibular joint

Fibula

Ant tibial a

Soleus m

Interosseous membrane

Patella

Lat inf genicular a

Lat meniscus, ant horn

Patellar lig

Infrapatellar fat body

Tibia

Tibialis ant m

Extensor digitorum longus m

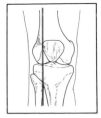

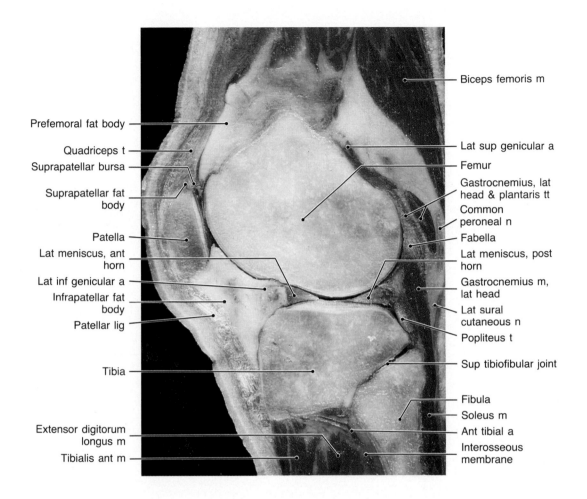

Prefemoral fat body

Quadriceps t

Suprapatellar bursa

Suprapatellar fat body

Patella

Lat meniscus, ant horn

Lat inf genicular a

Infrapatellar fat body

Patellar lig

Tibia

Extensor digitorum longus m

Tibialis ant m

Biceps femoris m

Lat sup genicular a

Femur

Gastrocnemius, lat head & plantaris tt

Common peroneal n

Fabella

Lat meniscus, post horn

Gastrocnemius m, lat head

Lat sural cutaneous n

Popliteus t

Sup tibiofibular joint

Fibula

Soleus m

Ant tibial a

Interosseous membrane

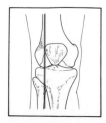

KNEE, SAGITTAL

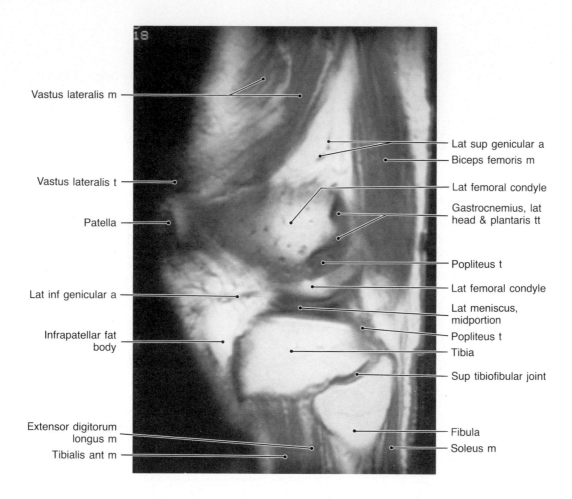

Vastus lateralis m

Vastus lateralis t

Patella

Lat inf genicular a

Infrapatellar fat body

Extensor digitorum longus m

Tibialis ant m

Lat sup genicular a

Biceps femoris m

Lat femoral condyle

Gastrocnemius, lat head & plantaris tt

Popliteus t

Lat femoral condyle

Lat meniscus, midportion

Popliteus t

Tibia

Sup tibiofibular joint

Fibula

Soleus m

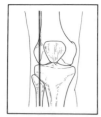

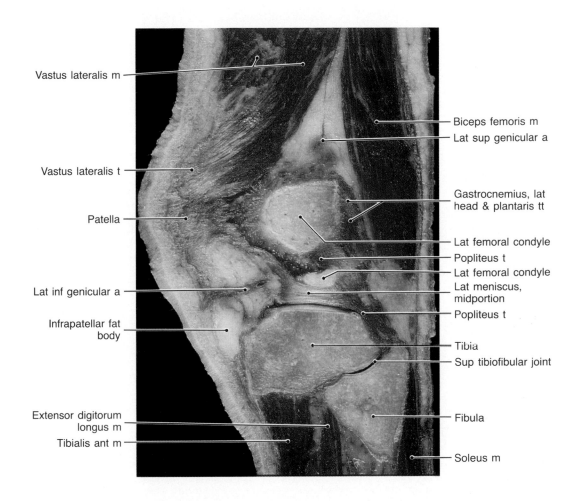

Vastus lateralis m

Vastus lateralis t

Patella

Lat inf genicular a

Infrapatellar fat body

Extensor digitorum longus m

Tibialis ant m

Biceps femoris m

Lat sup genicular a

Gastrocnemius, lat head & plantaris tt

Lat femoral condyle

Popliteus t

Lat femoral condyle

Lat meniscus, midportion

Popliteus t

Tibia

Sup tibiofibular joint

Fibula

Soleus m

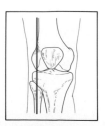

KNEE, SAGITTAL

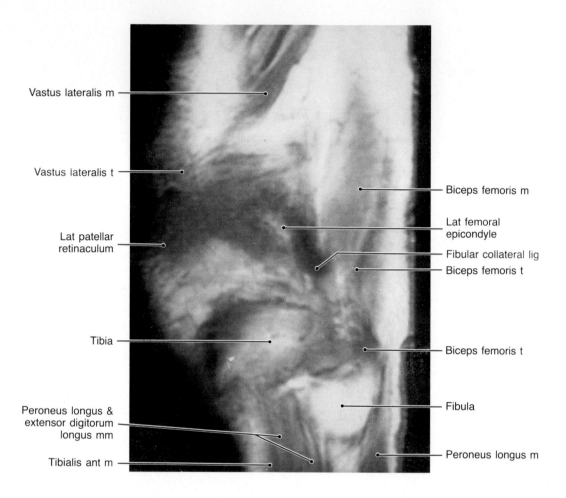

Vastus lateralis m

Vastus lateralis t

Lat patellar
retinaculum

Tibia

Peroneus longus &
extensor digitorum
longus mm

Tibialis ant m

Biceps femoris m

Lat femoral
epicondyle

Fibular collateral lig

Biceps femoris t

Biceps femoris t

Fibula

Peroneus longus m

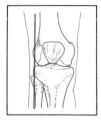

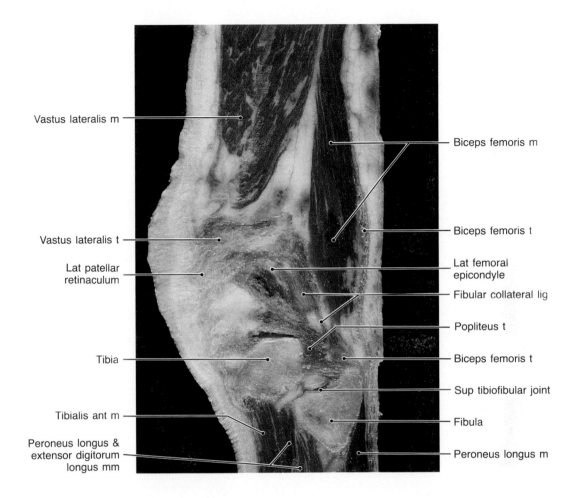

Vastus lateralis m

Vastus lateralis t

Lat patellar retinaculum

Tibia

Tibialis ant m

Peroneus longus & extensor digitorum longus mm

Biceps femoris m

Biceps femoris t

Lat femoral epicondyle

Fibular collateral lig

Popliteus t

Biceps femoris t

Sup tibiofibular joint

Fibula

Peroneus longus m

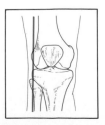

KNEE, SAGITTAL, INJECTED

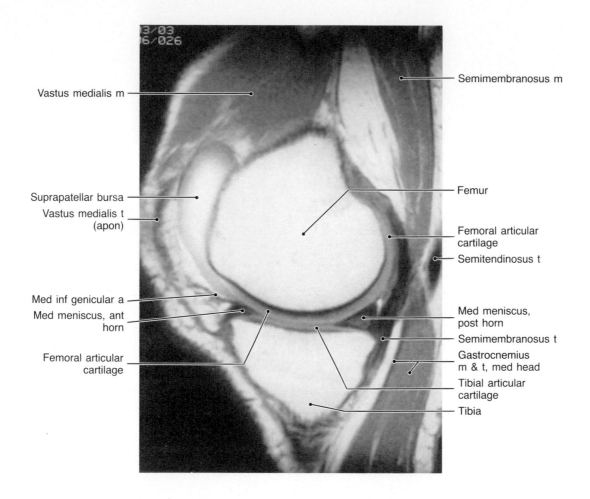

Vastus medialis m

Semimembranosus m

Suprapatellar bursa

Vastus medialis t
(apon)

Femur

Femoral articular
cartilage

Semitendinosus t

Med inf genicular a

Med meniscus, ant
horn

Femoral articular
cartilage

Med meniscus,
post horn

Semimembranosus t

Gastrocnemius
m & t, med head

Tibial articular
cartilage

Tibia

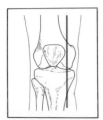

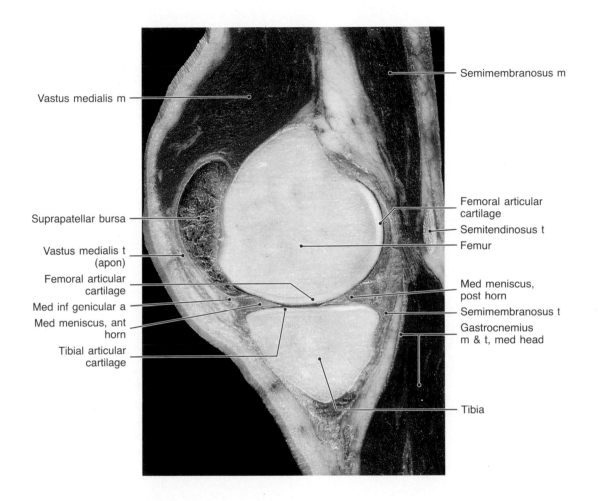

Vastus medialis m

Suprapatellar bursa

Vastus medialis t
(apon)

Femoral articular
cartilage

Med inf genicular a

Med meniscus, ant
horn

Tibial articular
cartilage

Semimembranosus m

Femoral articular
cartilage

Semitendinosus t

Femur

Med meniscus,
post horn

Semimembranosus t

Gastrocnemius
m & t, med head

Tibia

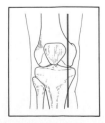

KNEE, SAGITTAL, INJECTED

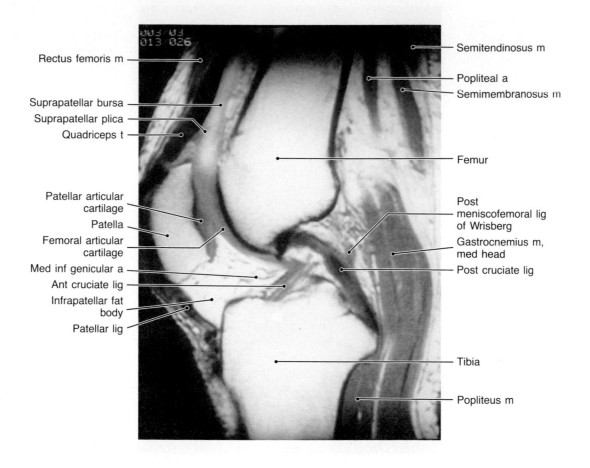

Rectus femoris m

Suprapatellar bursa

Suprapatellar plica

Quadriceps t

Patellar articular cartilage

Patella

Femoral articular cartilage

Med inf genicular a

Ant cruciate lig

Infrapatellar fat body

Patellar lig

Semitendinosus m

Popliteal a

Semimembranosus m

Femur

Post meniscofemoral lig of Wrisberg

Gastrocnemius m, med head

Post cruciate lig

Tibia

Popliteus m

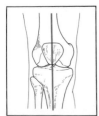

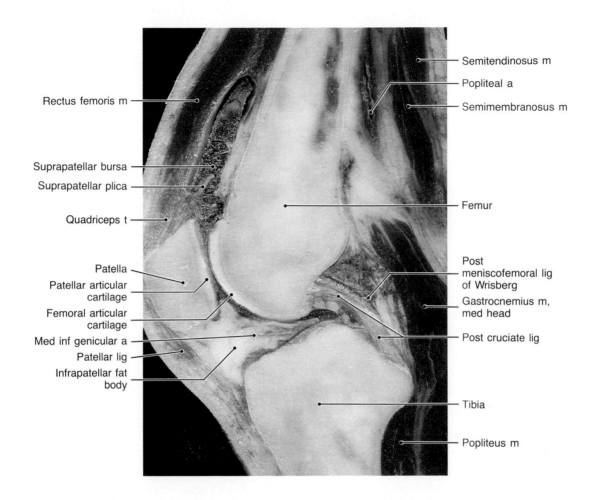

Rectus femoris m

Suprapatellar bursa

Suprapatellar plica

Quadriceps t

Patella

Patellar articular cartilage

Femoral articular cartilage

Med inf genicular a

Patellar lig

Infrapatellar fat body

Semitendinosus m

Popliteal a

Semimembranosus m

Femur

Post meniscofemoral lig of Wrisberg

Gastrocnemius m, med head

Post cruciate lig

Tibia

Popliteus m

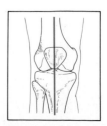

KNEE, SAGITTAL, INJECTED

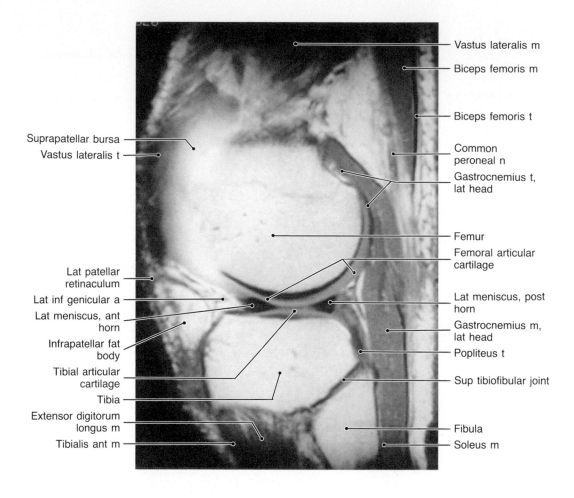

Vastus lateralis m

Biceps femoris m

Biceps femoris t

Suprapatellar bursa

Vastus lateralis t

Common peroneal n

Gastrocnemius t, lat head

Femur

Femoral articular cartilage

Lat patellar retinaculum

Lat inf genicular a

Lat meniscus, ant horn

Infrapatellar fat body

Tibial articular cartilage

Tibia

Extensor digitorum longus m

Tibialis ant m

Lat meniscus, post horn

Gastrocnemius m, lat head

Popliteus t

Sup tibiofibular joint

Fibula

Soleus m

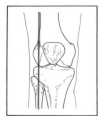

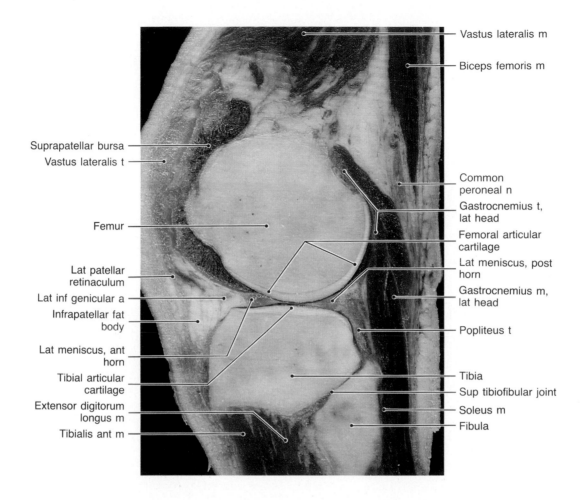

Vastus lateralis m

Biceps femoris m

Suprapatellar bursa

Vastus lateralis t

Common peroneal n

Gastrocnemius t, lat head

Femur

Femoral articular cartilage

Lat patellar retinaculum

Lat meniscus, post horn

Lat inf genicular a

Gastrocnemius m, lat head

Infrapatellar fat body

Popliteus t

Lat meniscus, ant horn

Tibial articular cartilage

Tibia

Sup tibiofibular joint

Extensor digitorum longus m

Soleus m

Tibialis ant m

Fibula

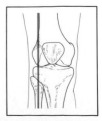

7 ANKLE AND FOOT

ANKLE AND FOOT, CORONAL

Peroneus brevis m

Flexor hallucis longus m & t

Sural n

Lesser saphenous v

Calcaneus

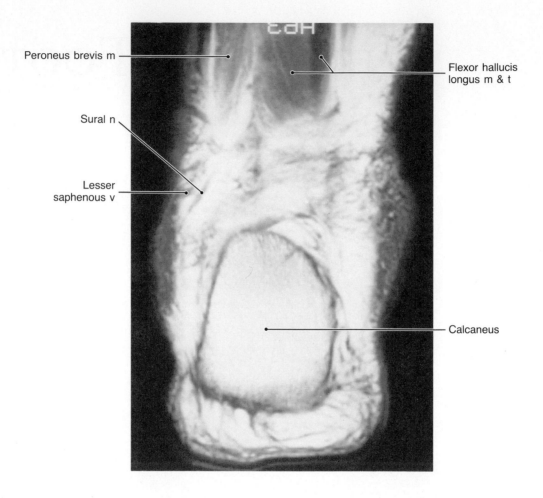

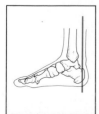

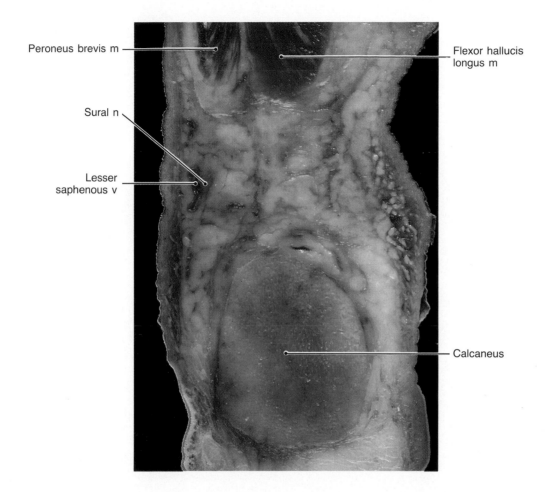

Peroneus brevis m

Flexor hallucis
longus m

Sural n

Lesser
saphenous v

Calcaneus

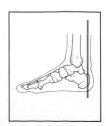

ANKLE AND FOOT, CORONAL

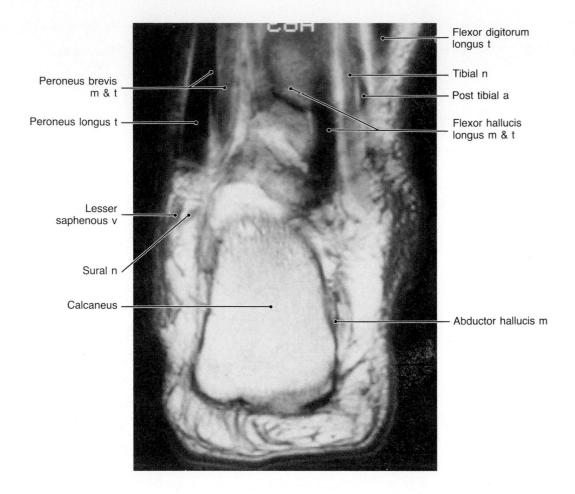

Peroneus brevis m & t

Peroneus longus t

Lesser saphenous v

Sural n

Calcaneus

Flexor digitorum longus t

Tibial n

Post tibial a

Flexor hallucis longus m & t

Abductor hallucis m

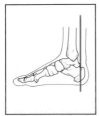

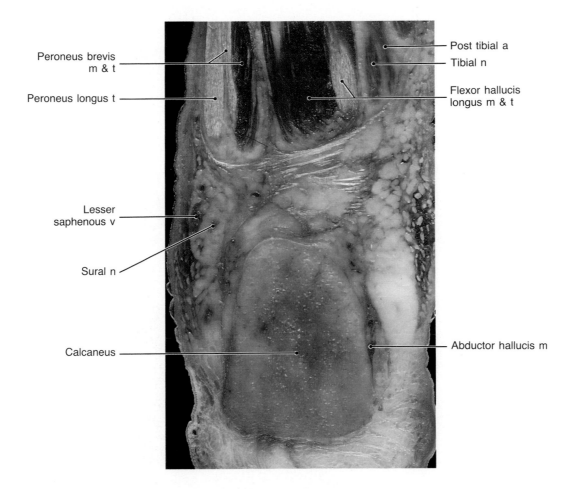

Peroneus brevis
m & t

Peroneus longus t

Lesser
saphenous v

Sural n

Calcaneus

Post tibial a

Tibial n

Flexor hallucis
longus m & t

Abductor hallucis m

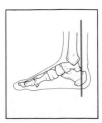

ANKLE AND FOOT, CORONAL

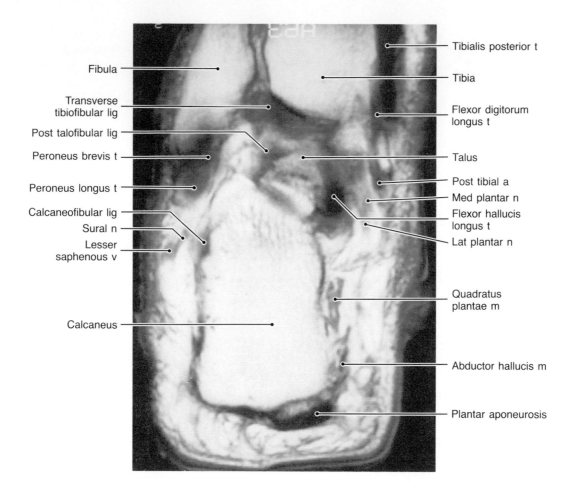

Fibula

Transverse
tibiofibular lig

Post talofibular lig

Peroneus brevis t

Peroneus longus t

Calcaneofibular lig

Sural n

Lesser
saphenous v

Calcaneus

Tibialis posterior t

Tibia

Flexor digitorum
longus t

Talus

Post tibial a

Med plantar n

Flexor hallucis
longus t

Lat plantar n

Quadratus
plantae m

Abductor hallucis m

Plantar aponeurosis

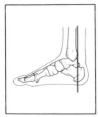

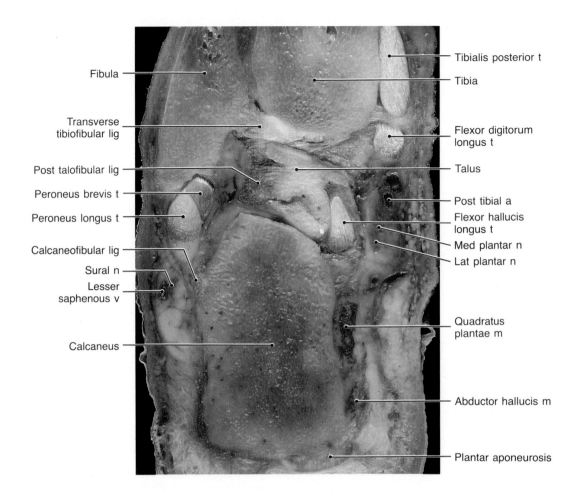

Fibula

Transverse
tibiofibular lig

Post talofibular lig

Peroneus brevis t

Peroneus longus t

Calcaneofibular lig

Sural n

Lesser
saphenous v

Calcaneus

Tibialis posterior t

Tibia

Flexor digitorum
longus t

Talus

Post tibial a

Flexor hallucis
longus t

Med plantar n

Lat plantar n

Quadratus
plantae m

Abductor hallucis m

Plantar aponeurosis

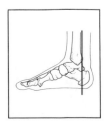

ANKLE AND FOOT, CORONAL

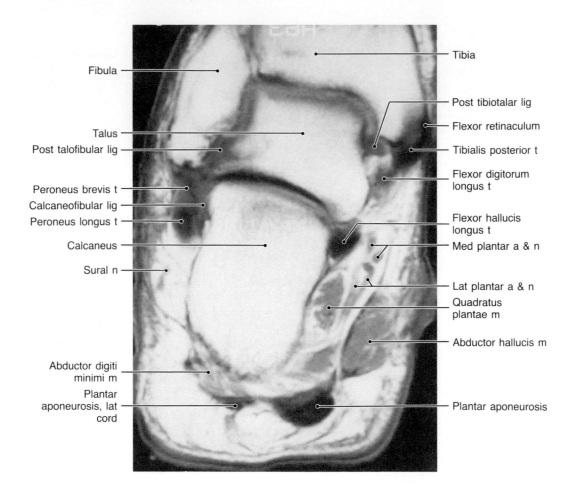

Fibula

Talus

Post talofibular lig

Peroneus brevis t

Calcaneofibular lig

Peroneus longus t

Calcaneus

Sural n

Abductor digiti
minimi m

Plantar
aponeurosis, lat
cord

Tibia

Post tibiotalar lig

Flexor retinaculum

Tibialis posterior t

Flexor digitorum
longus t

Flexor hallucis
longus t

Med plantar a & n

Lat plantar a & n

Quadratus
plantae m

Abductor hallucis m

Plantar aponeurosis

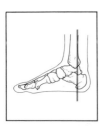

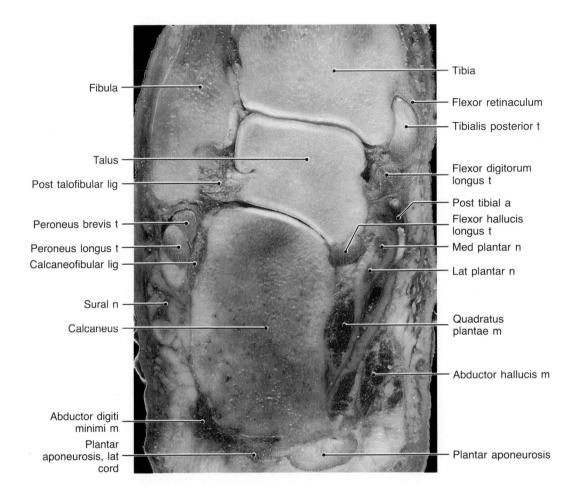

Fibula

Talus

Post talofibular lig

Peroneus brevis t

Peroneus longus t

Calcaneofibular lig

Sural n

Calcaneus

Abductor digiti minimi m

Plantar aponeurosis, lat cord

Tibia

Flexor retinaculum

Tibialis posterior t

Flexor digitorum longus t

Post tibial a

Flexor hallucis longus t

Med plantar n

Lat plantar n

Quadratus plantae m

Abductor hallucis m

Plantar aponeurosis

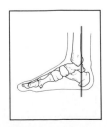

ANKLE AND FOOT, CORONAL

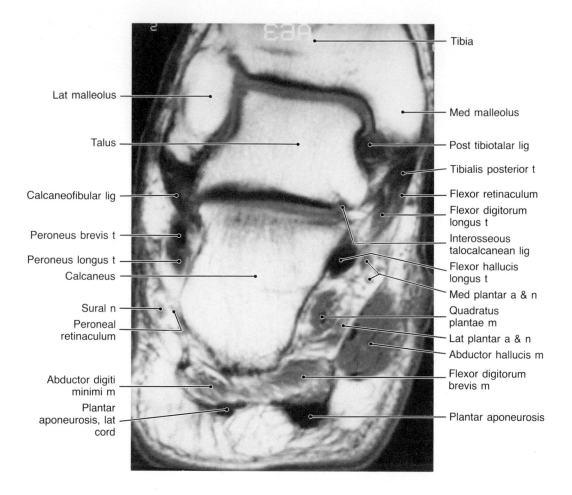

Lat malleolus

Talus

Calcaneofibular lig

Peroneus brevis t

Peroneus longus t

Calcaneus

Sural n

Peroneal retinaculum

Abductor digiti minimi m

Plantar aponeurosis, lat cord

Tibia

Med malleolus

Post tibiotalar lig

Tibialis posterior t

Flexor retinaculum

Flexor digitorum longus t

Interosseous talocalcanean lig

Flexor hallucis longus t

Med plantar a & n

Quadratus plantae m

Lat plantar a & n

Abductor hallucis m

Flexor digitorum brevis m

Plantar aponeurosis

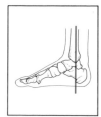

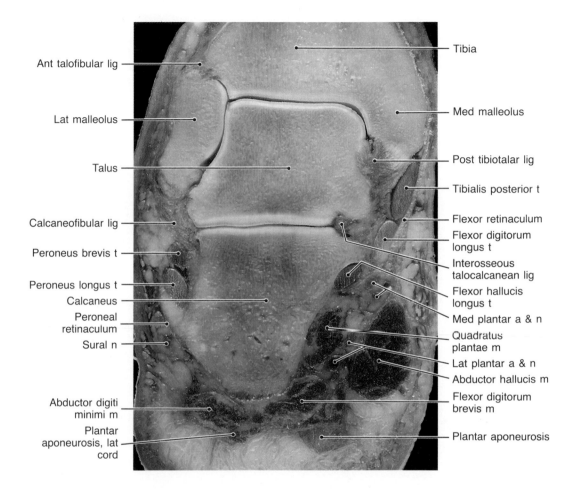

Ant talofibular lig

Lat malleolus

Talus

Calcaneofibular lig

Peroneus brevis t

Peroneus longus t

Calcaneus

Peroneal retinaculum

Sural n

Abductor digiti minimi m

Plantar aponeurosis, lat cord

Tibia

Med malleolus

Post tibiotalar lig

Tibialis posterior t

Flexor retinaculum

Flexor digitorum longus t

Interosseous talocalcanean lig

Flexor hallucis longus t

Med plantar a & n

Quadratus plantae m

Lat plantar a & n

Abductor hallucis m

Flexor digitorum brevis m

Plantar aponeurosis

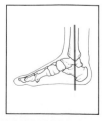

ANKLE AND FOOT, CORONAL

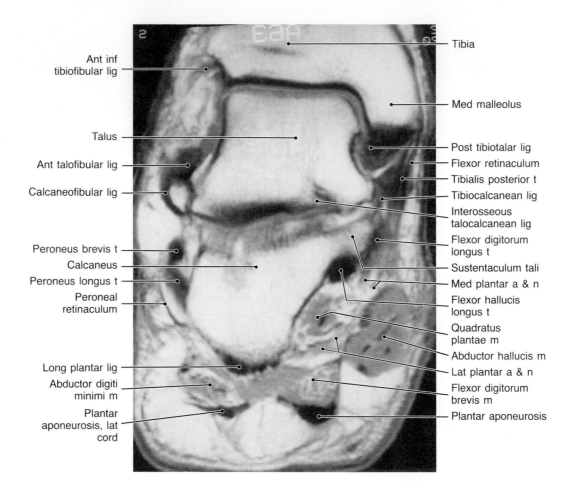

Ant inf tibiofibular lig

Talus

Ant talofibular lig

Calcaneofibular lig

Peroneus brevis t

Calcaneus

Peroneus longus t

Peroneal retinaculum

Long plantar lig

Abductor digiti minimi m

Plantar aponeurosis, lat cord

Tibia

Med malleolus

Post tibiotalar lig

Flexor retinaculum

Tibialis posterior t

Tibiocalcanean lig

Interosseous talocalcanean lig

Flexor digitorum longus t

Sustentaculum tali

Med plantar a & n

Flexor hallucis longus t

Quadratus plantae m

Abductor hallucis m

Lat plantar a & n

Flexor digitorum brevis m

Plantar aponeurosis

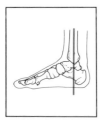

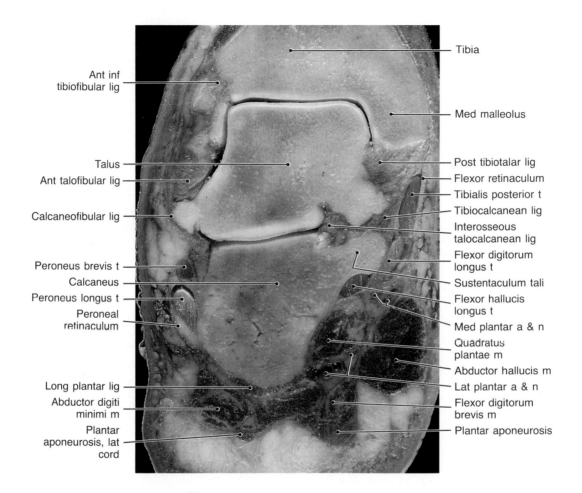

Ant inf tibiofibular lig

Talus

Ant talofibular lig

Calcaneofibular lig

Peroneus brevis t

Calcaneus

Peroneus longus t

Peroneal retinaculum

Long plantar lig

Abductor digiti minimi m

Plantar aponeurosis, lat cord

Tibia

Med malleolus

Post tibiotalar lig

Flexor retinaculum

Tibialis posterior t

Tibiocalcanean lig

Interosseous talocalcanean lig

Flexor digitorum longus t

Sustentaculum tali

Flexor hallucis longus t

Med plantar a & n

Quadratus plantae m

Abductor hallucis m

Lat plantar a & n

Flexor digitorum brevis m

Plantar aponeurosis

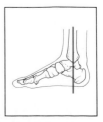

ANKLE AND FOOT, CORONAL

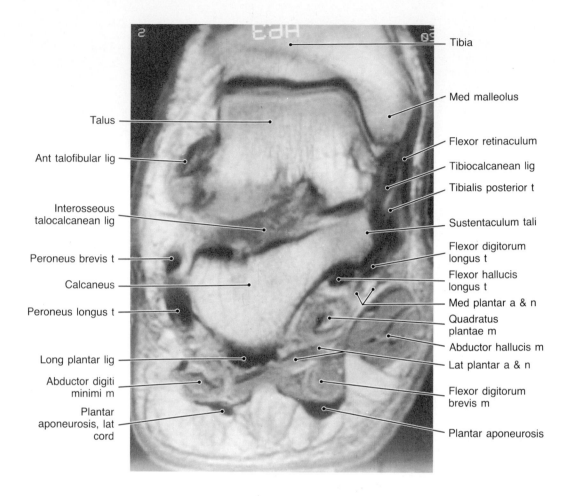

Talus

Ant talofibular lig

Interosseous talocalcanean lig

Peroneus brevis t

Calcaneus

Peroneus longus t

Long plantar lig

Abductor digiti minimi m

Plantar aponeurosis, lat cord

Tibia

Med malleolus

Flexor retinaculum

Tibiocalcanean lig

Tibialis posterior t

Sustentaculum tali

Flexor digitorum longus t

Flexor hallucis longus t

Med plantar a & n

Quadratus plantae m

Abductor hallucis m

Lat plantar a & n

Flexor digitorum brevis m

Plantar aponeurosis

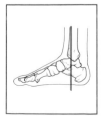

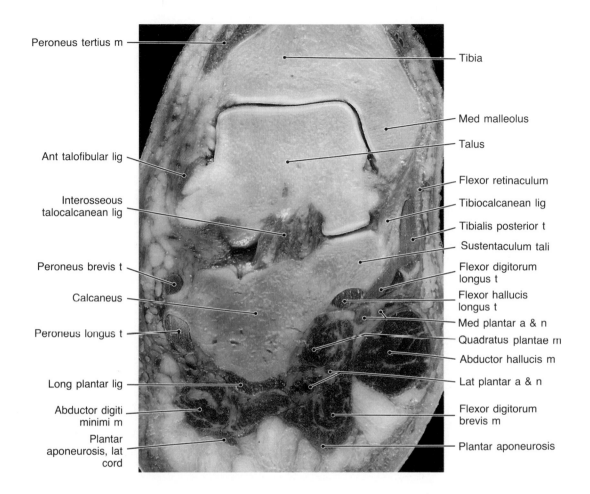

Peroneus tertius m

Ant talofibular lig

Interosseous talocalcanean lig

Peroneus brevis t

Calcaneus

Peroneus longus t

Long plantar lig

Abductor digiti minimi m

Plantar aponeurosis, lat cord

Tibia

Med malleolus

Talus

Flexor retinaculum

Tibiocalcanean lig

Tibialis posterior t

Sustentaculum tali

Flexor digitorum longus t

Flexor hallucis longus t

Med plantar a & n

Quadratus plantae m

Abductor hallucis m

Lat plantar a & n

Flexor digitorum brevis m

Plantar aponeurosis

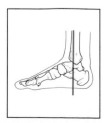

ANKLE AND FOOT, CORONAL

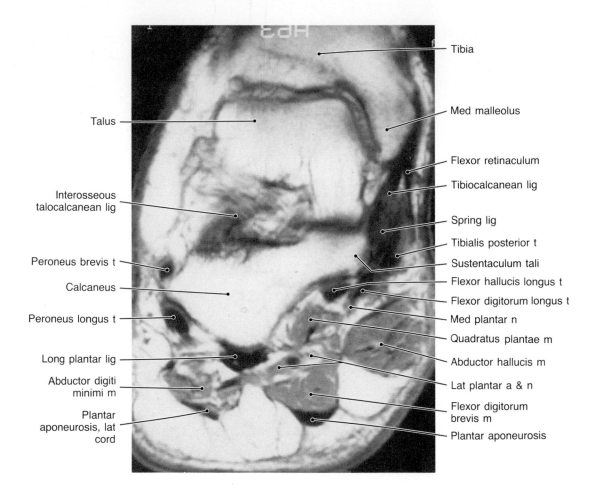

- Tibia
- Talus
- Med malleolus
- Flexor retinaculum
- Tibiocalcanean lig
- Interosseous talocalcanean lig
- Spring lig
- Tibialis posterior t
- Peroneus brevis t
- Sustentaculum tali
- Calcaneus
- Flexor hallucis longus t
- Flexor digitorum longus t
- Peroneus longus t
- Med plantar n
- Quadratus plantae m
- Long plantar lig
- Abductor hallucis m
- Abductor digiti minimi m
- Lat plantar a & n
- Flexor digitorum brevis m
- Plantar aponeurosis, lat cord
- Plantar aponeurosis

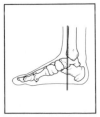

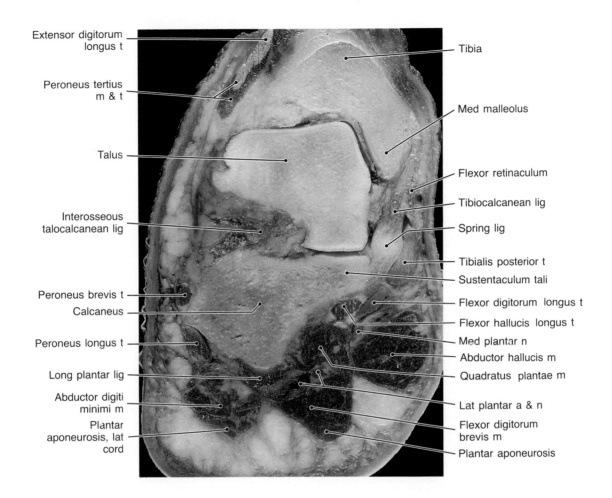

Extensor digitorum longus t

Peroneus tertius m & t

Talus

Interosseous talocalcanean lig

Peroneus brevis t

Calcaneus

Peroneus longus t

Long plantar lig

Abductor digiti minimi m

Plantar aponeurosis, lat cord

Tibia

Med malleolus

Flexor retinaculum

Tibiocalcanean lig

Spring lig

Tibialis posterior t

Sustentaculum tali

Flexor digitorum longus t

Flexor hallucis longus t

Med plantar n

Abductor hallucis m

Quadratus plantae m

Lat plantar a & n

Flexor digitorum brevis m

Plantar aponeurosis

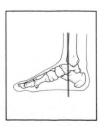

ANKLE AND FOOT, CORONAL

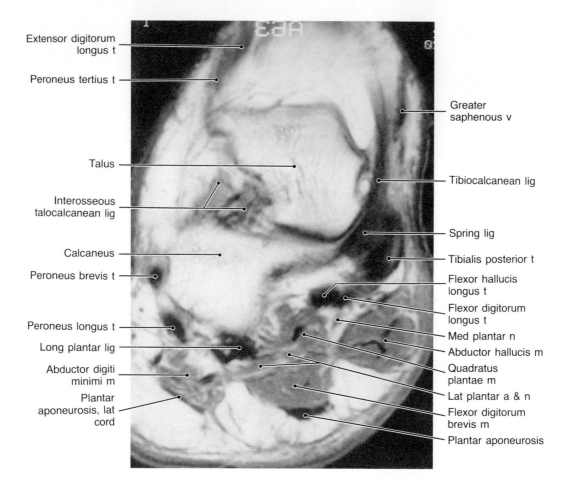

Extensor digitorum longus t

Peroneus tertius t

Greater saphenous v

Talus

Tibiocalcanean lig

Interosseous talocalcanean lig

Spring lig

Calcaneus

Tibialis posterior t

Peroneus brevis t

Flexor hallucis longus t

Flexor digitorum longus t

Peroneus longus t

Med plantar n

Long plantar lig

Abductor hallucis m

Abductor digiti minimi m

Quadratus plantae m

Plantar aponeurosis, lat cord

Lat plantar a & n

Flexor digitorum brevis m

Plantar aponeurosis

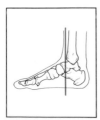

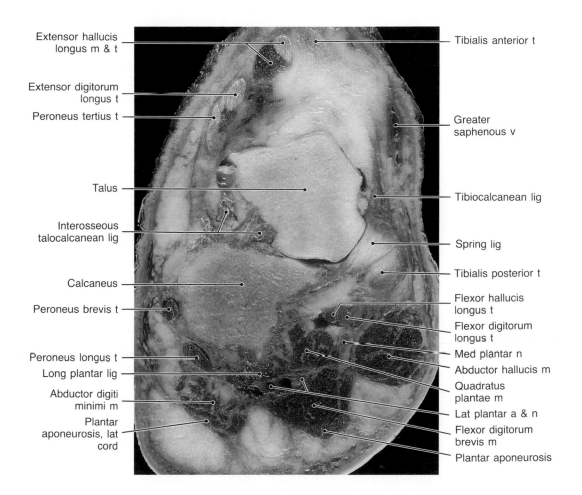

Extensor hallucis longus m & t

Extensor digitorum longus t

Peroneus tertius t

Talus

Interosseous talocalcanean lig

Calcaneus

Peroneus brevis t

Peroneus longus t

Long plantar lig

Abductor digiti minimi m

Plantar aponeurosis, lat cord

Tibialis anterior t

Greater saphenous v

Tibiocalcanean lig

Spring lig

Tibialis posterior t

Flexor hallucis longus t

Flexor digitorum longus t

Med plantar n

Abductor hallucis m

Quadratus plantae m

Lat plantar a & n

Flexor digitorum brevis m

Plantar aponeurosis

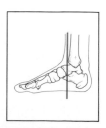

ANKLE AND FOOT, CORONAL

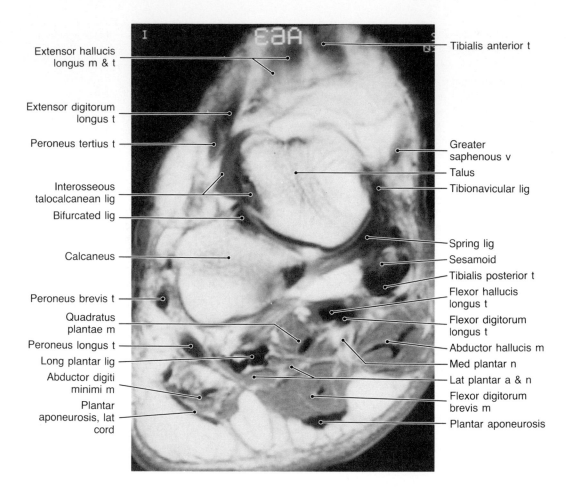

Extensor hallucis longus m & t

Extensor digitorum longus t

Peroneus tertius t

Interosseous talocalcanean lig

Bifurcated lig

Calcaneus

Peroneus brevis t

Quadratus plantae m

Peroneus longus t

Long plantar lig

Abductor digiti minimi m

Plantar aponeurosis, lat cord

Tibialis anterior t

Greater saphenous v

Talus

Tibionavicular lig

Spring lig

Sesamoid

Tibialis posterior t

Flexor hallucis longus t

Flexor digitorum longus t

Abductor hallucis m

Med plantar n

Lat plantar a & n

Flexor digitorum brevis m

Plantar aponeurosis

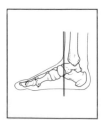

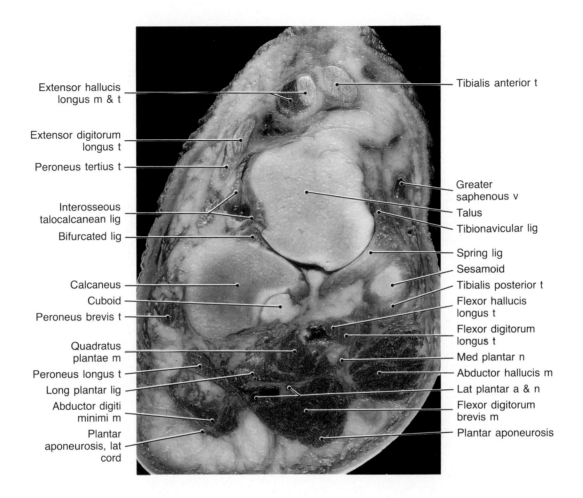

Extensor hallucis longus m & t

Extensor digitorum longus t

Peroneus tertius t

Interosseous talocalcanean lig

Bifurcated lig

Calcaneus

Cuboid

Peroneus brevis t

Quadratus plantae m

Peroneus longus t

Long plantar lig

Abductor digiti minimi m

Plantar aponeurosis, lat cord

Tibialis anterior t

Greater saphenous v

Talus

Tibionavicular lig

Spring lig

Sesamoid

Tibialis posterior t

Flexor hallucis longus t

Flexor digitorum longus t

Med plantar n

Abductor hallucis m

Lat plantar a & n

Flexor digitorum brevis m

Plantar aponeurosis

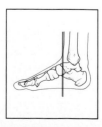

ANKLE AND FOOT, CORONAL

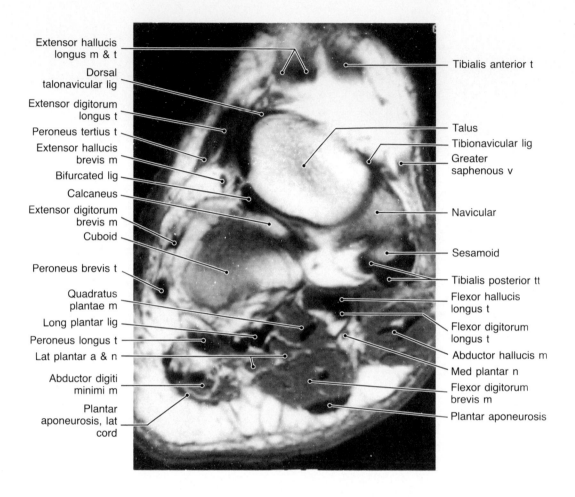

Extensor hallucis longus m & t

Dorsal talonavicular lig

Extensor digitorum longus t

Peroneus tertius t

Extensor hallucis brevis m

Bifurcated lig

Calcaneus

Extensor digitorum brevis m

Cuboid

Peroneus brevis t

Quadratus plantae m

Long plantar lig

Peroneus longus t

Lat plantar a & n

Abductor digiti minimi m

Plantar aponeurosis, lat cord

Tibialis anterior t

Talus

Tibionavicular lig

Greater saphenous v

Navicular

Sesamoid

Tibialis posterior tt

Flexor hallucis longus t

Flexor digitorum longus t

Abductor hallucis m

Med plantar n

Flexor digitorum brevis m

Plantar aponeurosis

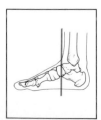

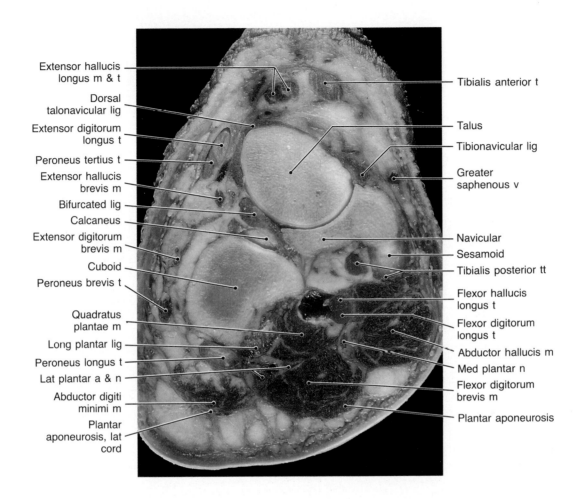

Extensor hallucis longus m & t

Dorsal talonavicular lig

Extensor digitorum longus t

Peroneus tertius t

Extensor hallucis brevis m

Bifurcated lig

Calcaneus

Extensor digitorum brevis m

Cuboid

Peroneus brevis t

Quadratus plantae m

Long plantar lig

Peroneus longus t

Lat plantar a & n

Abductor digiti minimi m

Plantar aponeurosis, lat cord

Tibialis anterior t

Talus

Tibionavicular lig

Greater saphenous v

Navicular

Sesamoid

Tibialis posterior tt

Flexor hallucis longus t

Flexor digitorum longus t

Abductor hallucis m

Med plantar n

Flexor digitorum brevis m

Plantar aponeurosis

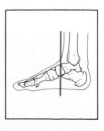

ANKLE AND FOOT, CORONAL

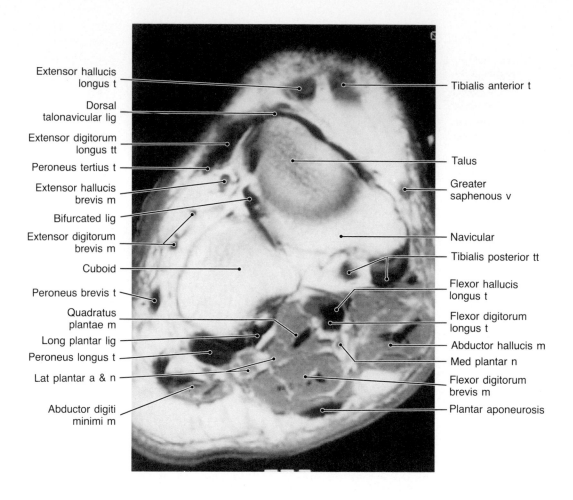

Extensor hallucis longus t

Dorsal talonavicular lig

Extensor digitorum longus tt

Peroneus tertius t

Extensor hallucis brevis m

Bifurcated lig

Extensor digitorum brevis m

Cuboid

Peroneus brevis t

Quadratus plantae m

Long plantar lig

Peroneus longus t

Lat plantar a & n

Abductor digiti minimi m

Tibialis anterior t

Talus

Greater saphenous v

Navicular

Tibialis posterior tt

Flexor hallucis longus t

Flexor digitorum longus t

Abductor hallucis m

Med plantar n

Flexor digitorum brevis m

Plantar aponeurosis

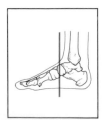

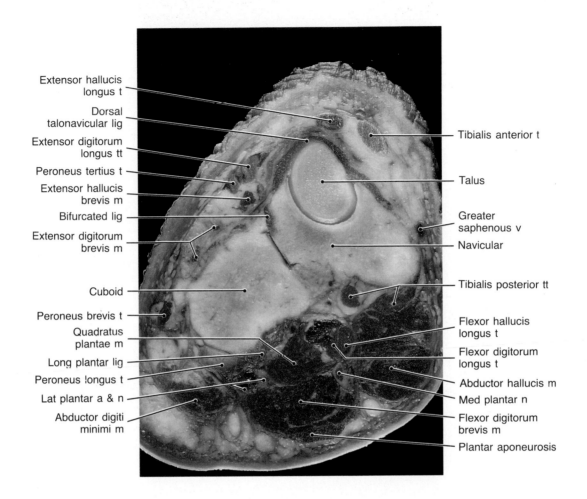

Extensor hallucis longus t

Dorsal talonavicular lig

Extensor digitorum longus tt

Peroneus tertius t

Extensor hallucis brevis m

Bifurcated lig

Extensor digitorum brevis m

Cuboid

Peroneus brevis t

Quadratus plantae m

Long plantar lig

Peroneus longus t

Lat plantar a & n

Abductor digiti minimi m

Tibialis anterior t

Talus

Greater saphenous v

Navicular

Tibialis posterior tt

Flexor hallucis longus t

Flexor digitorum longus t

Abductor hallucis m

Med plantar n

Flexor digitorum brevis m

Plantar aponeurosis

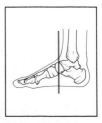

ANKLE AND FOOT, CORONAL

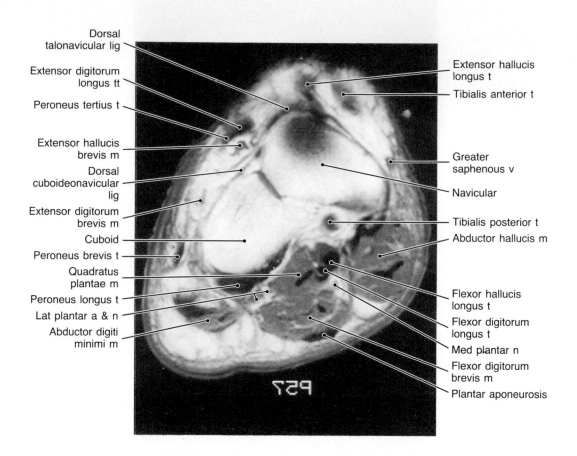

Dorsal talonavicular lig

Extensor digitorum longus tt

Peroneus tertius t

Extensor hallucis brevis m

Dorsal cuboideonavicular lig

Extensor digitorum brevis m

Cuboid

Peroneus brevis t

Quadratus plantae m

Peroneus longus t

Lat plantar a & n

Abductor digiti minimi m

Extensor hallucis longus t

Tibialis anterior t

Greater saphenous v

Navicular

Tibialis posterior t

Abductor hallucis m

Flexor hallucis longus t

Flexor digitorum longus t

Med plantar n

Flexor digitorum brevis m

Plantar aponeurosis

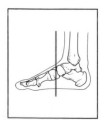

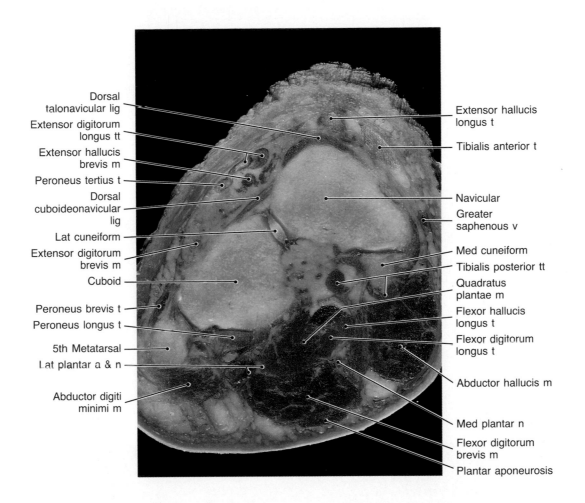

Dorsal talonavicular lig

Extensor digitorum longus tt

Extensor hallucis brevis m

Peroneus tertius t

Dorsal cuboideonavicular lig

Lat cuneiform

Extensor digitorum brevis m

Cuboid

Peroneus brevis t

Peroneus longus t

5th Metatarsal

Lat plantar a & n

Abductor digiti minimi m

Extensor hallucis longus t

Tibialis anterior t

Navicular

Greater saphenous v

Med cuneiform

Tibialis posterior tt

Quadratus plantae m

Flexor hallucis longus t

Flexor digitorum longus t

Abductor hallucis m

Med plantar n

Flexor digitorum brevis m

Plantar aponeurosis

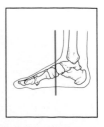

ANKLE AND FOOT, CORONAL

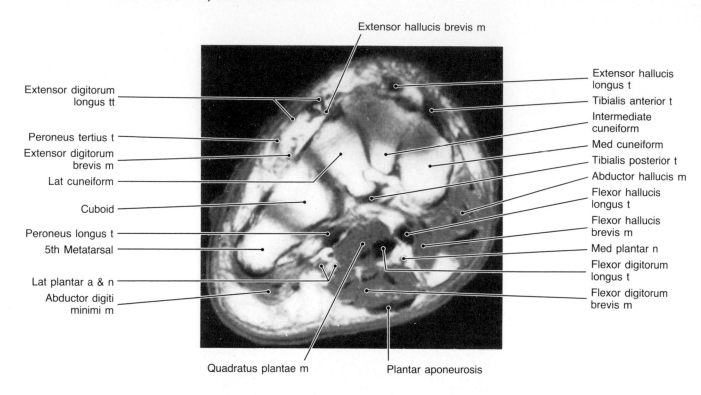

Extensor hallucis brevis m

Extensor digitorum longus tt

Peroneus tertius t

Extensor digitorum brevis m

Lat cuneiform

Cuboid

Peroneus longus t

5th Metatarsal

Lat plantar a & n

Abductor digiti minimi m

Extensor hallucis longus t

Tibialis anterior t

Intermediate cuneiform

Med cuneiform

Tibialis posterior t

Abductor hallucis m

Flexor hallucis longus t

Flexor hallucis brevis m

Med plantar n

Flexor digitorum longus t

Flexor digitorum brevis m

Quadratus plantae m

Plantar aponeurosis

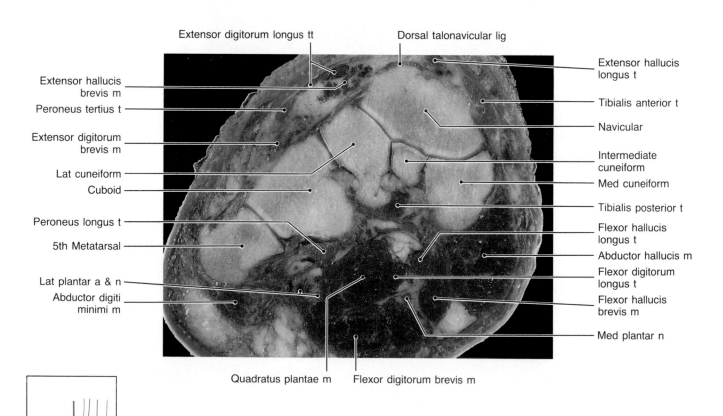

Extensor digitorum longus tt

Dorsal talonavicular lig

Extensor hallucis brevis m

Peroneus tertius t

Extensor digitorum brevis m

Lat cuneiform

Cuboid

Peroneus longus t

5th Metatarsal

Lat plantar a & n

Abductor digiti minimi m

Extensor hallucis longus t

Tibialis anterior t

Navicular

Intermediate cuneiform

Med cuneiform

Tibialis posterior t

Flexor hallucis longus t

Abductor hallucis m

Flexor digitorum longus t

Flexor hallucis brevis m

Med plantar n

Quadratus plantae m   Flexor digitorum brevis m

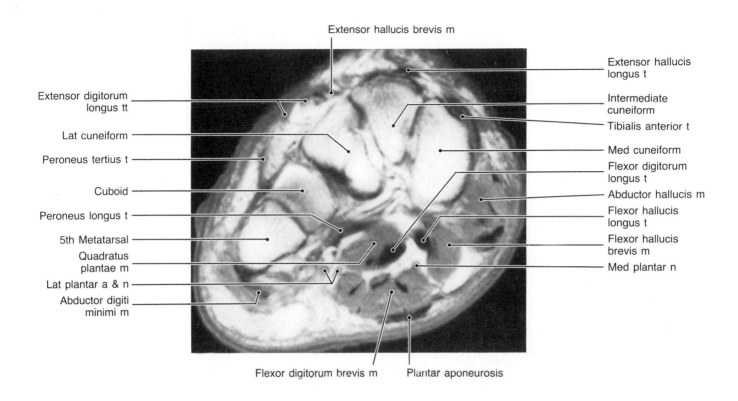

Extensor hallucis brevis m

Extensor digitorum longus tt

Lat cuneiform

Peroneus tertius t

Cuboid

Peroneus longus t

5th Metatarsal

Quadratus plantae m

Lat plantar a & n

Abductor digiti minimi m

Extensor hallucis longus t

Intermediate cuneiform

Tibialis anterior t

Med cuneiform

Flexor digitorum longus t

Abductor hallucis m

Flexor hallucis longus t

Flexor hallucis brevis m

Med plantar n

Flexor digitorum brevis m   Plantar aponeurosis

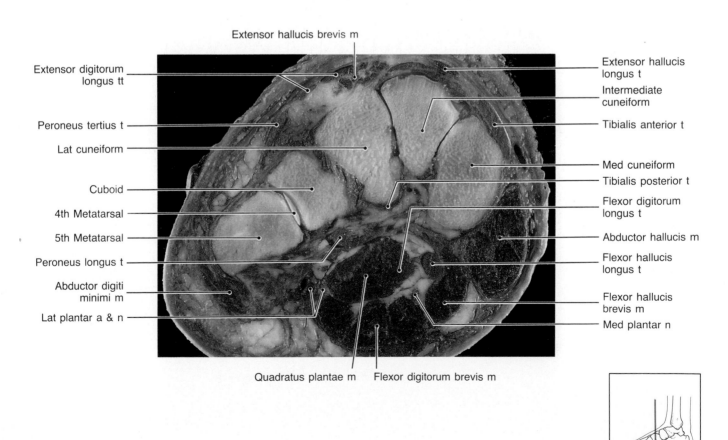

Extensor hallucis brevis m

Extensor digitorum longus tt

Peroneus tertius t

Lat cuneiform

Cuboid

4th Metatarsal

5th Metatarsal

Peroneus longus t

Abductor digiti minimi m

Lat plantar a & n

Extensor hallucis longus t

Intermediate cuneiform

Tibialis anterior t

Med cuneiform

Tibialis posterior t

Flexor digitorum longus t

Abductor hallucis m

Flexor hallucis longus t

Flexor hallucis brevis m

Med plantar n

Quadratus plantae m   Flexor digitorum brevis m

ANKLE AND FOOT, CORONAL

Extensor hallucis brevis m

Extensor hallucis longus t

Extensor digitorum longus tt

Intermediate cuneiform

Lat cuneiform

Tibialis anterior t

Peroneus tertius t

Med cuneiform

4th Metatarsal

Peroneus longus t

Abductor hallucis m

5th Metatarsal

Flexor hallucis longus t

Adductor hallucis m, oblique head

Flexor hallucis brevis m

Abductor digiti minimi m

Flexor digitorum longus tt

Flexor digiti minimi brevis m

Med plantar n

Lat plantar a & n

Plantar aponeurosis

Quadratus plantae m   Flexor digitorum brevis m

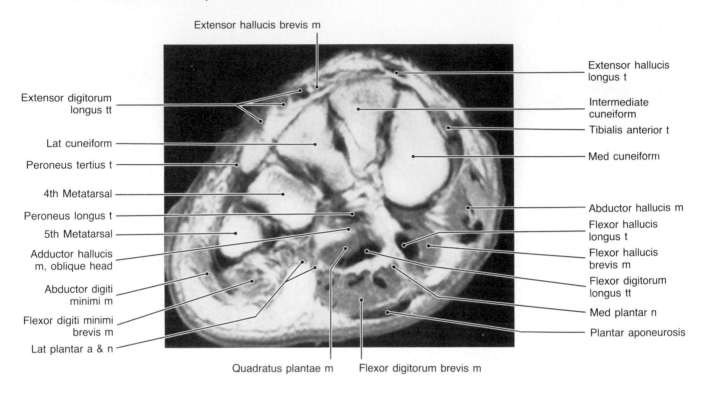

Extensor hallucis brevis m

Extensor digitorum longus tt

Extensor hallucis longus t

Intermediate cuneiform

Lat cuneiform

Tibialis anterior t

Peroneus tertius t

Med cuneiform

4th Metatarsal

Peroneus longus t

5th Metatarsal

Abductor hallucis m

Adductor hallucis m, oblique head

Flexor digitorum longus t

Abductor digiti minimi m

Flexor hallucis longus t

Flexor digiti minimi brevis m

Flexor hallucis brevis m

Lat plantar a & n

Med plantar n

Quadratus plantae m   Flexor digitorum brevis m

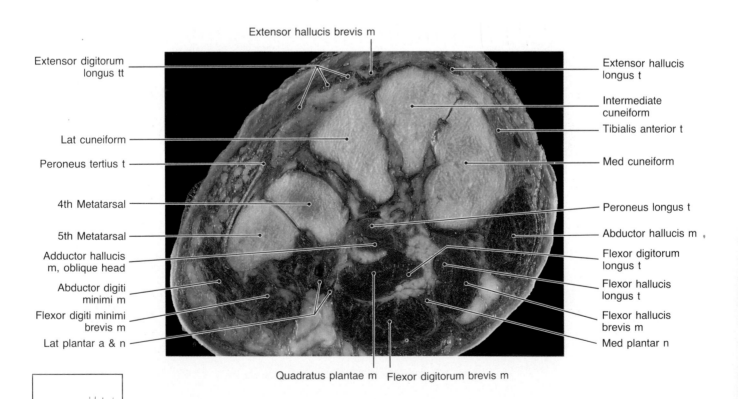

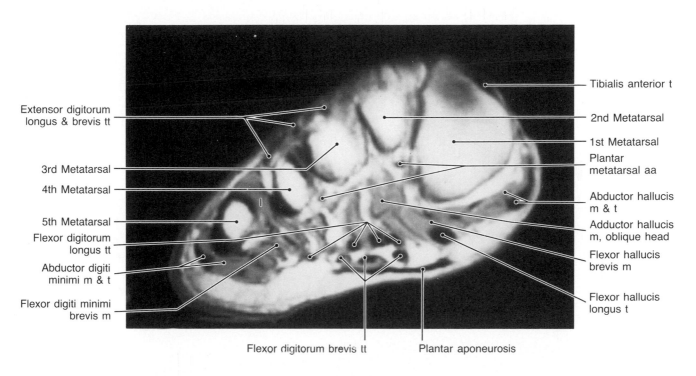

Extensor digitorum longus & brevis tt

3rd Metatarsal

4th Metatarsal

5th Metatarsal

Flexor digitorum longus tt

Abductor digiti minimi m & t

Flexor digiti minimi brevis m

Tibialis anterior t

2nd Metatarsal

1st Metatarsal

Plantar metatarsal aa

Abductor hallucis m & t

Adductor hallucis m, oblique head

Flexor hallucis brevis m

Flexor hallucis longus t

Flexor digitorum brevis tt

Plantar aponeurosis

I: Interosseous m

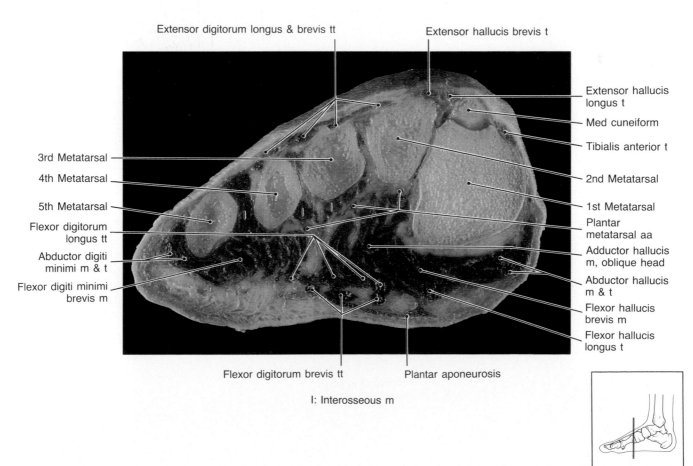

Extensor digitorum longus & brevis tt

Extensor hallucis brevis t

Extensor hallucis longus t

Med cuneiform

Tibialis anterior t

2nd Metatarsal

1st Metatarsal

Plantar metatarsal aa

Adductor hallucis m, oblique head

Abductor hallucis m & t

Flexor hallucis brevis m

Flexor hallucis longus t

3rd Metatarsal

4th Metatarsal

5th Metatarsal

Flexor digitorum longus tt

Abductor digiti minimi m & t

Flexor digiti minimi brevis m

Flexor digitorum brevis tt

Plantar aponeurosis

I: Interosseous m

ANKLE AND FOOT, CORONAL

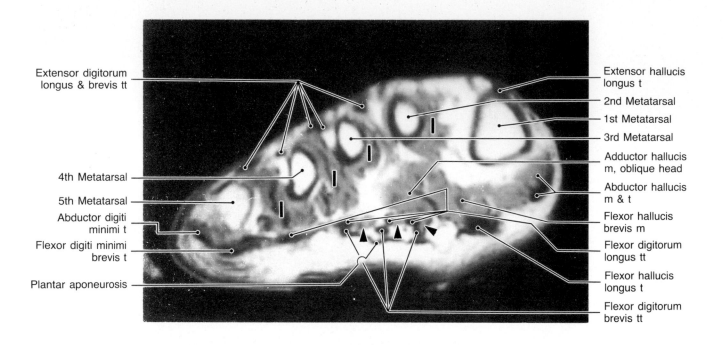

Extensor digitorum longus & brevis tt

Extensor hallucis longus t

2nd Metatarsal

1st Metatarsal

3rd Metatarsal

4th Metatarsal

Adductor hallucis m, oblique head

5th Metatarsal

Abductor hallucis m & t

Abductor digiti minimi t

Flexor hallucis brevis m

Flexor digiti minimi brevis t

Flexor digitorum longus tt

Plantar aponeurosis

Flexor hallucis longus t

Flexor digitorum brevis tt

I: Interosseous m

Arrowhead: Lumbrical m

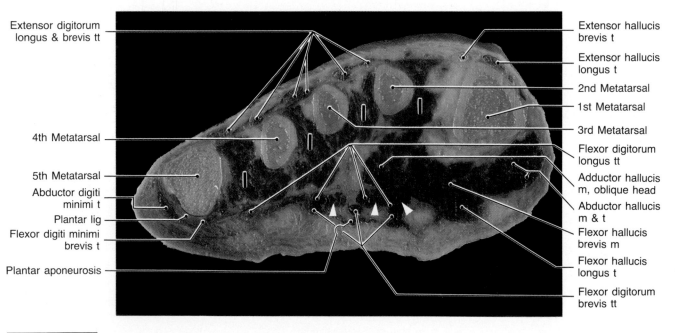

Extensor digitorum longus & brevis tt

Extensor hallucis brevis t

Extensor hallucis longus t

2nd Metatarsal

1st Metatarsal

4th Metatarsal

3rd Metatarsal

Flexor digitorum longus tt

5th Metatarsal

Adductor hallucis m, oblique head

Abductor digiti minimi t

Abductor hallucis m & t

Plantar lig

Flexor hallucis brevis m

Flexor digiti minimi brevis t

Flexor hallucis longus t

Plantar aponeurosis

Flexor digitorum brevis tt

I: Interosseous m

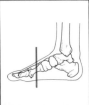

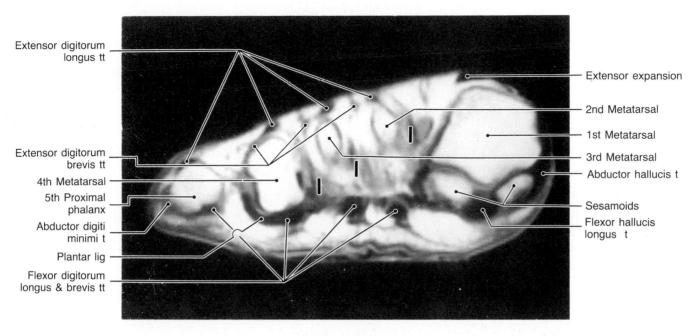

Extensor digitorum longus tt

Extensor digitorum brevis tt

4th Metatarsal

5th Proximal phalanx

Abductor digiti minimi t

Plantar lig

Flexor digitorum longus & brevis tt

Extensor expansion

2nd Metatarsal

1st Metatarsal

3rd Metatarsal

Abductor hallucis t

Sesamoids

Flexor hallucis longus t

I: Interosseous m

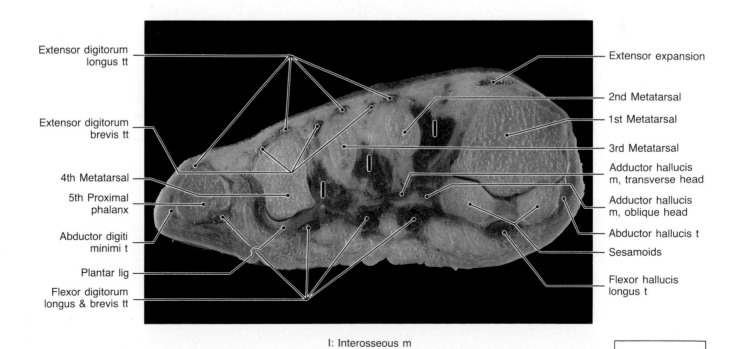

Extensor digitorum longus tt

Extensor digitorum brevis tt

4th Metatarsal

5th Proximal phalanx

Abductor digiti minimi t

Plantar lig

Flexor digitorum longus & brevis tt

Extensor expansion

2nd Metatarsal

1st Metatarsal

3rd Metatarsal

Adductor hallucis m, transverse head

Adductor hallucis m, oblique head

Abductor hallucis t

Sesamoids

Flexor hallucis longus t

I: Interosseous m

ANKLE AND FOOT, CORONAL

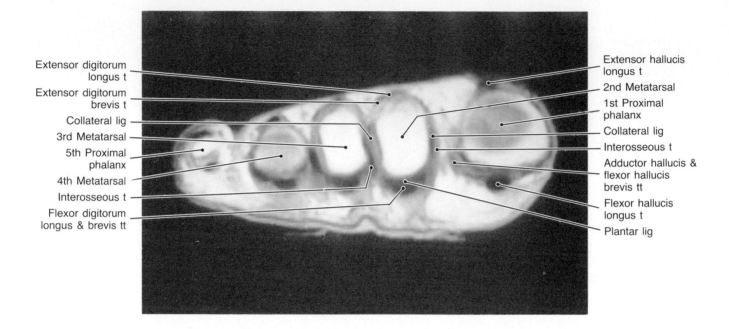

Extensor digitorum longus t

Extensor digitorum brevis t

Collateral lig

3rd Metatarsal

5th Proximal phalanx

4th Metatarsal

Interosseous t

Flexor digitorum longus & brevis tt

Extensor hallucis longus t

2nd Metatarsal

1st Proximal phalanx

Collateral lig

Interosseous t

Adductor hallucis & flexor hallucis brevis tt

Flexor hallucis longus t

Plantar lig

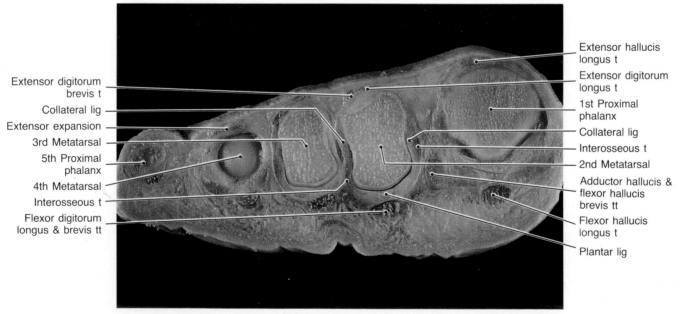

Extensor digitorum brevis t

Collateral lig

Extensor expansion

3rd Metatarsal

5th Proximal phalanx

4th Metatarsal

Interosseous t

Flexor digitorum longus & brevis tt

Extensor hallucis longus t

Extensor digitorum longus t

1st Proximal phalanx

Collateral lig

Interosseous t

2nd Metatarsal

Adductor hallucis & flexor hallucis brevis tt

Flexor hallucis longus t

Plantar lig

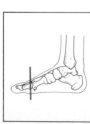

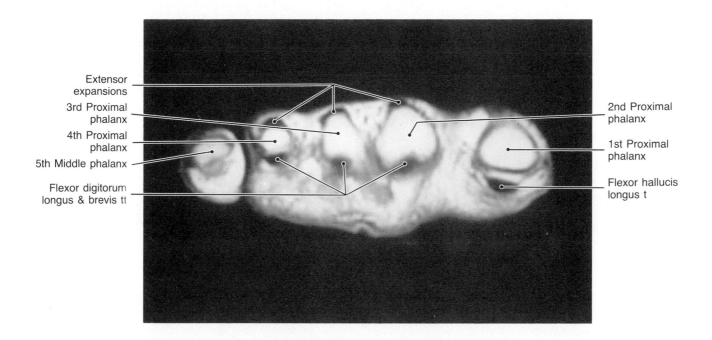

Extensor expansions

3rd Proximal phalanx

4th Proximal phalanx

5th Middle phalanx

Flexor digitorum longus & brevis tt

2nd Proximal phalanx

1st Proximal phalanx

Flexor hallucis longus t

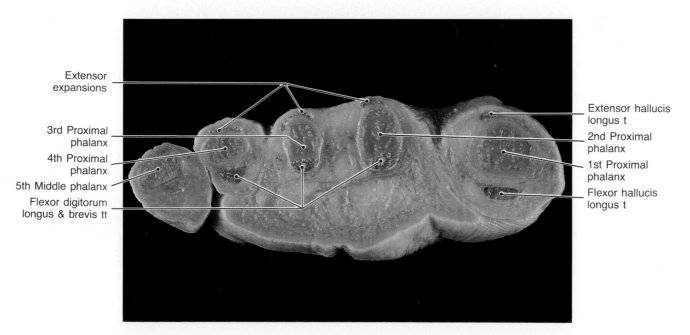

Extensor expansions

3rd Proximal phalanx

4th Proximal phalanx

5th Middle phalanx

Flexor digitorum longus & brevis tt

Extensor hallucis longus t

2nd Proximal phalanx

1st Proximal phalanx

Flexor hallucis longus t

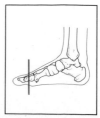

ANKLE AND FOOT, TRANSVERSE

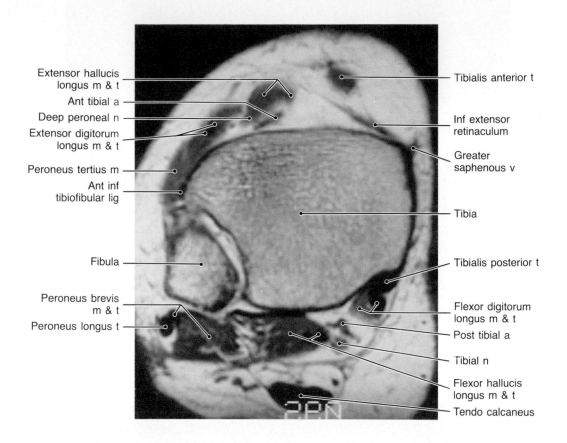

Extensor hallucis longus m & t

Ant tibial a

Deep peroneal n

Extensor digitorum longus m & t

Peroneus tertius m

Ant inf tibiofibular lig

Fibula

Peroneus brevis m & t

Peroneus longus t

Tibialis anterior t

Inf extensor retinaculum

Greater saphenous v

Tibia

Tibialis posterior t

Flexor digitorum longus m & t

Post tibial a

Tibial n

Flexor hallucis longus m & t

Tendo calcaneus

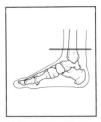

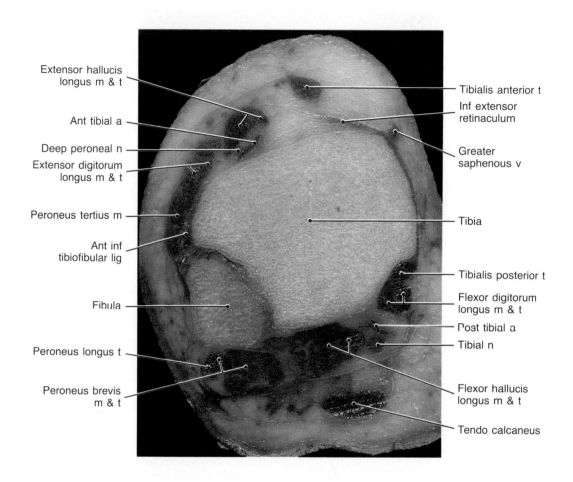

Extensor hallucis longus m & t

Ant tibial a

Deep peroneal n

Extensor digitorum longus m & t

Peroneus tertius m

Ant inf tibiofibular lig

Fibula

Peroneus longus t

Peroneus brevis m & t

Tibialis anterior t

Inf extensor retinaculum

Greater saphenous v

Tibia

Tibialis posterior t

Flexor digitorum longus m & t

Post tibial a

Tibial n

Flexor hallucis longus m & t

Tendo calcaneus

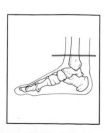

ANKLE AND FOOT, TRANSVERSE

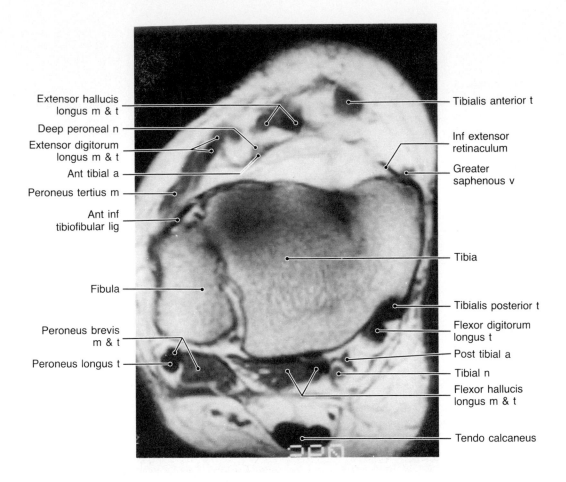

Extensor hallucis longus m & t

Deep peroneal n

Extensor digitorum longus m & t

Ant tibial a

Peroneus tertius m

Ant inf tibiofibular lig

Fibula

Peroneus brevis m & t

Peroneus longus t

Tibialis anterior t

Inf extensor retinaculum

Greater saphenous v

Tibia

Tibialis posterior t

Flexor digitorum longus t

Post tibial a

Tibial n

Flexor hallucis longus m & t

Tendo calcaneus

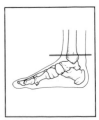

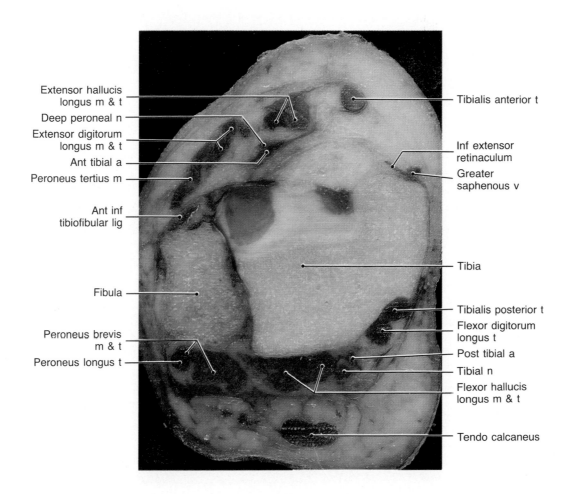

Extensor hallucis longus m & t

Deep peroneal n

Extensor digitorum longus m & t

Ant tibial a

Peroneus tertius m

Ant inf tibiofibular lig

Fibula

Peroneus brevis m & t

Peroneus longus t

Tibialis anterior t

Inf extensor retinaculum

Greater saphenous v

Tibia

Tibialis posterior t

Flexor digitorum longus t

Post tibial a

Tibial n

Flexor hallucis longus m & t

Tendo calcaneus

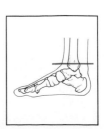

ANKLE AND FOOT, TRANSVERSE

Extensor hallucis longus m & t

Deep peroneal n

Extensor digitorum longus m & t

Ant tibial a

Peroneus tertius m

Talus

Lat malleolus

Post inf tibiofibular lig

Peroneus brevis m & t

Peroneus longus t

Tibialis anterior t

Greater saphenous v

Tibionavicular lig

Med malleolus

Tibialis posterior t

Flexor digitorum longus t

Post tibial a

Tibial n

Flexor hallucis longus m & t

Tendo calcaneus

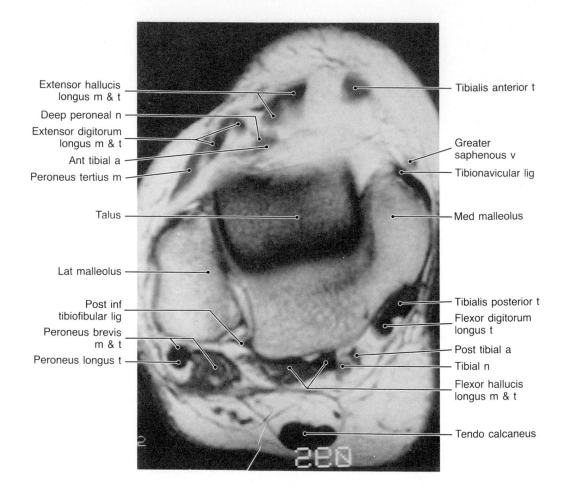

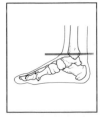

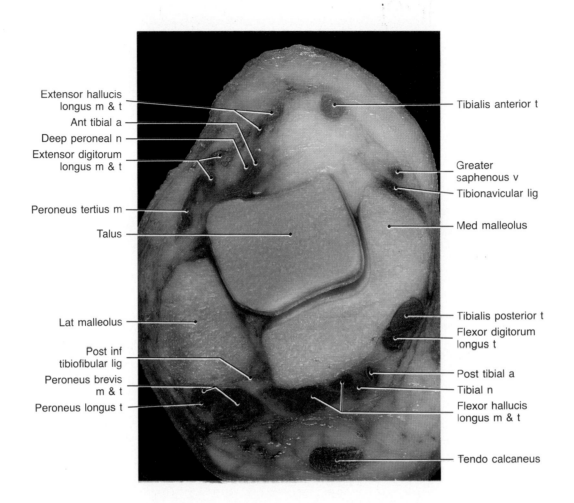

Extensor hallucis longus m & t

Ant tibial a

Deep peroneal n

Extensor digitorum longus m & t

Peroneus tertius m

Talus

Lat malleolus

Post inf tibiofibular lig

Peroneus brevis m & t

Peroneus longus t

Tibialis anterior t

Greater saphenous v

Tibionavicular lig

Med malleolus

Tibialis posterior t

Flexor digitorum longus t

Post tibial a

Tibial n

Flexor hallucis longus m & t

Tendo calcaneus

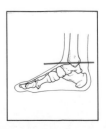

ANKLE AND FOOT, TRANSVERSE

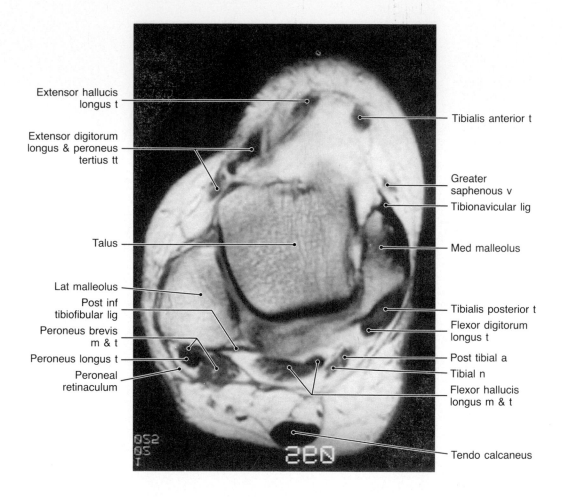

Extensor hallucis longus t

Extensor digitorum longus & peroneus tertius tt

Talus

Lat malleolus

Post inf tibiofibular lig

Peroneus brevis m & t

Peroneus longus t

Peroneal retinaculum

Tibialis anterior t

Greater saphenous v

Tibionavicular lig

Med malleolus

Tibialis posterior t

Flexor digitorum longus t

Post tibial a

Tibial n

Flexor hallucis longus m & t

Tendo calcaneus

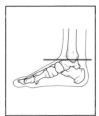

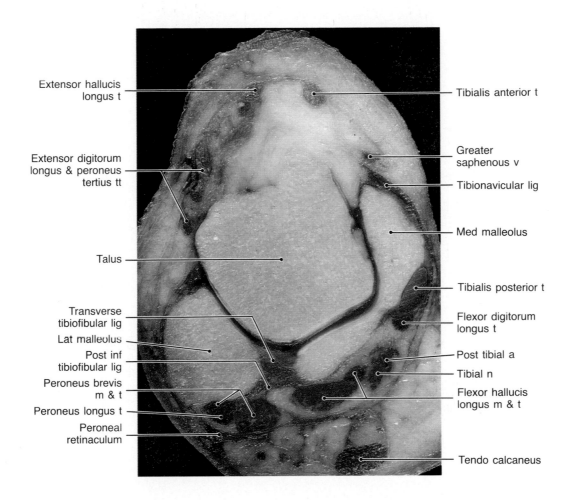

Extensor hallucis longus t

Tibialis anterior t

Extensor digitorum longus & peroneus tertius tt

Greater saphenous v

Tibionavicular lig

Talus

Med malleolus

Tibialis posterior t

Transverse tibiofibular lig

Flexor digitorum longus t

Lat malleolus

Post inf tibiofibular lig

Post tibial a

Tibial n

Peroneus brevis m & t

Flexor hallucis longus m & t

Peroneus longus t

Peroneal retinaculum

Tendo calcaneus

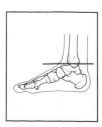

ANKLE AND FOOT, TRANSVERSE

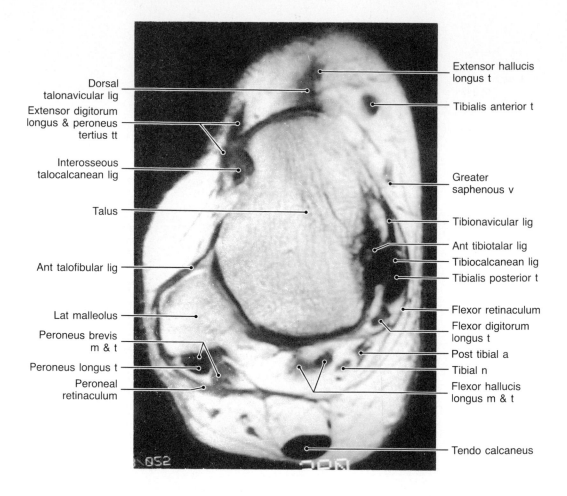

Dorsal talonavicular lig

Extensor digitorum longus & peroneus tertius tt

Interosseous talocalcanean lig

Talus

Ant talofibular lig

Lat malleolus

Peroneus brevis m & t

Peroneus longus t

Peroneal retinaculum

Extensor hallucis longus t

Tibialis anterior t

Greater saphenous v

Tibionavicular lig

Ant tibiotalar lig

Tibiocalcanean lig

Tibialis posterior t

Flexor retinaculum

Flexor digitorum longus t

Post tibial a

Tibial n

Flexor hallucis longus m & t

Tendo calcaneus

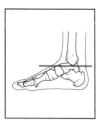

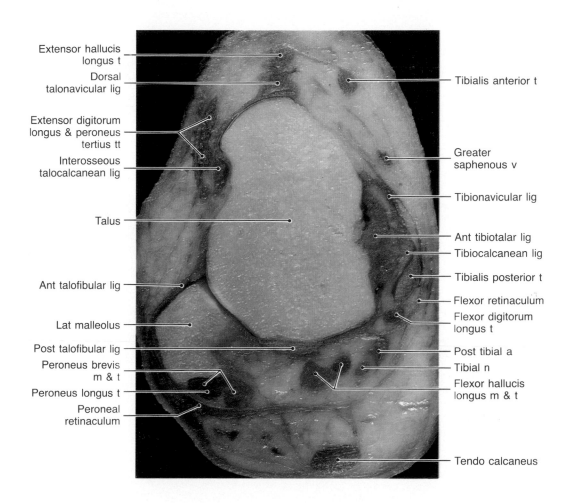

Extensor hallucis longus t

Dorsal talonavicular lig

Extensor digitorum longus & peroneus tertius tt

Interosseous talocalcanean lig

Talus

Ant talofibular lig

Lat malleolus

Post talofibular lig

Peroneus brevis m & t

Peroneus longus t

Peroneal retinaculum

Tibialis anterior t

Greater saphenous v

Tibionavicular lig

Ant tibiotalar lig

Tibiocalcanean lig

Tibialis posterior t

Flexor retinaculum

Flexor digitorum longus t

Post tibial a

Tibial n

Flexor hallucis longus m & t

Tendo calcaneus

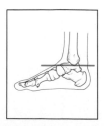

ANKLE AND FOOT, TRANSVERSE

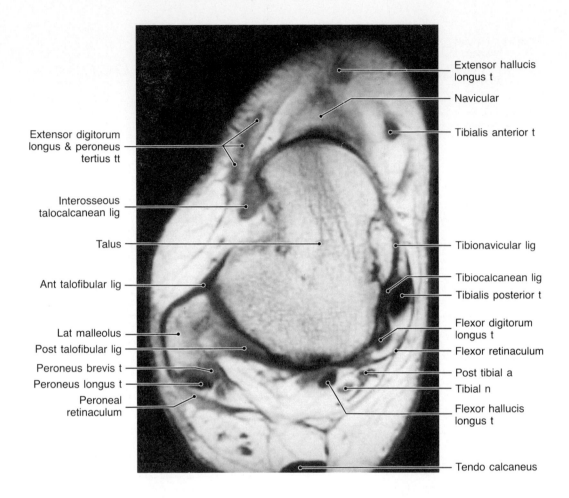

Extensor hallucis longus t

Navicular

Tibialis anterior t

Extensor digitorum longus & peroneus tertius tt

Interosseous talocalcanean lig

Talus

Ant talofibular lig

Lat malleolus

Post talofibular lig

Peroneus brevis t

Peroneus longus t

Peroneal retinaculum

Tibionavicular lig

Tibiocalcanean lig

Tibialis posterior t

Flexor digitorum longus t

Flexor retinaculum

Post tibial a

Tibial n

Flexor hallucis longus t

Tendo calcaneus

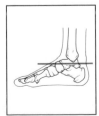

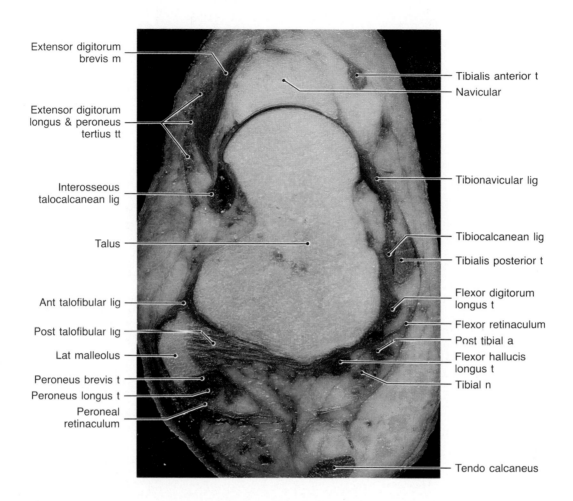

Extensor digitorum brevis m

Extensor digitorum longus & peroneus tertius tt

Interosseous talocalcanean lig

Talus

Ant talofibular lig

Post talofibular lig

Lat malleolus

Peroneus brevis t

Peroneus longus t

Peroneal retinaculum

Tibialis anterior t

Navicular

Tibionavicular lig

Tibiocalcanean lig

Tibialis posterior t

Flexor digitorum longus t

Flexor retinaculum

Post tibial a

Flexor hallucis longus t

Tibial n

Tendo calcaneus

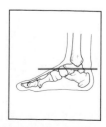

ANKLE AND FOOT, TRANSVERSE

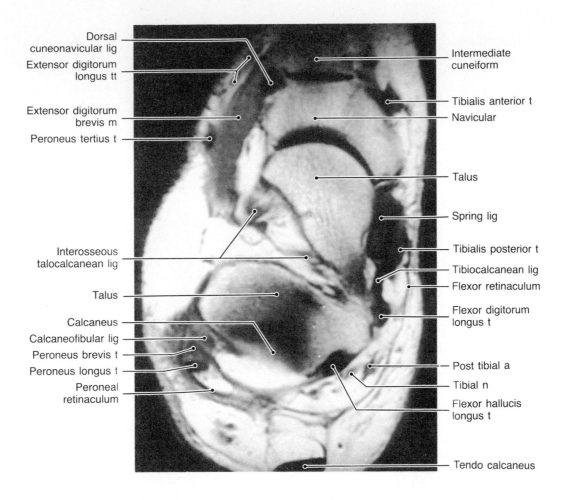

Dorsal cuneonavicular lig

Extensor digitorum longus tt

Extensor digitorum brevis m

Peroneus tertius t

Interosseous talocalcanean lig

Talus

Calcaneus

Calcaneofibular lig

Peroneus brevis t

Peroneus longus t

Peroneal retinaculum

Intermediate cuneiform

Tibialis anterior t

Navicular

Talus

Spring lig

Tibialis posterior t

Tibiocalcanean lig

Flexor retinaculum

Flexor digitorum longus t

Post tibial a

Tibial n

Flexor hallucis longus t

Tendo calcaneus

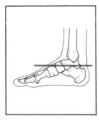

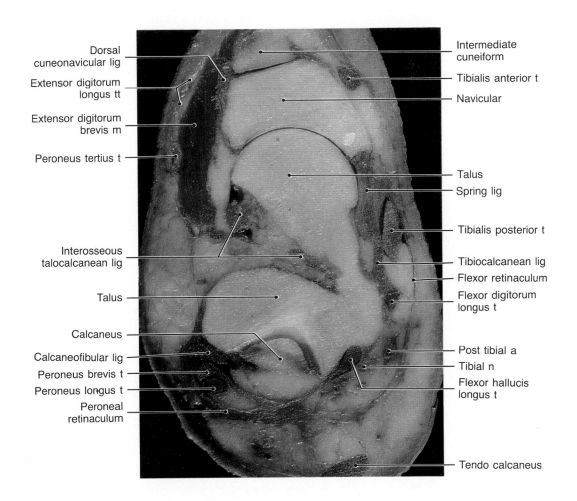

Dorsal cuneonavicular lig

Extensor digitorum longus tt

Extensor digitorum brevis m

Peroneus tertius t

Interosseous talocalcanean lig

Talus

Calcaneus

Calcaneofibular lig

Peroneus brevis t

Peroneus longus t

Peroneal retinaculum

Intermediate cuneiform

Tibialis anterior t

Navicular

Talus

Spring lig

Tibialis posterior t

Tibiocalcanean lig

Flexor retinaculum

Flexor digitorum longus t

Post tibial a

Tibial n

Flexor hallucis longus t

Tendo calcaneus

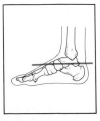

ANKLE AND FOOT, TRANSVERSE

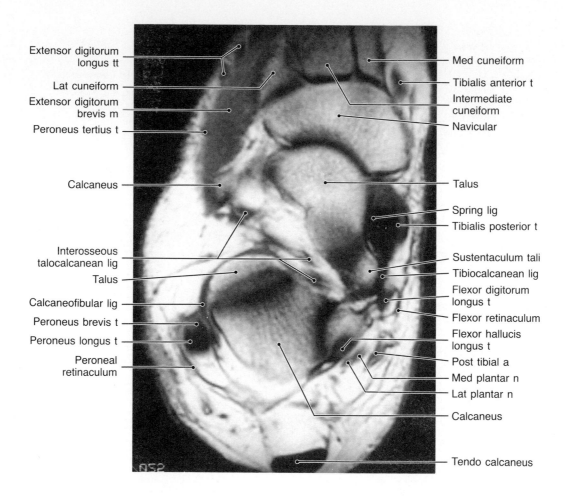

Extensor digitorum longus tt

Lat cuneiform

Extensor digitorum brevis m

Peroneus tertius t

Calcaneus

Interosseous talocalcanean lig

Talus

Calcaneofibular lig

Peroneus brevis t

Peroneus longus t

Peroneal retinaculum

Med cuneiform

Tibialis anterior t

Intermediate cuneiform

Navicular

Talus

Spring lig

Tibialis posterior t

Sustentaculum tali

Tibiocalcanean lig

Flexor digitorum longus t

Flexor retinaculum

Flexor hallucis longus t

Post tibial a

Med plantar n

Lat plantar n

Calcaneus

Tendo calcaneus

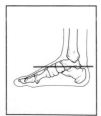

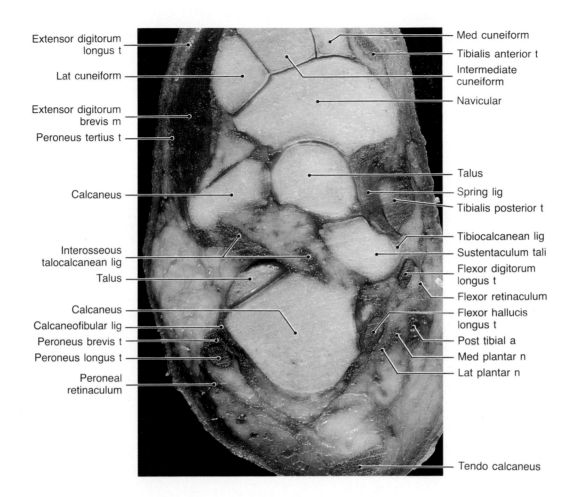

Extensor digitorum longus t

Lat cuneiform

Extensor digitorum brevis m

Peroneus tertius t

Calcaneus

Interosseous talocalcanean lig

Talus

Calcaneus

Calcaneofibular lig

Peroneus brevis t

Peroneus longus t

Peroneal retinaculum

Med cuneiform

Tibialis anterior t

Intermediate cuneiform

Navicular

Talus

Spring lig

Tibialis posterior t

Tibiocalcanean lig

Sustentaculum tali

Flexor digitorum longus t

Flexor retinaculum

Flexor hallucis longus t

Post tibial a

Med plantar n

Lat plantar n

Tendo calcaneus

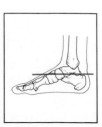

ANKLE AND FOOT, TRANSVERSE

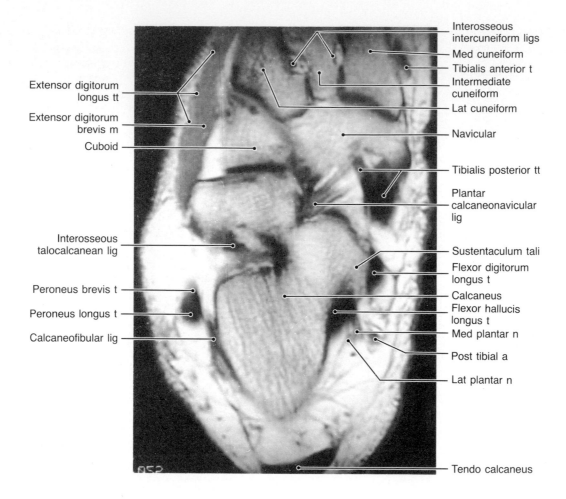

Extensor digitorum longus tt

Extensor digitorum brevis m

Cuboid

Interosseous talocalcanean lig

Peroneus brevis t

Peroneus longus t

Calcaneofibular lig

Interosseous intercuneiform ligs

Med cuneiform

Tibialis anterior t

Intermediate cuneiform

Lat cuneiform

Navicular

Tibialis posterior tt

Plantar calcaneonavicular lig

Sustentaculum tali

Flexor digitorum longus t

Calcaneus

Flexor hallucis longus t

Med plantar n

Post tibial a

Lat plantar n

Tendo calcaneus

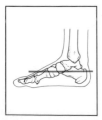

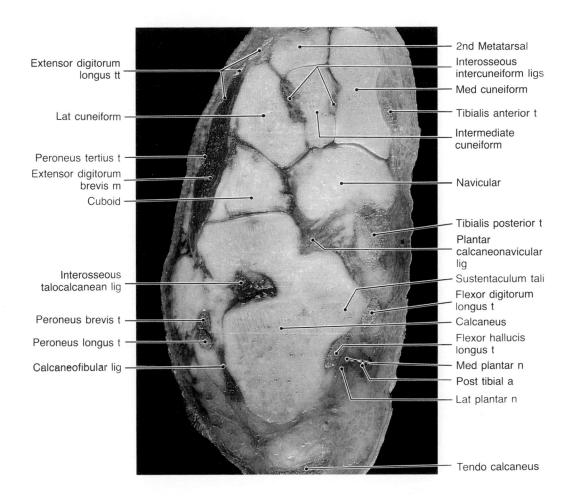

Extensor digitorum longus tt

Lat cuneiform

Peroneus tertius t

Extensor digitorum brevis m

Cuboid

Interosseous talocalcanean lig

Peroneus brevis t

Peroneus longus t

Calcaneofibular lig

2nd Metatarsal

Interosseous intercuneiform ligs

Med cuneiform

Tibialis anterior t

Intermediate cuneiform

Navicular

Tibialis posterior t

Plantar calcaneonavicular lig

Sustentaculum tali

Flexor digitorum longus t

Calcaneus

Flexor hallucis longus t

Med plantar n

Post tibial a

Lat plantar n

Tendo calcaneus

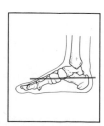

ANKLE AND FOOT, TRANSVERSE

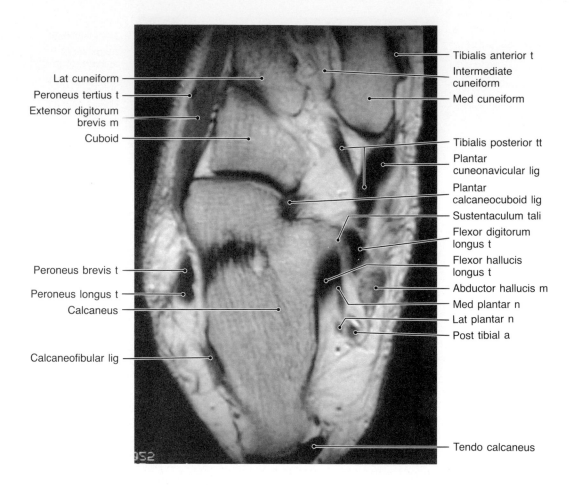

Lat cuneiform
Peroneus tertius t
Extensor digitorum brevis m
Cuboid

Peroneus brevis t
Peroneus longus t
Calcaneus

Calcaneofibular lig

Tibialis anterior t
Intermediate cuneiform
Med cuneiform

Tibialis posterior tt
Plantar cuneonavicular lig
Plantar calcaneocuboid lig
Sustentaculum tali
Flexor digitorum longus t
Flexor hallucis longus t
Abductor hallucis m
Med plantar n
Lat plantar n
Post tibial a

Tendo calcaneus

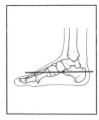

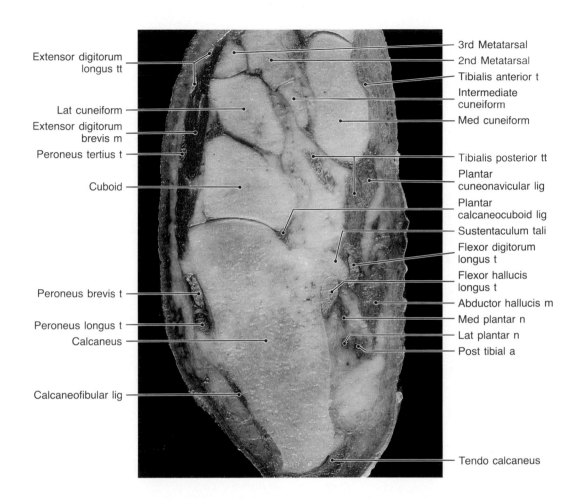

Extensor digitorum longus tt

Lat cuneiform

Extensor digitorum brevis m

Peroneus tertius t

Cuboid

Peroneus brevis t

Peroneus longus t

Calcaneus

Calcaneofibular lig

3rd Metatarsal

2nd Metatarsal

Tibialis anterior t

Intermediate cuneiform

Med cuneiform

Tibialis posterior tt

Plantar cuneonavicular lig

Plantar calcaneocuboid lig

Sustentaculum tali

Flexor digitorum longus t

Flexor hallucis longus t

Abductor hallucis m

Med plantar n

Lat plantar n

Post tibial a

Tendo calcaneus

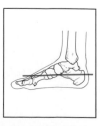

ANKLE AND FOOT, TRANSVERSE

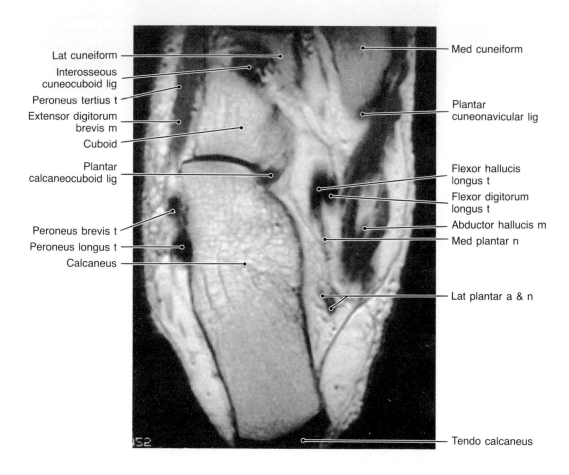

Lat cuneiform

Interosseous cuneocuboid lig

Peroneus tertius t

Extensor digitorum brevis m

Cuboid

Plantar calcaneocuboid lig

Peroneus brevis t

Peroneus longus t

Calcaneus

Med cuneiform

Plantar cuneonavicular lig

Flexor hallucis longus t

Flexor digitorum longus t

Abductor hallucis m

Med plantar n

Lat plantar a & n

Tendo calcaneus

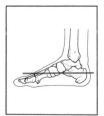

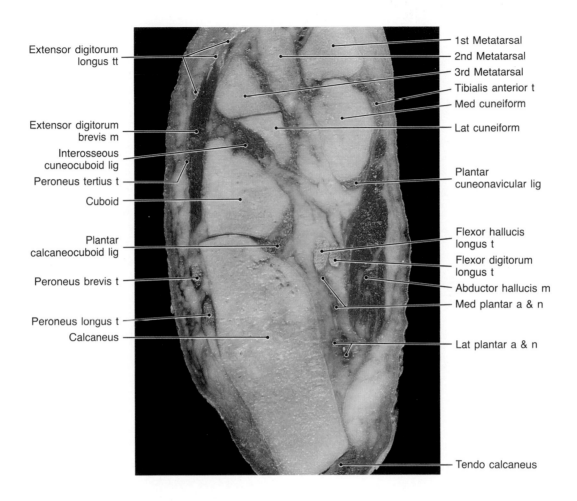

Extensor digitorum longus tt

Extensor digitorum brevis m

Interosseous cuneocuboid lig

Peroneus tertius t

Cuboid

Plantar calcaneocuboid lig

Peroneus brevis t

Peroneus longus t

Calcaneus

1st Metatarsal

2nd Metatarsal

3rd Metatarsal

Tibialis anterior t

Med cuneiform

Lat cuneiform

Plantar cuneonavicular lig

Flexor hallucis longus t

Flexor digitorum longus t

Abductor hallucis m

Med plantar a & n

Lat plantar a & n

Tendo calcaneus

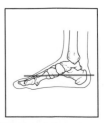

ANKLE AND FOOT, TRANSVERSE

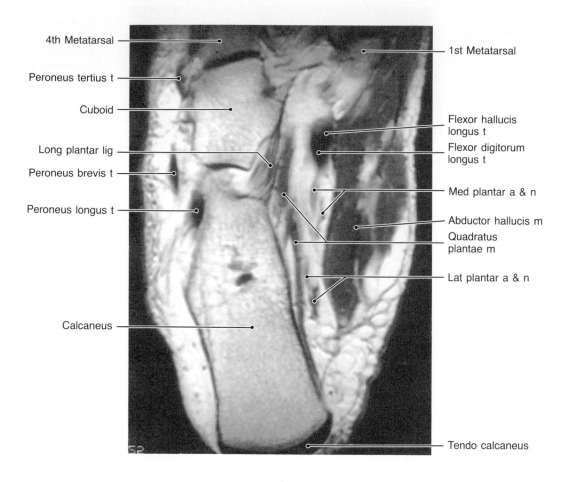

4th Metatarsal

Peroneus tertius t

Cuboid

Long plantar lig

Peroneus brevis t

Peroneus longus t

Calcaneus

1st Metatarsal

Flexor hallucis longus t

Flexor digitorum longus t

Med plantar a & n

Abductor hallucis m

Quadratus plantae m

Lat plantar a & n

Tendo calcaneus

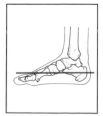

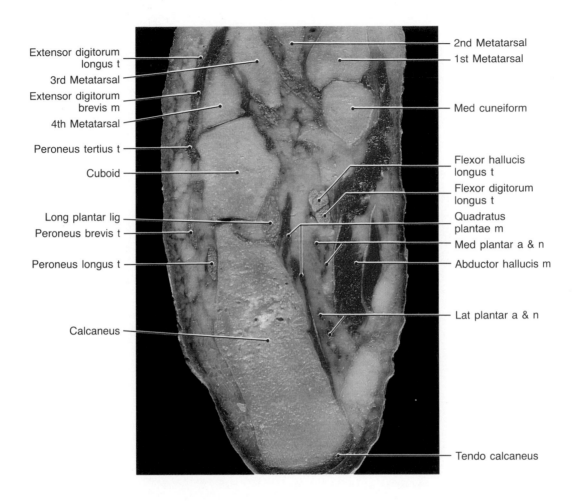

Extensor digitorum longus t

3rd Metatarsal

Extensor digitorum brevis m

4th Metatarsal

Peroneus tertius t

Cuboid

Long plantar lig

Peroneus brevis t

Peroneus longus t

Calcaneus

2nd Metatarsal

1st Metatarsal

Med cuneiform

Flexor hallucis longus t

Flexor digitorum longus t

Quadratus plantae m

Med plantar a & n

Abductor hallucis m

Lat plantar a & n

Tendo calcaneus

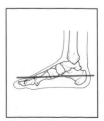

ANKLE AND FOOT, TRANSVERSE

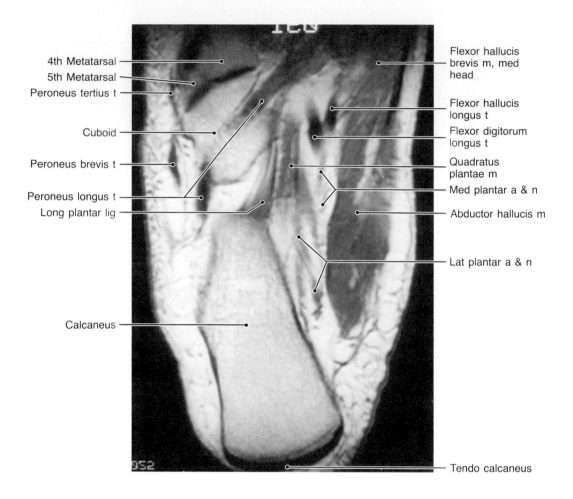

4th Metatarsal

5th Metatarsal

Peroneus tertius t

Cuboid

Peroneus brevis t

Peroneus longus t

Long plantar lig

Calcaneus

Flexor hallucis brevis m, med head

Flexor hallucis longus t

Flexor digitorum longus t

Quadratus plantae m

Med plantar a & n

Abductor hallucis m

Lat plantar a & n

Tendo calcaneus

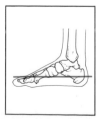

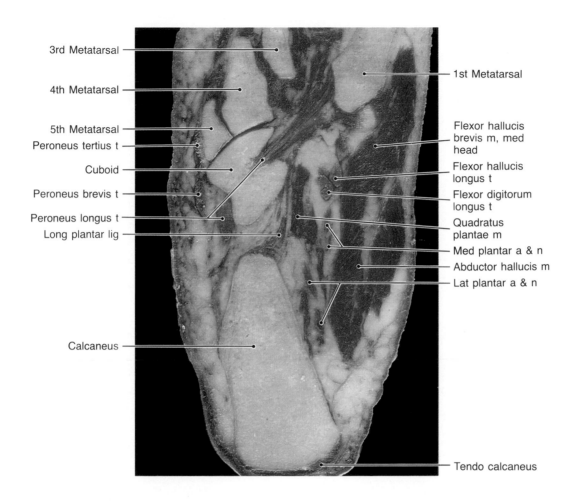

3rd Metatarsal

4th Metatarsal

5th Metatarsal

Peroneus tertius t

Cuboid

Peroneus brevis t

Peroneus longus t

Long plantar lig

Calcaneus

1st Metatarsal

Flexor hallucis brevis m, med head

Flexor hallucis longus t

Flexor digitorum longus t

Quadratus plantae m

Med plantar a & n

Abductor hallucis m

Lat plantar a & n

Tendo calcaneus

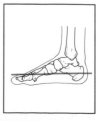

ANKLE AND FOOT, TRANSVERSE

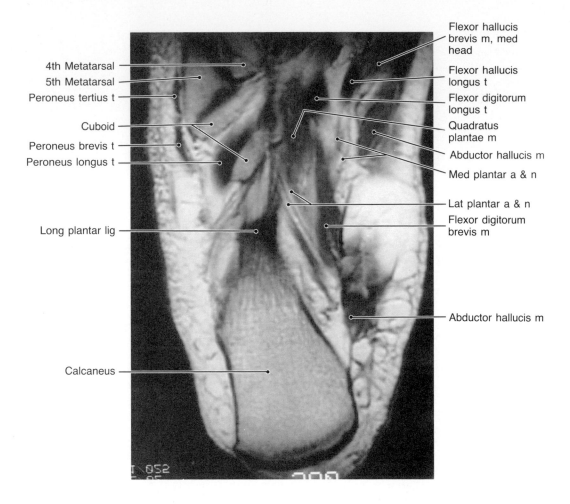

4th Metatarsal

5th Metatarsal

Peroneus tertius t

Cuboid

Peroneus brevis t

Peroneus longus t

Long plantar lig

Calcaneus

Flexor hallucis brevis m, med head

Flexor hallucis longus t

Flexor digitorum longus t

Quadratus plantae m

Abductor hallucis m

Med plantar a & n

Lat plantar a & n

Flexor digitorum brevis m

Abductor hallucis m

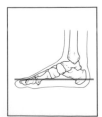

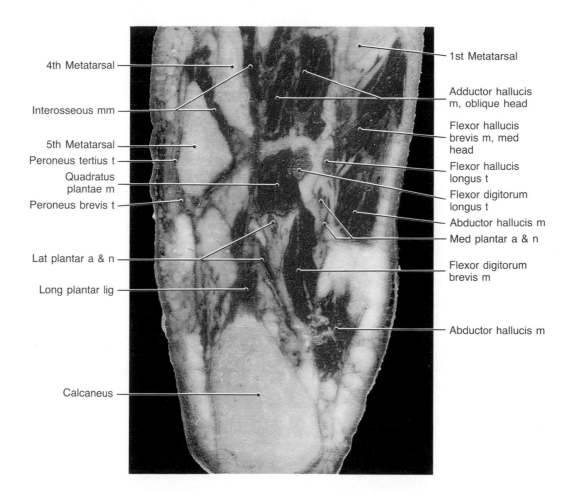

4th Metatarsal

Interosseous mm

5th Metatarsal
Peroneus tertius t
Quadratus
plantae m
Peroneus brevis t

Lat plantar a & n

Long plantar lig

Calcaneus

1st Metatarsal

Adductor hallucis
m, oblique head

Flexor hallucis
brevis m, med
head

Flexor hallucis
longus t

Flexor digitorum
longus t

Abductor hallucis m

Med plantar a & n

Flexor digitorum
brevis m

Abductor hallucis m

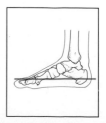

ANKLE AND FOOT, TRANSVERSE

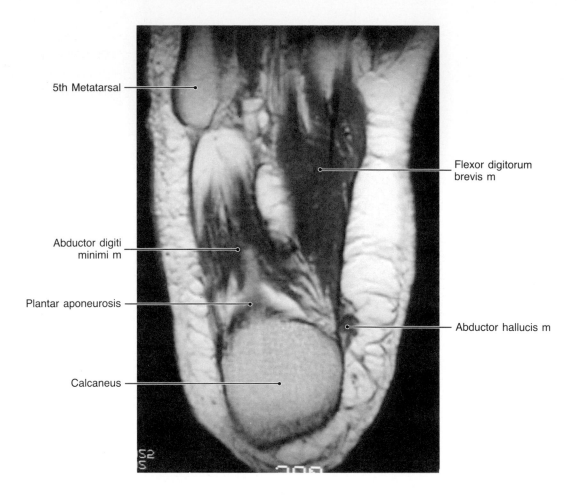

5th Metatarsal

Flexor digitorum brevis m

Abductor digiti minimi m

Plantar aponeurosis

Abductor hallucis m

Calcaneus

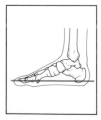

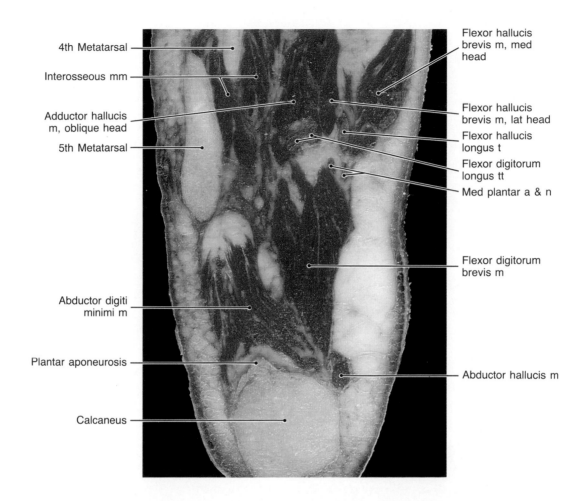

4th Metatarsal

Interosseous mm

Adductor hallucis m, oblique head

5th Metatarsal

Abductor digiti minimi m

Plantar aponeurosis

Calcaneus

Flexor hallucis brevis m, med head

Flexor hallucis brevis m, lat head

Flexor hallucis longus t

Flexor digitorum longus tt

Med plantar a & n

Flexor digitorum brevis m

Abductor hallucis m

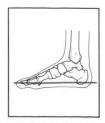

ANKLE AND FOOT, SAGITTAL

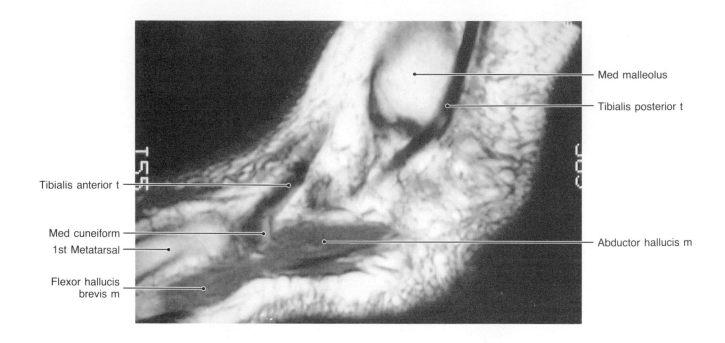

Med malleolus

Tibialis posterior t

Tibialis anterior t

Med cuneiform

1st Metatarsal

Flexor hallucis brevis m

Abductor hallucis m

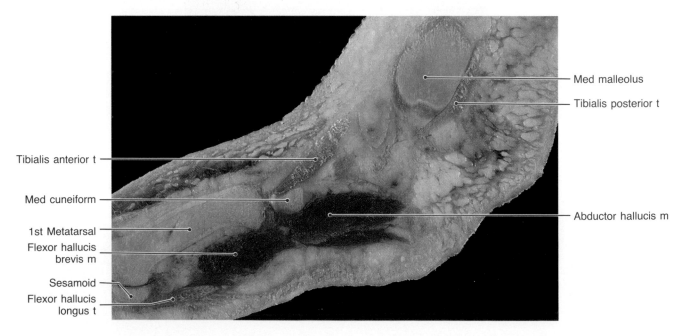

Med malleolus

Tibialis posterior t

Tibialis anterior t

Med cuneiform

1st Metatarsal

Flexor hallucis brevis m

Sesamoid

Flexor hallucis longus t

Abductor hallucis m

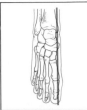

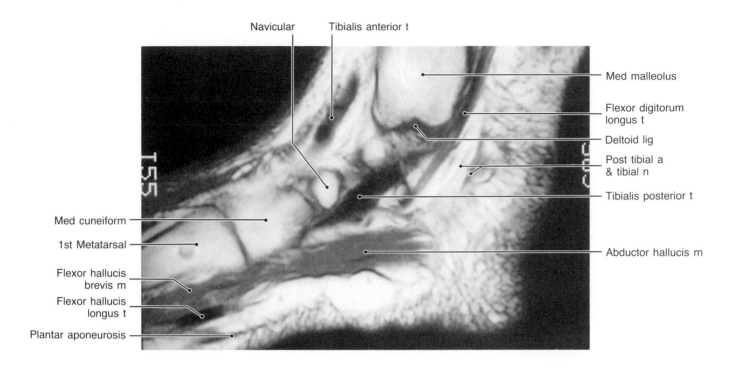

Navicular — Tibialis anterior t

Med malleolus

Flexor digitorum longus t

Deltoid lig

Post tibial a & tibial n

Tibialis posterior t

Abductor hallucis m

Med cuneiform

1st Metatarsal

Flexor hallucis brevis m

Flexor hallucis longus t

Plantar aponeurosis

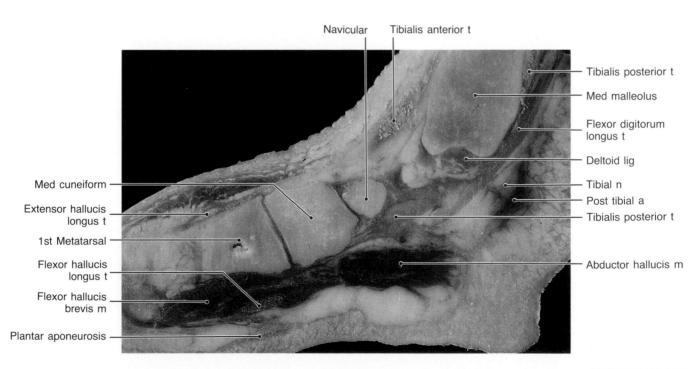

Navicular — Tibialis anterior t

Tibialis posterior t

Med malleolus

Flexor digitorum longus t

Deltoid lig

Tibial n

Post tibial a

Tibialis posterior t

Abductor hallucis m

Med cuneiform

Extensor hallucis longus t

1st Metatarsal

Flexor hallucis longus t

Flexor hallucis brevis m

Plantar aponeurosis

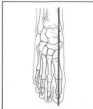

ANKLE AND FOOT, SAGITTAL

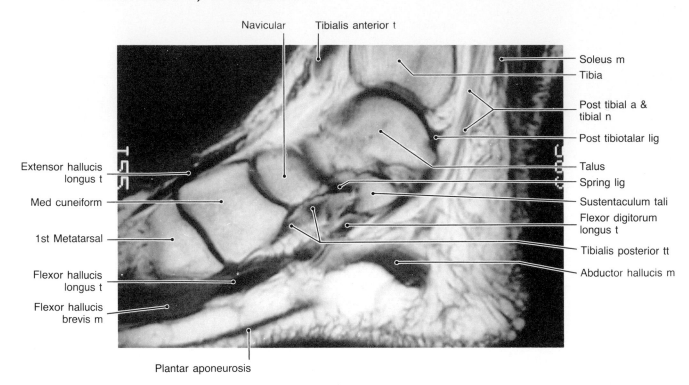

Navicular
Tibialis anterior t
Soleus m
Tibia
Post tibial a & tibial n
Post tibiotalar lig
Talus
Spring lig
Sustentaculum tali
Flexor digitorum longus t
Tibialis posterior tt
Abductor hallucis m
Extensor hallucis longus t
Med cuneiform
1st Metatarsal
Flexor hallucis longus t
Flexor hallucis brevis m
Plantar aponeurosis

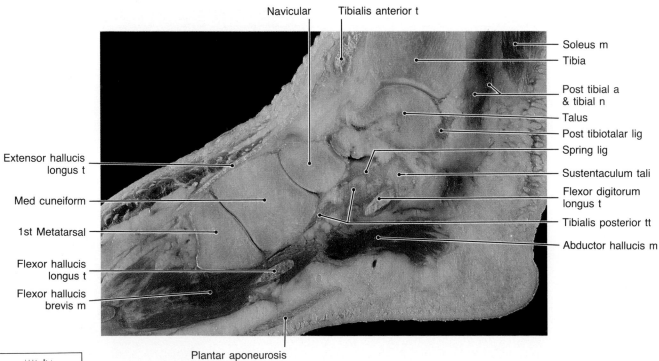

Navicular
Tibialis anterior t
Soleus m
Tibia
Post tibial a & tibial n
Talus
Post tibiotalar lig
Spring lig
Sustentaculum tali
Flexor digitorum longus t
Tibialis posterior tt
Abductor hallucis m
Extensor hallucis longus t
Med cuneiform
1st Metatarsal
Flexor hallucis longus t
Flexor hallucis brevis m
Plantar aponeurosis

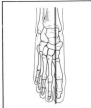

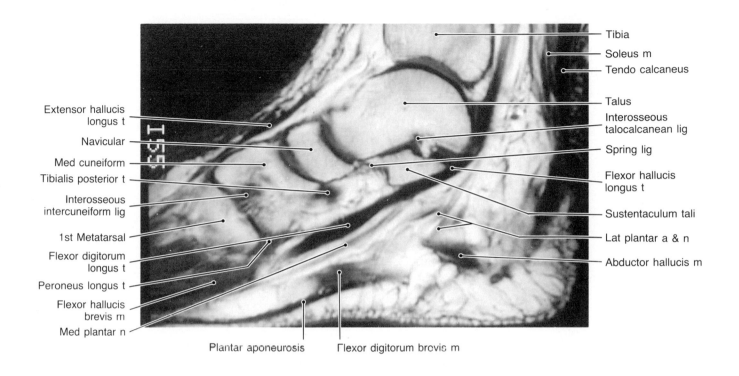

Tibia
Soleus m
Tendo calcaneus
Talus
Interosseous talocalcanean lig
Spring lig
Flexor hallucis longus t
Sustentaculum tali
Lat plantar a & n
Abductor hallucis m

Extensor hallucis longus t
Navicular
Med cuneiform
Tibialis posterior t
Interosseous intercuneiform lig
1st Metatarsal
Flexor digitorum longus t
Peroneus longus t
Flexor hallucis brevis m
Med plantar n

Plantar aponeurosis   Flexor digitorum brevis m

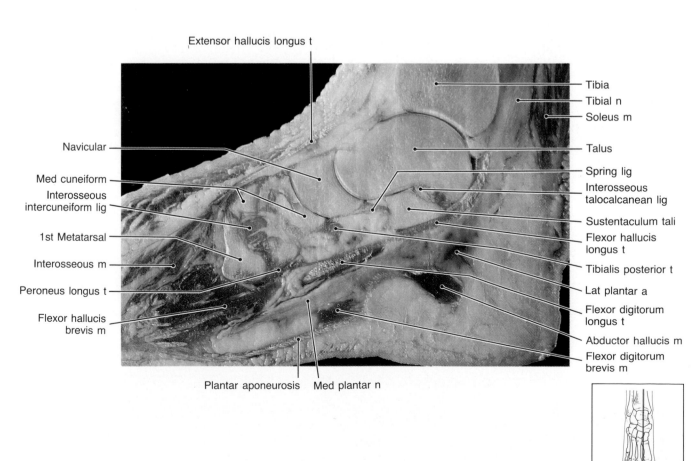

Extensor hallucis longus t

Tibia
Tibial n
Soleus m
Talus
Spring lig
Interosseous talocalcanean lig
Sustentaculum tali
Flexor hallucis longus t
Tibialis posterior t
Lat plantar a
Flexor digitorum longus t
Abductor hallucis m
Flexor digitorum brevis m

Navicular
Med cuneiform
Interosseous intercuneiform lig
1st Metatarsal
Interosseous m
Peroneus longus t
Flexor hallucis brevis m

Plantar aponeurosis   Med plantar n

ANKLE AND FOOT, SAGITTAL

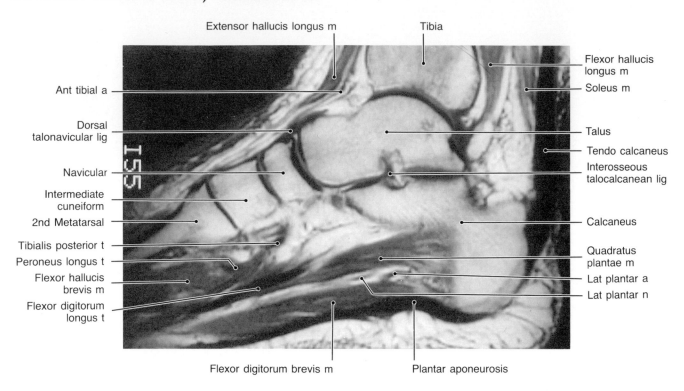

Extensor hallucis longus m — Tibia

Ant tibial a

Dorsal talonavicular lig

Navicular

Intermediate cuneiform

2nd Metatarsal

Tibialis posterior t

Peroneus longus t

Flexor hallucis brevis m

Flexor digitorum longus t

Flexor hallucis longus m

Soleus m

Talus

Tendo calcaneus

Interosseous talocalcanean lig

Calcaneus

Quadratus plantae m

Lat plantar a

Lat plantar n

Flexor digitorum brevis m — Plantar aponeurosis

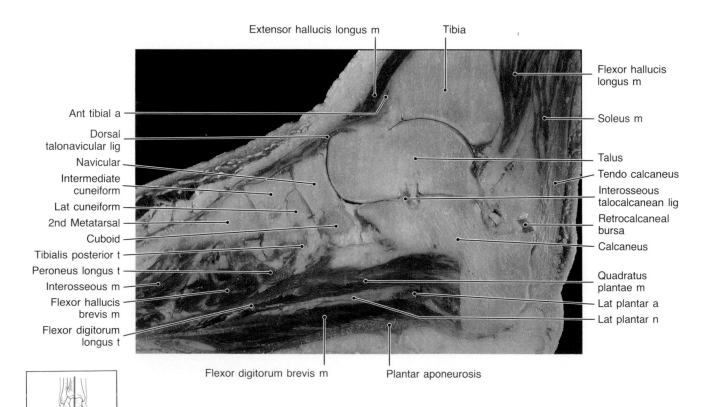

Extensor hallucis longus m — Tibia

Ant tibial a

Dorsal talonavicular lig

Navicular

Intermediate cuneiform

Lat cuneiform

2nd Metatarsal

Cuboid

Tibialis posterior t

Peroneus longus t

Interosseous m

Flexor hallucis brevis m

Flexor digitorum longus t

Flexor hallucis longus m

Soleus m

Talus

Tendo calcaneus

Interosseous talocalcanean lig

Retrocalcaneal bursa

Calcaneus

Quadratus plantae m

Lat plantar a

Lat plantar n

Flexor digitorum brevis m — Plantar aponeurosis

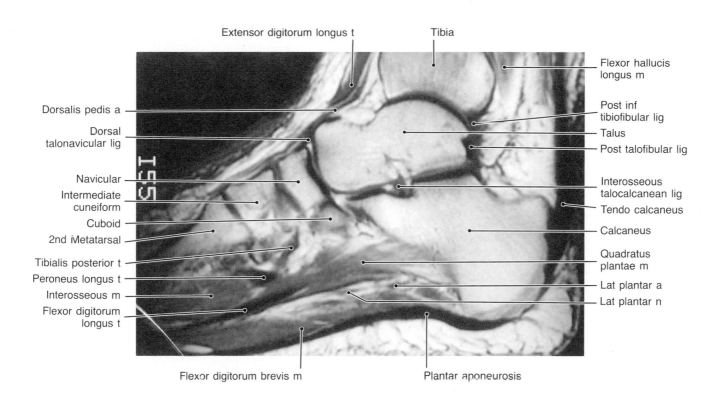

Extensor digitorum longus t — Tibia

Flexor hallucis longus m

Dorsalis pedis a

Dorsal talonavicular lig

Post inf tibiofibular lig

Talus

Post talofibular lig

Navicular

Intermediate cuneiform

Interosseous talocalcanean lig

Tendo calcaneus

Cuboid

2nd Metatarsal

Calcaneus

Tibialis posterior t

Quadratus plantae m

Peroneus longus t

Interosseous m

Lat plantar a

Flexor digitorum longus t

Lat plantar n

Flexor digitorum brevis m — Plantar aponeurosis

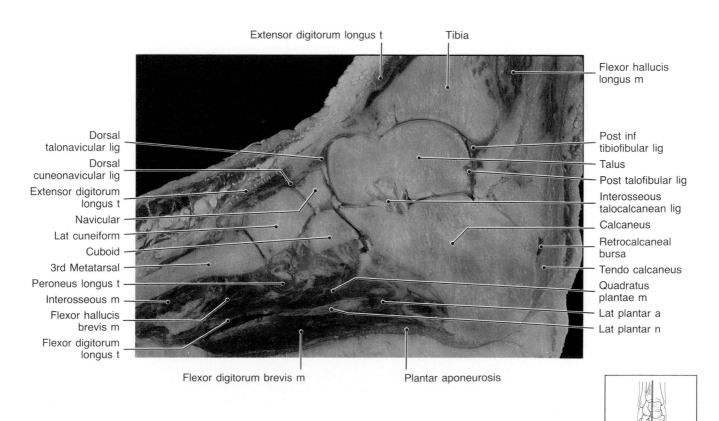

Extensor digitorum longus t — Tibia

Flexor hallucis longus m

Dorsal talonavicular lig

Dorsal cuneonavicular lig

Post inf tibiofibular lig

Talus

Post talofibular lig

Extensor digitorum longus t

Navicular

Interosseous talocalcanean lig

Calcaneus

Lat cuneiform

Cuboid

Retrocalcaneal bursa

3rd Metatarsal

Tendo calcaneus

Peroneus longus t

Interosseous m

Quadratus plantae m

Flexor hallucis brevis m

Lat plantar a

Flexor digitorum longus t

Lat plantar n

Flexor digitorum brevis m — Plantar aponeurosis

ANKLE AND FOOT, SAGITTAL

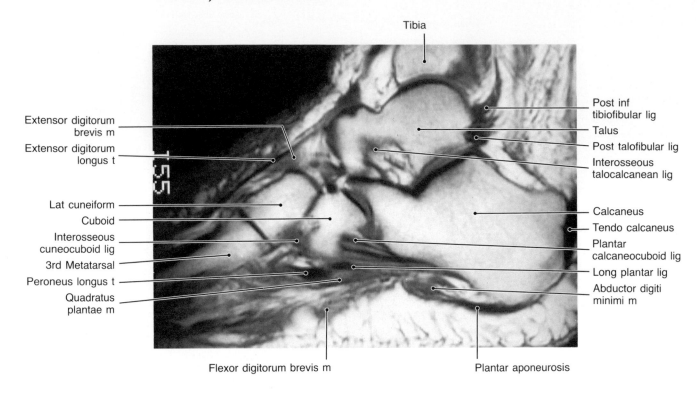

Tibia

Extensor digitorum
brevis m

Extensor digitorum
longus t

Post inf
tibiofibular lig

Talus

Post talofibular lig

Interosseous
talocalcanean lig

Lat cuneiform

Cuboid

Interosseous
cuneocuboid lig

3rd Metatarsal

Peroneus longus t

Quadratus
plantae m

Calcaneus

Tendo calcaneus

Plantar
calcaneocuboid lig

Long plantar lig

Abductor digiti
minimi m

Flexor digitorum brevis m

Plantar aponeurosis

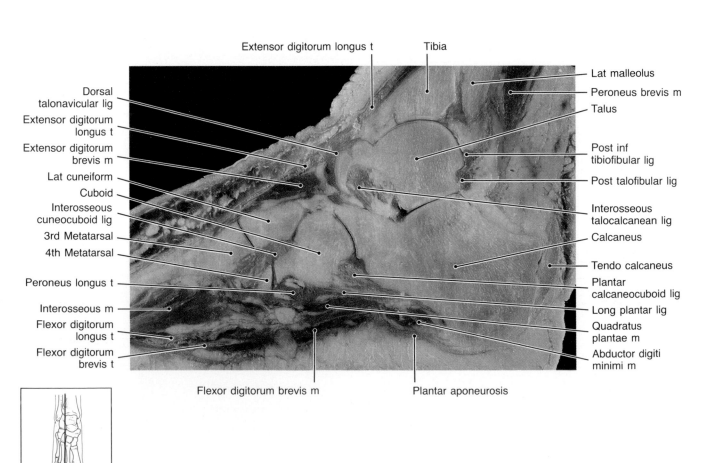

Extensor digitorum longus t   Tibia

Dorsal
talonavicular lig

Extensor digitorum
longus t

Extensor digitorum
brevis m

Lat cuneiform

Cuboid

Interosseous
cuneocuboid lig

3rd Metatarsal

4th Metatarsal

Peroneus longus t

Interosseous m

Flexor digitorum
longus t

Flexor digitorum
brevis t

Lat malleolus

Peroneus brevis m

Talus

Post inf
tibiofibular lig

Post talofibular lig

Interosseous
talocalcanean lig

Calcaneus

Tendo calcaneus

Plantar
calcaneocuboid lig

Long plantar lig

Quadratus
plantae m

Abductor digiti
minimi m

Flexor digitorum brevis m   Plantar aponeurosis

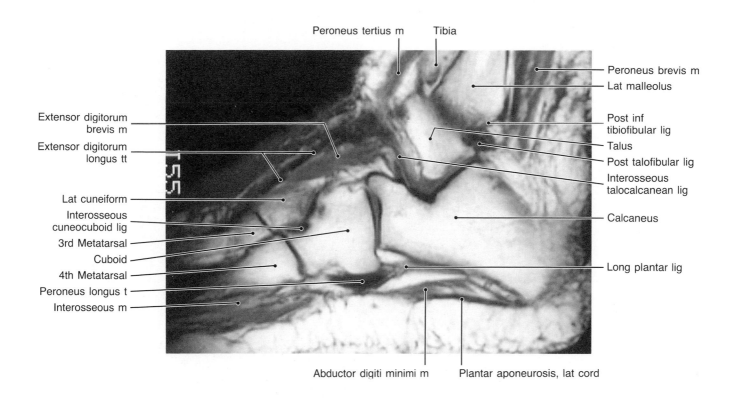

Peroneus tertius m   Tibia

Peroneus brevis m
Lat malleolus

Extensor digitorum brevis m

Extensor digitorum longus tt

Post inf tibiofibular lig
Talus
Post talofibular lig
Interosseous talocalcanean lig

Lat cuneiform

Interosseous cuneocuboid lig

3rd Metatarsal

Cuboid

4th Metatarsal

Peroneus longus t

Interosseous m

Calcaneus

Long plantar lig

Abductor digiti minimi m   Plantar aponeurosis, lat cord

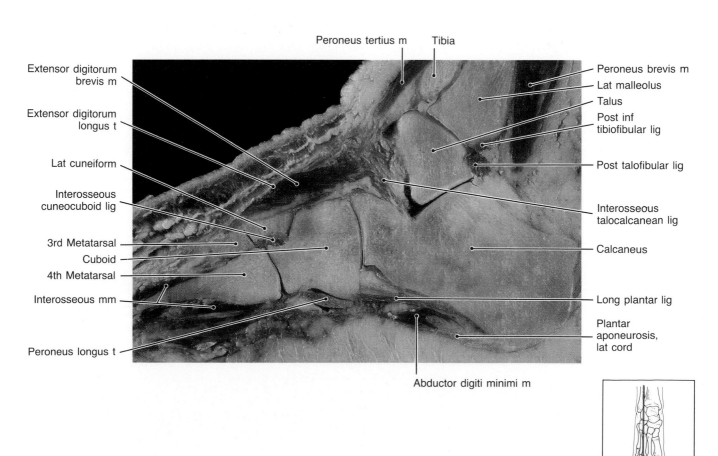

Peroneus tertius m   Tibia

Extensor digitorum brevis m

Extensor digitorum longus t

Peroneus brevis m
Lat malleolus
Talus
Post inf tibiofibular lig

Lat cuneiform

Post talofibular lig

Interosseous cuneocuboid lig

Interosseous talocalcanean lig

3rd Metatarsal

Cuboid

4th Metatarsal

Interosseous mm

Peroneus longus t

Calcaneus

Long plantar lig

Plantar aponeurosis, lat cord

Abductor digiti minimi m

ANKLE AND FOOT, SAGITTAL

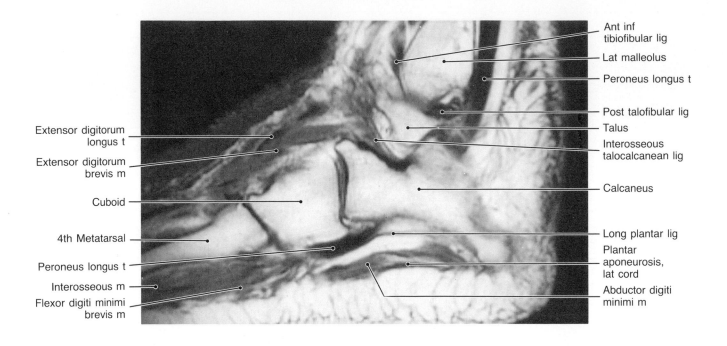

Ant inf tibiofibular lig
Lat malleolus
Peroneus longus t
Post talofibular lig
Talus
Interosseous talocalcanean lig
Calcaneus
Long plantar lig
Plantar aponeurosis, lat cord
Abductor digiti minimi m

Extensor digitorum longus t
Extensor digitorum brevis m
Cuboid
4th Metatarsal
Peroneus longus t
Interosseous m
Flexor digiti minimi brevis m

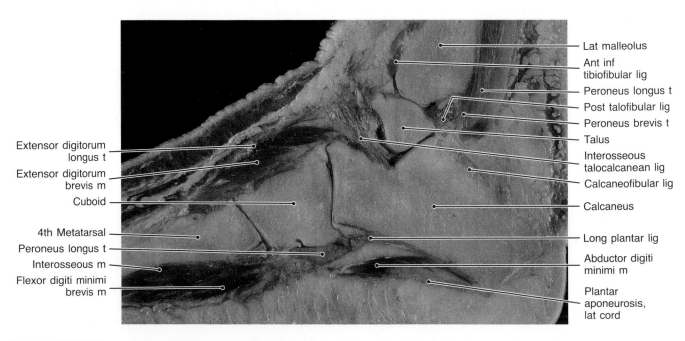

Lat malleolus
Ant inf tibiofibular lig
Peroneus longus t
Post talofibular lig
Peroneus brevis t
Talus
Interosseous talocalcanean lig
Calcaneofibular lig
Calcaneus
Long plantar lig
Abductor digiti minimi m
Plantar aponeurosis, lat cord

Extensor digitorum longus t
Extensor digitorum brevis m
Cuboid
4th Metatarsal
Peroneus longus t
Interosseous m
Flexor digiti minimi brevis m

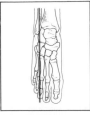

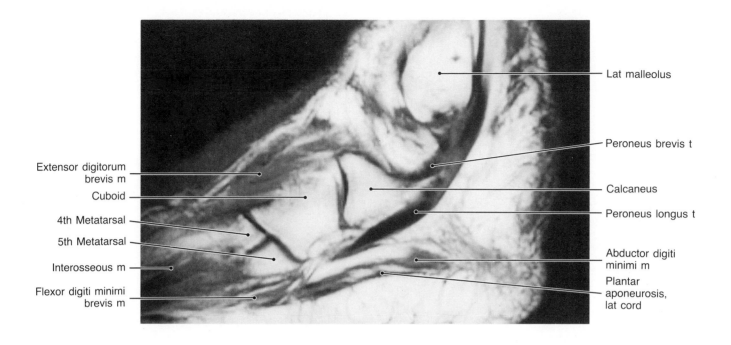

Extensor digitorum
brevis m

Cuboid

4th Metatarsal

5th Metatarsal

Interosseous m

Flexor digiti minimi
brevis m

Lat malleolus

Peroneus brevis t

Calcaneus

Peroneus longus t

Abductor digiti
minimi m

Plantar
aponeurosis,
lat cord

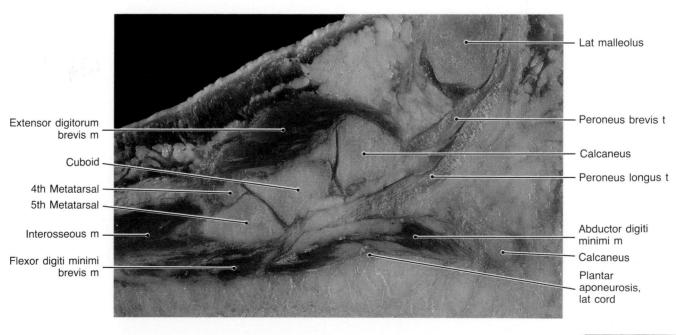

Extensor digitorum
brevis m

Cuboid

4th Metatarsal

5th Metatarsal

Interosseous m

Flexor digiti minimi
brevis m

Lat malleolus

Peroneus brevis t

Calcaneus

Peroneus longus t

Abductor digiti
minimi m

Calcaneus

Plantar
aponeurosis,
lat cord

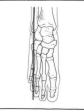

ANKLE AND FOOT, SAGITTAL

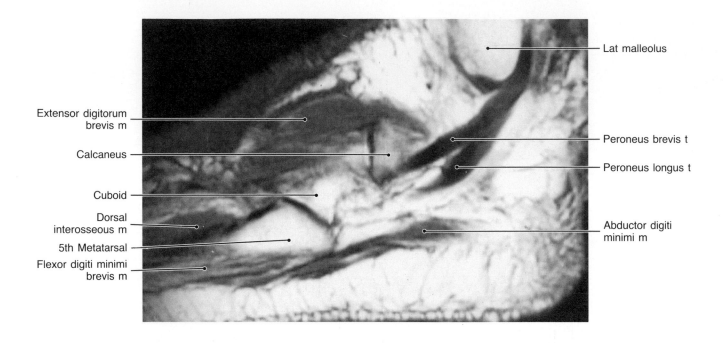

Lat malleolus

Extensor digitorum
brevis m

Peroneus brevis t

Calcaneus

Peroneus longus t

Cuboid

Dorsal
interosseous m

Abductor digiti
minimi m

5th Metatarsal

Flexor digiti minimi
brevis m

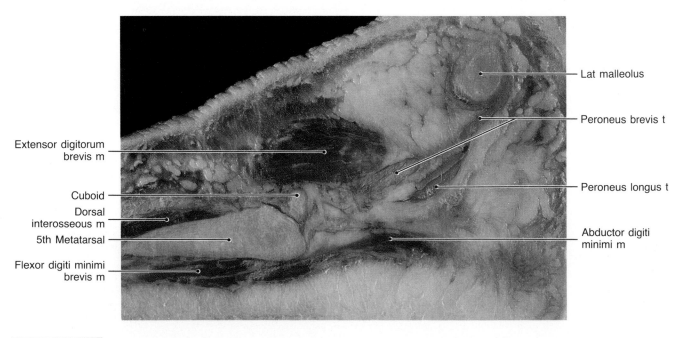

Lat malleolus

Peroneus brevis t

Extensor digitorum
brevis m

Peroneus longus t

Cuboid

Dorsal
interosseous m

5th Metatarsal

Abductor digiti
minimi m

Flexor digiti minimi
brevis m

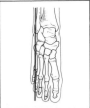

INDEX